Critical Care of the Cancer Patient & Geriatric Critical Care

Editors

STEPHEN M. PASTORES
WENDY R. GREENE
MAXWELL A. HOCKSTEIN

CRITICAL CARE CLINICS

www.criticalcare.theclinics.com

Consulting Editor
JOHN A. KELLUM

January 2021 • Volume 37 • Number 1

ELSEVIER

1600 John F. Kennedy Boulevard • Suite 1800 • Philadelphia, Pennsylvania, 19103-2899

http://www.theclinics.com

CRITICAL CARE CLINICS Volume 37, Number 1
January 2021 ISSN 0749-0704, ISBN-13: 978-0-323-75512-2

Editor: Kerry Holland
Developmental Editor: Casey Potter

Critical Care Clinics (ISSN: 0749-0704) is published quarterly by Elsevier Inc., 360 Park Avenue South, New York, NY 10010-1710. Months of issue are January, April, July, and October. Business and Editorial Offices: 1600 John F. Kennedy Blvd., Suite 1800, Philadelphia, PA 19103-2899. Customer Service Office: 6277 Sea Harbor Drive, Orlando, FL 32887-4800. Periodicals postage paid at New York, NY and additional mailing offices. Subscription prices are $258.00 per year for US individuals, $890.00 per year for US institutions, $100.00 per year for US students and residents, $287.00 per year for Canadian individuals, $952.00 per year for Canadian institutions, $328.00 per year for international individuals, $952.00 per year for international institutions, $100.00 per year for Canadian students/residents, and $150.00 per year for foreign students/residents. To receive student/resident rate, orders must be accompanied by name of affiliated institution, date of term, and the signature of program/residency coordinator on institution letterhead. Orders will be billed at individual rate until proof of status is received. Foreign air speed delivery is included in all *Clinics* subscription prices. All prices are subject to change without notice. POSTMASTER: Send address changes to *Critical Care Clinics*, Elsevier Periodicals Customer Service, 11830 Westline Industrial Drive, St. Louis, MO 63146. **Customer Service: 1-800-654-2452 (US). From outside of the US, call 1-314-447-8871. Fax: 1-314-447-8029. E-mail: journalscustomerservice-usa@elsevier.com (for print support) or journalsonlinesupport-usa@elsevier.com (for online support).**

Reprints. For copies of 100 or more of articles in this publication, please contact the Commercial Reprints Department, Elsevier Inc., 360 Park Avenue South, New York, NY 10010-1710. Tel.: 212-633-3874; Fax: 212-633-3820; E-mail: reprints@elsevier.com.

Critical Care Clinics is also published in Spanish by Editorial Inter-Medica, Junin 917, 1er A, 1113, Buenos Aires, Argentina.

Critical Care Clinics is covered in *MEDLINE/PubMed (Index Medicus), EMBASE/Excerpta Medica, Current Concepts/ Clinical Medicine, ISI/BIOMED, and Chemical Abstracts.*

Contributors

CONSULTING EDITOR

JOHN A. KELLUM, MD, MCCM
Professor, Critical Care Medicine, Medicine, Bioengineering and Clinical and Translational
Science, Director, Center for Critical Care Nephrology, The Clinical Research Investigation
and Systems Modeling of Acute Illness (CRISMA) Center, Vice Chair for Research,
Department of Critical Care Medicine, University of Pittsburgh School of Medicine,
Pittsburgh, Pennsylvania, USA

EDITORS

STEPHEN M. PASTORES, MD, MACP, FCCP, FCCM
Program Director, Critical Care Medicine, Vice Chair of Education, Department of
Anesthesiology and Critical Care Medicine, Memorial Sloan Kettering Cancer Center,
Professor of Medicine and Anesthesiology, Weill Cornell Medical College, New York, New
York, USA

WENDY R. GREENE, MD, FACS, FCCM
Department of Surgery, Emory University College of Medicine, Atlanta, Georgia, USA

MAXWELL A. HOCKSTEIN, MD
Department of Critical Care, MedStar Washington Hospital Center, Washington, DC,
USA

AUTHORS

STEPHEN D. ANTON, PhD
Department of Aging and Geriatric Research, University of Florida College of Medicine,
Gainesville, Florida, USA

CHERISSE BERRY, MD, FACS
Assistant Professor, Department of Surgery, Division of Acute Care Surgery, NYU
Grossman School of Medicine, New York, New York, USA

GREGORY H. BOTZ, MD, FCCM
Professor of Critical Care, Department of Critical Care and Respiratory Care, Division of
Anesthesiology, Critical Care and Pain Medicine, The University of Texas MD Anderson
Cancer Center, Houston, Texas, USA

SCOTT C. BRAKENRIDGE, MD, MSCS, FACS
Department of Surgery, University of Florida College of Medicine, Gainesville, Florida, USA

EMILY P. BRIGHAM, MD, MHS
Assistant Professor of Medicine, Oncology Intensive Care Unit, Division of Pulmonary and
Critical Care Medicine, Department of Medicine, Johns Hopkins University, Baltimore,
Maryland, USA

JIYEON CHOI, PhD, RN
Assistant Professor, Yonsei University College of Nursing, Mo-Im Kim Nursing Research Institute, Seoul, Korea

ZARA COOPER, MD, MSc, FACS
Kessler Director, Center for Surgery and Public Health, Associate Professor of Surgery, Harvard Medical School, Division of Trauma, Burn, and Critical Care, Department of Surgery, Brigham and Women's Hospital, Boston, Massachusetts, USA

KIMBERLY CURSEEN, MD
Associate Professor of Medicine, Director, Supportive and Palliative Care Outpatient Services, Division of Palliative Medicine, Department of Medicine, Emory Healthcare, Emory University School of Medicine, Atlanta, Georgia, USA

SANJEET S. DADWAL, MD, FACP
Clinical Professor, Division of Infectious Diseases, Department of Medicine, City of Hope National Medical Center, Duarte, California, USA

DIJOIA B. DARDEN, MD
Department of Surgery, University of Florida College of Medicine, Gainesville, Florida, USA

JOSE J. DIAZ Jr, MD, CNS, FACS, FCCM
Professor of Surgery, Epidemiology, and Public Health, Surgery Quality Officer, Department of Surgery, Chief, Division Acute Care Surgery and Program Director Acute Care Surgery Fellowship, Program in Trauma, R Adams Cowley Shock Trauma Center, The University of Maryland Medical Center, Baltimore, Maryland, USA

MARIA C. DUGGAN, MD, MPH
Assistant Professor of Medicine, Division of Geriatric Medicine, Vanderbilt University School of Medicine, Department of Veteran Affairs, Geriatric Research Education and Clinical Center (GRECC), Tennessee Valley Healthcare System, Nashville, Tennessee, USA

PHILIP A. EFRON, MD, FACS, FCCM
Department of Surgery, University of Florida College of Medicine, Gainesville, Florida, USA

EUGENE WESLEY ELY, MD, MPH
Professor of Medicine, Department of Veteran Affairs, Geriatric Research Education and Clinical Center (GRECC), Tennessee Valley Healthcare System, Division of Allergy, Pulmonary, and Critical Care Medicine, Vanderbilt University School of Medicine, Center for Health Services Research (HSR), Vanderbilt University Medical Center, Nashville, Tennessee, USA

RACHAEL A. FORNWALT, RN, MSN, ACNP
Oncology Intensive Care Unit, Johns Hopkins Sidney Kimmel Comprehensive Cancer Center, Johns Hopkins Hospital, Baltimore, Maryland, USA

MIRA GHNEIM, MD, MS, FACS
Assistant Professor of Trauma and Acute Care Surgery, R Adams Cowley Shock Trauma Center, The University of Maryland Medical Center, Baltimore, Maryland, USA

CRISTINA GUTIERREZ, MD
Associate Professor of Medicine, Department of Critical Care Medicine, The University of Texas MD Anderson Cancer Center, Houston, Texas, USA

RANDEEP S. JAWA, MD, FACS, FCCM
Professor of Clinical Surgery, Division of Trauma, Surgical Critical Care, and Emergency Surgery, Department of Surgery, Stony Brook University Renaissance School of Medicine, Stony Brook, New York, USA

CHRISTIAAN LEEUWENBURGH, PhD
Department of Aging and Geriatric Research, University of Florida College of Medicine, Gainesville, Florida, USA

CATHERINE LIU, MD, FIDSA
Associate Professor, Vaccine and Infectious Disease Division, Fred Hutchison Cancer Research Center, Department of Medicine, University of Washington, Seattle, Washington, USA

ROBERT T. MANKOWSKI, PhD
Department of Aging and Geriatric Research, University of Florida, Gainesville, Florida, USA

CHRISTINA A. MINAMI, MD, MS
Division of Breast Surgery, Department of Surgery, Brigham and Women's Hospital, Breast Oncology Program, Dana-Farber Cancer Institute, Boston, Massachusetts, USA

ALICIA M. MOHR, MD, FACS, FCCM
Department of Surgery, University of Florida College of Medicine, Gainesville, Florida, USA

LYLE L. MOLDAWER, PhD
Department of Surgery, University of Florida College of Medicine, Gainesville, Florida, USA

FREDERICK A. MOORE, MD, FACS, MCCM
Department of Surgery, University of Florida College of Medicine, Gainesville, Florida, USA

LAVEENA MUNSHI, MD, MSc
Interdepartmental Division of Critical Care Medicine, Department of Medicine, University of Toronto, Sinai Health System and University Health Network, Mount Sinai Hospital, Toronto, Ontario, Canada

EDUARDO B. NAVARRO, BHS
Department of Surgery, University of Florida College of Medicine, Gainesville, Florida, USA

BRITTANY NOWAK, MD
Department of Surgery, Division of Acute Care Surgery, NYU Grossman School of Medicine, New York, New York, USA

STEPHEN M. PASTORES, MD, MACP, FCCP, FCCM
Program Director, Critical Care Medicine, Vice Chair of Education, Department of Anesthesiology and Critical Care Medicine, Memorial Sloan Kettering Cancer Center, Professor of Medicine and Anesthesiology, Weill Cornell Medical College, New York, New York, USA

RAJEEV B. PATEL, MD
Assistant Professor of Medicine, Division of Pulmonary, Critical Care, and Sleep Medicine, Department of Medicine, Stony Brook University Renaissance School of Medicine, Stony Brook, New York, USA

PRABALINI RAJENDRAM, MD
Assistant Professor of Medicine, Department of Critical Care, Respiratory Institute, Cleveland Clinic, Cleveland, Ohio, USA

DEREDDI RAJA SHEKAR REDDY, MD, FACP, FCCP
Assistant Professor of Critical Care, Department of Critical Care and Respiratory Care, Division of Anesthesiology, Critical Care and Pain Medicine, The University of Texas MD Anderson Cancer Center, Houston, Texas, USA

JAMIE C. RICHES, DO
Memorial Sloan Kettering Cancer Center, New York, New York, USA

R. SCOTT STEPHENS, MD
Director, Oncology and Bone Marrow Transplant Critical Care, Oncology Intensive Care Unit, Division of Pulmonary and Critical Care Medicine, Assistant Professor, Departments of Medicine and Oncology, Johns Hopkins University, Baltimore, Maryland, USA

SUSAN K. SEO, MD, FACP, FIDSA
Clinical Member, Infectious Disease Service, Department of Medicine, Memorial Sloan Kettering Cancer, Professor of Clinical Medicine, Department of Medicine, Weill Cornell Medical College, New York, New York, USA

ALEXANDER SHIMABUKURO-VORNHAGEN, MD
Department I of Internal Medicine, University Hospital of Cologne, Cologne, Germany

JENNA SPRING, MD
Interdepartmental Division of Critical Care Medicine, Department of Medicine, University of Toronto, Sinai Health System and University Health Network, Sunnybrook Health Sciences Centre, Toronto, Ontario, Canada

COREY X. TAPPER, MD, MS
Assistant Professor of Medicine, Associate Program Director, Hospice and Palliative Medicine Fellowship, Division of General Internal Medicine, Section of Palliative Medicine, Johns Hopkins School of Medicine, Baltimore, Maryland, USA

JUDITH A. TATE, PhD, RN
Assistant Professor, Center of Healthy Aging, Self-Management and Complex Care, Director, Undergraduate Nursing Honors Program, The Ohio State University College of Nursing, Columbus, Ohio, USA

JULIE VAN
Doctoral Student, Division of Allergy, Pulmonary, and Critical Care Medicine, Vanderbilt University School of Medicine, Center for Health Services Research (HSR), Vanderbilt University Medical Center, Nashville, Tennessee, USA

LOUIS P. VOIGT, MD, FCCP, MBE
Memorial Sloan Kettering Cancer Center, New York, New York, USA

DAVID H. YOUNG, MD, FCCM
Associate Professor of Surgery (Retired), Division of Trauma/Critical Care, Department of Surgery, University of Nebraska Medical Center, Omaha, Nebraska, USA

Contents

Triage and Prognostication of Cancer Patients Admitted to the Intensive Care Unit   1

Dereddi Raja Shekar Reddy and Gregory H. Botz

> Cancer remains a leading cause of morbidity and mortality. Advances in cancer screening, early detection, targeted therapies, and supportive care have led to improvements in outcomes and quality of life. The rapid increase in novel cancer therapies can cause life-threatening adverse events. The need for intensive care unit (ICU) care is projected to increase. Until 2 decades ago, cancer diagnosis often precluded ICU admission. Recently, substantial cancer survival has been achieved; therefore, ICU denial is not recommended. ICU resources are limited and expensive; hence, appropriate utilization is needed. This review focuses on triage and prognosis in critically ill cancer patients requiring ICU admission.

Intensive Care Unit Organization and Interdisciplinary Care for Critically Ill Patients with Cancer   19

Alexander Shimabukuro-Vornhagen

> Patients with cancer are at high risk of developing acute critical illness requiring intensive care unit (ICU) admission. Critically ill patients with cancer have complex medical needs that can best be served by a multidisciplinary ICU care team. This article provides an overview of the current state-of-the-art in multidisciplinary care for critically ill patients with cancer. Better integration of multidisciplinary critical care into the continuum of care for patients with cancer offers the prospect of further improvements in the outcomes of patients with cancer.

Critical Care of Hematopoietic Stem Cell Transplant Patients   29

Rachael A. Fornwalt, Emily P. Brigham, and R. Scott Stephens

> Life-threatening complications are frequent after hematopoietic stem cell transplant (HSCT), and optimum critical care is essential to ensuring good outcomes. The immunologic consequences of HSCT result in a markedly different host response to critical illness. Infection is the most common cause of critical illness but noninfectious complications are frequent. Respiratory failure or sepsis are the typical presentations but the sequelae of HSCT can affect nearly any organ system. Pattern recognition can facilitate anticipation and early intervention in post-HSCT critical illness. HSCT critical care is a multidisciplinary endeavor. Continued investigation and focus on process improvement will continue to improve outcomes.

surrogates to share the burdens of decision, and institutional support for early integration of palliative care can foster an ethical climate.

Elderly patients who are critically ill have unique challenges that must be considered when attempting to prognosticate survival and determine expectations for physical rehabilitation and meaningful recovery. Furthermore, frail elderly patients present unique rehabilitation and clinical challenges when suffering from critical illness. There are multiple symptoms and syndromes that affect morbidity and mortality of elderly patients who require intensive care unit management including delirium, dementia, pain, and constipation. Rehabilitation goals should be based on patient values, clinical course, and functional status. Patients and families need accurate prognostic information to choose the appropriate level of care needed after critical illness.

Older patients experience a decline in their physiologic reserves as well as chronic low-grade inflammation named "inflammaging." Both of these contribute significantly to aging-related factors that alter the acute, subacute, and chronic response of these patients to critical illness, such as sepsis. Unfortunately, this altered response to stressors can lead to chronic critical illness followed by dismal outcomes and death. The primary goal of this review is to briefly highlight age-specific changes in physiologic systems majorly affected in critical illness, especially because it pertains to sepsis and trauma, which can lead to chronic critical illness and describe implications in clinical management.

The number of older adults with cancer is growing in the United States, and there is a relative paucity of data relating the presence of frailty with its outcomes of interest. The authors present the surgical oncology, radiation oncology, and medical oncology literature with respect to the presence of frailty in older adults with cancer. More research is needed to understand how the presence of frailty should be used by surgical, radiation, and medical oncologists to guide patient counseling and treatment planning.

Rehabilitation is critical in improving quality of life by maximizing physical, cognitive, and psychological recovery from injury or disease.

JiYeon Choi and Judith A. Tate

Communication is a critical component of patient-centered care. Critically ill, mechanically ventilated patients are unable to speak and this condition is frightening, frustrating, and stressful. Impaired communication in the intensive care unit (ICU) contributes to poor symptom identification and restricts effective patient engagement. Older adults are at higher risk for communication impairments in the ICU because of pre-illness communication disorders and cognitive dysfunction that often accompanies or precedes critical illness. Assessing communication disorders and developing patient-centered strategies to enhance communication can lessen communication difficulty and increase patient satisfaction.

CRITICAL CARE CLINICS

SERIES OF RELATED INTEREST

Medical Clinics
Cardiology Clinics

THE CLINICS ARE AVAILABLE ONLINE!
Access your subscription at:
www.theclinics.com

Dedication

To my wife Maria Teresa De Sancho, MD, MSc, and 2 children, Steven Michael and Monica Cristina, for their loving support, and to the medical, nursing, and ancillary staff at Memorial Sloan Kettering Cancer Center for their tireless work ethic, compassion, and skill in caring for our oncology patients.

Stephen M. Pastores, MACP, FCCP, FCCM
Memorial Sloan Kettering Cancer Center
1275 York Avenue C-1179
New York, NY 10065, USA

E-mail address:
pastores@mskcc.org

Crit Care Clin 37 (2021) xiii
https://doi.org/10.1016/j.ccc.2020.10.003
0749-0704/21/© 2020 Published by Elsevier Inc.

Section 1: Critical Care of the Cancer Patient

Preface

Critical Care and Oncology

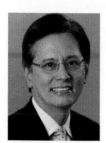

Stephen M. Pastores, MD, MACP, FCCP, FCCM
Editor

Cancer remains a leading health care challenge worldwide, including the United States, where 1.8 million new cases of cancer and 606,520 deaths from cancer are estimated in 2020. Over the past few decades, our understanding of the biology of cancer has grown rapidly, leading to major therapeutic advances in oncology, including the use of targeted agents, immune checkpoint blockade, and chimeric antigen receptor T-cell therapy, as well as innovations in cancer surgery and radiotherapy. These developments have improved not only patient outcomes but also their quality of life. However, oncology patients remain vulnerable and at high risk of developing acute critical illness requiring admission to the intensive care unit (ICU). Oncology patients account for up to 20% of all ICU patients. Many of these patients are admitted to the ICU due to either the malignancy itself, cancer treatment-related side effects or complications, or an underlying medical condition unrelated to the cancer.

Given the complex care needs of oncology patients who become critically ill, it has become increasingly clear that expert knowledge from specialists of several disciplines working collaboratively with ICU clinicians is mandatory to ensure the best possible outcomes and appropriate use of available critical care resources.

In this issue of *Critical Care Clinics*, an excellent group of highly regarded and practicing clinicians in the field of critical care oncology and supportive care has been assembled to provide their expertise on the care of the critically ill cancer patient. This issue leads off with important articles on the triage and prognostication of cancer patients admitted to the ICU and the key aspects of ICU organization and interdisciplinary care of these patients. The articles that follow highlight critical care issues in hematopoietic stem cell transplant recipients, diagnostic and management strategies of toxicities associated with immunotherapy and cardiotoxicity in the era of novel cancer therapies, infectious disease complications, and oncologic emergencies necessitating ICU care. The final article discusses the scope of the ethical conundrums that arise in the provision of end-of-life care to adult patients with cancer and the need for early

Crit Care Clin 37 (2021) xv–xvi
https://doi.org/10.1016/j.ccc.2020.10.001
0749-0704/21/© 2020 Published by Elsevier Inc.

criticalcare.theclinics.com

involvement of palliative care teams in the critical care setting. It was a privilege and honor for me to work with them on this issue.

I would like to express my sincere appreciation and gratitude to all of the contributing authors and to Casey Marie Potter, Kerry Holland, Joanna Collett, and Nicholas Henderson at Elsevier for their assistance in getting this work product completed in the midst of the COVID-19 global pandemic.

Stephen M. Pastores, MD, MACP, FCCP, FCCM
Memorial Sloan Kettering Cancer Center
1275 York Avenue C-1179
New York, NY 10065, USA

E-mail address:
pastores@mskcc.org

Triage and Prognostication of Cancer Patients Admitted to the Intensive Care Unit

Dereddi Raja Shekar Reddy, MD, FCCP, Gregory H. Botz, MD, FCCM*

KEYWORDS

- Critical care • Intensive care • Critically ill • Triage • Prognosis • Admission
- ICU utilization • Cancer

KEY POINTS

- Critically ill cancer patients increasingly require intensive care unit (ICU) admission.
- Malignancy or metastasis should not be used as a triage criterion for ICU admission.
- Short-term outcomes in critically ill cancer patients have improved.

CRITICAL CARE IN CANCER PATIENTS

Cancer is the second leading cause of death in the United States, exceeded only by heart disease. In 2018, there were an estimated 1,735,350 new cases of cancer, with 609,640 deaths in the United States. For every 100,000 people, there are 439 new cancer cases, with reported 164 deaths. One of every 4 deaths in the United States is due to cancer.[1] In 1999, the American College of Critical Care Medicine Guidelines for Intensive Care Unit Admission, Discharge, and Triage stated that patients with hematological or metastasized oncological malignancies are poor candidates for ICU admission, with a mortality rate of up to 90%. Therefore, ICU admission refusal in cancer patients was common.[2] With advances in cancer screening and early detection as well as improvements in therapeutics and supportive care, however, cancer mortality has decreased by 23% since the 1990s. The American Association for Cancer Research recently reported that cancer survivorship has increased from 1 in 69 (1.4%) to 1 in 21 (4.8%) people.[3,4] There will be an estimated 26 million cancer survivors by 2040, a majority of whom will be in their 60s, 70s, and 80s.[5]

Financial Support: None.

Department of Critical Care and Respiratory Care, Division of Anesthesiology, Critical Care and Pain Medicine, University of Texas MD Anderson Cancer Center, 1515 Holcombe Boulevard, Unit 112, Houston, TX 77030, USA

* Corresponding author.

E-mail address: gbotz@mdanderson.org

Crit Care Clin 37 (2021) 1–18
https://doi.org/10.1016/j.ccc.2020.08.001
0749-0704/21/© 2020 Elsevier Inc. All rights reserved.

In the past 2 decades, the development of targeted immunotherapy led to significantly improved outcomes and quality of life in cancer patients. These therapies can manifest, however, severe life-threatening adverse effects requiring ICU admission.[6] With the rapid proliferation of novel therapies, the need for ICU care is projected to accelerate. For instance, cytokine-release syndromes in chimeric antigen receptor T-cell therapy has led to an increased need for life support measures.[7] ICU therapies generally are offered to patients with potentially reversible conditions (**Table 1**). Patients with advanced cancer have a terminal disease; ICU admission may not be offered. Many patients with potentially "irreversible" diseases, however, such as end-stage heart failure, end-stage liver failure, and end-stage lung disease, often are offered ICU admission. The in-hospital mortality for critically ill cancer patients is not higher compared with their counterparts with these comorbidities.[8] Recent studies suggest that substantial survival can be achieved even in severely ill cancer patients.[9–11] According to expert consensus, it is not recommended to deny ICU admission to those with advanced malignancies in the earliest disease phase because this is a time when response to therapy is unknown.[12]

Five major changes in the care of critically ill cancer patients have occurred over the past 2 decades.[13] (1) ICU care for cancer patients has increased, with approximately 15% of ICU beds occupied by cancer patients.[14,15] (2) Patients with hematological malignancies have improved ICU and in-hospital survival rates. The hospital, 90-day, and 1-year survival rates were 60.7%, 52.5%, and 43.3%, respectively. ICU survivors achieve disease remission and good quality of life that is comparable to non-ICU patients.[16,17] (3) Neutropenia, autologous bone marrow transplantation, and type of malignancy no longer are associated with excessive hospital mortality after ICU admission.[18] (4) New noninvasive diagnostic and therapeutic strategies have permitted new clinical approaches for high-risk cancer patients.[19] These strategies have supported early ICU admission, avoiding risky procedures and offering earlier monitoring. (5) Traditional ICU admission triage criteria have shown poor reliability. Newer ICU admission strategies have been applied to cancer patients.[12]

TRIAGE

Triage comes from the French verb, *trier*, which means, "to sort, separate, shift or select." It originally was used to describe the sorting of agricultural products.[20,21] Dominique-Jean Larrey, a surgeon in Napoleon Bonaparte's Imperial Guard, invented modern medical triage. He prioritized the rapid evacuation of wounded soldiers from the battlefield by establishing a categorical rule for the triage of war casualties. It focused on treating the wounded according to the observed gravity of their injuries and the urgency for medical care, regardless of their rank or nationality.[22,23] French doctors implemented triage during World War I when treating the battlefield wounded at the aid stations behind the front. The wounded were divided into 3 categories: (1) those likely to live, regardless of what care they receive; (2) those unlikely to live, regardless of what care they receive; and (3) those for whom immediate care might improve outcome.[24]

When the demands for medical treatment surpass the available resources, the thoughtful distribution of scarce resources is essential. Not all needs are satisfied immediately, and some may not be satisfied at all. Triage is the process of sorting patients into the most appropriate level of care, based on their medical needs. In many hospitals, limited ICU bed availability makes triage essential. The challenge has been to identify those patients who are too sick to benefit and those who are too well to benefit from ICU care. In 1999, the American College of Critical Care Medicine

Table 1		
Diagnosis at intensive care unit admission in cancer patients		
	Common Indications	**Rare Indications**
Malignancy related	• Pulmonary embolism • Hypercalcemia • TLS • Superior vena cava syndrome • Disseminated intravascular coagulation • Adrenal insufficiency/crisis	• Spinal cord compression • Hyperuricemia with resulting oliguria • Lambert-Eaton syndrome • Hyponatremia • Seizures • Posterior reversible encephalopathy syndrome • Upper airway obstruction • Malignant pericardial tamponade • Hyperviscosity syndrome • Hyperleukocytic syndrome • Thrombocytopenia • Hemorrhage
Cancer therapy related	• Neutropenic fever • Anaphylaxis • Cytokine release syndrome • Arrhythmias • Pulmonary thromboembolism • TLS • Congestive heart failure	• Drug-induced organ failure • All-trans retinoic acid syndrome • Thrombocytopenia/hemorrhage • Thrombotic microangiopathy
Noninfectious	• Transfusion-associated lung injury • Pneumonitis • Transfusion-associated circulatory overload	• Alveolar hemorrhage • Polymyositis • Engraftment syndrome
Infectious	• Neutropenic fever • Pneumonia • Sepsis	

Data from Biskup E, Cai F, Vetter M, Marsch S. Oncological patients in the intensive care unit: prognosis, decision-making, therapies and end-of-life care. *Swiss Med Wkly.* 2017;147:w14481. Published 2017 Aug 14. https://doi.org/10.4414/smw.2017.14481 (Does not require permission).

Guidelines for Intensive Care Unit Admission, Discharge, and Triage included a list of diagnoses and a list of physiologic or hemodynamic conditions that might justify ICU admission.[2]

ICU TRIAL

The ICU Trial evaluated a new ICU admission policy to improve the chances of survival in critically ill cancer patients who could receive life-extending cancer treatment if they survive an acute illness episode.[10] Bedridden patients or those with no available life span–extending cancer treatment were excluded. These patients received full ICU management for a limited period of 3 days to 7 days followed by a reappraisal of the appropriate level of care (**Figs. 1** and **2, Table 2**).

The overall survival rate in 188 patients was 21.8% (41 of 188). The ICU Trial was seen an alternative to ICU refusal in cancer patients. Patients with poor survival potential were easier to identify after ICU Trial. Organ failure scores at ICU admission performed poorly, indicating that they should not be used for ICU triage. After adjusting

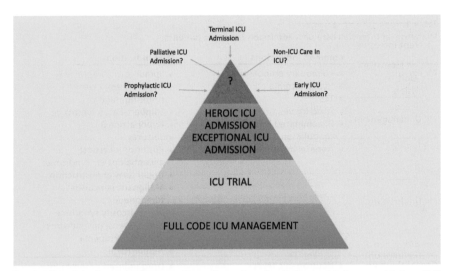

Fig. 1. ICU Trial schematic diagram. (*Data from*: Azoulay E, Soares M, Darmon M, Benoit D, Pastores S, Afessa B. Intensive care of the cancer patient: recent achievements and remaining challenges. *Ann Intensive Care*. 2011;1(1):5. Published 2011 Mar 23. https://doi.org/10.1186/2110-5820-1-5 (Does not require permission.)

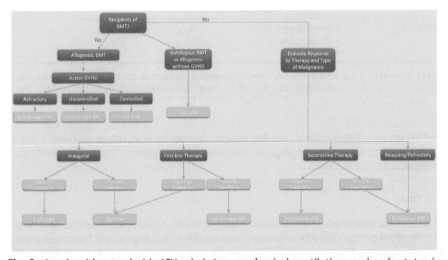

Fig. 2. An algorithm to decide ICU admission, mechanical ventilation, and code status in cancer patients. Good life expectancy refers to a malignancy where complete remission and long term survival are possible outcomes. Poor life expectancy refers to a malignancy where median life expectancy is below one year. BMT, bone marrow transplant; GVHD, graft versus host disease; MV, mechanical ventilation. (*Data from*: Azoulay E, Soares M, Darmon M, Benoit D, Pastores S, Afessa B. Intensive care of the cancer patient: recent achievements and remaining challenges. *Ann Intensive Care*. 2011;1(1):5. Published 2011 Mar 23. https://doi.org/10.1186/2110-5820-1-5 (Does not require permission.)

Table 2
Different intensive care unit admission policies

Type of Intensive Care Unit Admission	Code Status	Clinical Situation
1. Full code ICU management	Full code	Newly diagnosed malignancies Malignancies in complete remission
2. ICU Trial	Unlimited for a limited timeperiod—at least 3–5 d	Clinical response to therapy not available or undetermined
3. Exceptional ICU admission	Same as ICU Trial	Newly available effective therapy that should be tested in a patient who becomes critically ill
4. Heroic ICU admission	ICU management until conflict resolution	Both hematologists/oncologists and intensivists agree that ICU admission is not appropriate, but patients or relatives disagree with the appropriate level of care
5. Other admission modalities that are performed but not yet formally evaluated		
a. Prophylactic ICU admission	Full code; intensive clinical and biological monitoring; invasive procedures under safer conditions	Earliest phase of high-risk malignancies. Admission to the ICU is warranted to avoid development of organ dysfunction (ARF, TLS, and so forth)
b. Early ICU admission	Full code; intensive clinical and biological monitoring; invasive procedures under safe conditions; no life-sustaining therapies	Admission to the ICU in patients with no organ dysfunction but physiologic disturbances. ICU is warranted to avoid late ICU admission (condition associated with higher mortality)
c. Palliative ICU admission	Noninvasive strategies only	Admission to the ICU for the purpose of undergoing noninvasive mechanical ventilation as the ceiling of therapy
d. In-ICU non-ICU care	No life-sustaining therapies	Short ICU admission to help for optimal and prompt management (catheter withdrawal, early antibiotics, and so forth)
e. Terminal ICU admission	No life-sustaining therapies	ICU admission is required to best provide palliative care and symptom control. Controversial issue

Data from: Azoulay E, Soares M, Darmon M, Benoit D, Pastores S, Afessa B. Intensive care of the cancer patient: recent achievements and remaining challenges. Ann Intensive Care. 2011;1(1):5. Published 2011 Mar 23. https://doi.org/10.1186/2110-5820-1-5 (Does not require permission).

for age and severity of illness (SIL), the 3-day survival was higher in ICU patients than those admitted elsewhere in the hospital. There was no difference, however, in survival thereafter. There may be a window of critical opportunity, much like the golden hour in trauma, that is lost if access to ICU is not timely.[25] Triage decisions rely on a variety of factors, such as written admission criteria and available resources, with inherent interpersonal and interhospital biases.[26,27] The Guidelines for Intensive Care Unit Admission, Discharge, and Triage recommend that patients admitted to the ICU should meet 1 or more of the following criteria[28]:

- Require specialized ICU care that is not widely available elsewhere in the hospital (eg, invasive mechanical ventilation, management of shock, extracorporeal membrane oxygenation, or intra-aortic balloon pump).
- Have clinical instability (eg, status epilepticus, hypoxemia, and hypotension).
- Be at high risk for imminent decline (eg, impending intubation).

TRIAGE DECISION MAKERS

In general, ICU triage decisions are made by intensivists. But in some hospitals, these decisions can be made by hospitalists (or other physicians), advanced practice providers, or nursing leadership. An intensivist-led ICU triage service can have a favorable impact on ICU admission and discharge wait times, as well as surgical ICU length of stay.[29] When hospitalists made ICU triage decisions, facilitated patient transfers, made ICU bed management rounds twice a day, and regularly visited the emergency department to assess flow, the transfer time from the emergency department to the ICU decreased.[30] A multicenter randomized controlled trial that focused on the prioritization of ICU admission showed poor agreement among practitioners from 18 countries. Despite clear guidelines, practitioners often disagreed.[31] Consensus guidelines recommend that a designated person or service, with control over ICU resources, be responsible for ICU triage decisions during normal or emergency operations.[28]

FACTORS THAT AFFECT TRIAGE DECISIONS

For many years, the decision to admit cancer patients to the ICU was based on the cancer diagnosis and any complications from underlying disease and associated treatments. More recent data have shown, however, that the underlying malignancy or stage no longer is associated with increased mortality during or after an ICU stay.[15,32] One study showed that heart rate greater than 111 beats/min, oxygen saturation as measured by pulse oximetry less than 89%, and Glasgow Coma Scale score less than 8 were significantly associated with adverse outcome.[33] In another study, physicians used age, admitting diagnosis, SIL, number of available ICU beds, and operative status to make triage decisions. They found that ICU admission was associated with lower hospital mortality (14%) compared with refused admission (36%) and never admitted (46%).[34] A large prospective multicenter study found that ICU triage recommendations rarely are followed, particularly when the ICU is full or triage is done by telephone.[27] Active advance directives influence the triage decision process, often leading to refusal.[35] ICU admission refusal does not necessarily imply that death is considered inevitable. Rather, it reflects that other patients likely will benefit more from scarce ICU resources, based on distributive justice. Guidelines recommend that some over-triage is more acceptable than and preferable to under-triage.[28]

PROGNOSTICATION OF CRITICALLY ILL CANCER PATIENT
Short-Term and Long-Term Outcomes of Cancer Intensive Care Unit Patients

Niskanen and colleagues[36] studied 12,180 patients admitted to Finnish ICUs and showed that short-term survival was similar between cancer and noncancer patients but depended on the SIL. Survival rates between cancer and trauma patients with Acute Physiology and Chronic Health Evaluation (APACHE) II scores greater than 24 also was similar. Newer mortality prediction models show burn patients with 50% full-thickness surface area burns and APACHE III scores of 120 have a predicted mortality rate between 40% and 60%.[37] In comparison, breast cancer patients with liver metastases have a 50% 5-year survival.[38] ICU admission in cancer patients should be based on SIL and long-term prognosis rather than the presence of a malignancy or metastasis. Overall survival in medical oncology patients was 10.6 months, with ICU and hospital mortality rates at 5% and 22%, respectively.[39] This observation suggests that cancer patients can achieve favorable short-term outcomes after ICU admission. In the largest study to date, Pastores and colleagues[40] evaluated the short-term and long-term outcomes of adult patients with hematologic malignancies who received chemotherapy in the ICU. Their reported ICU and hospital mortality rates were 25% and 42% for chemotherapy patients, respectively, and 22% and 33% for nonchemotherapy patients, respectively. The 6-month and 12-month posthospital discharge survival estimates were 58% and 50%, respectively. Those who received chemotherapy in the ICU had a trend toward a higher risk of dying by 12 months (hazard ratio 1.45). The short-term outcomes in ICU patients with hematological malignancies who did and did not receive chemotherapy in the ICU were similar but with increased resource utilization.[40] In a series of postoperative gynecologic cancer patients, ICU survival and long-term survival rates were 81% and 33%, respectively, suggesting benefit from ICU admission after cancer surgery.[41]

General Predictors of Outcomes

The validity of appropriate ICU utilization criteria has not been well documented in cancer patient subgroups. Therefore, the precise indications for ICU admissions and/or continuation of care remain ambiguous.[2,28,31] In a study evaluating ICU admission in cancer patients, 20% of patients not admitted because they were considered "too well" died before hospital discharge, and 25% of patients who were not admitted because they were considered "too sick" survived.[42] Clinical judgment alone may be inaccurate and general triage criteria unreliable. A broader ICU admission policy based on reliable outcome predictors is needed (**Table 3**).

Outcomes vary in patients with solid and hematological malignancies. Critically ill hematopoietic stem cell transplantation (HSCT) recipients admitted to ICU have shorter survival, with 1-year, 3-year, and 5-year survival rates of 38%, 22%, and 18%, respectively, whereas similar patients who did not require ICU admission showed 1-year, 3-year, and 5-year better survival rates of 78%, 65%, and 60%, respectively.[43] In contrast, surgical ICU patients with solid tumors had ICU and hospital mortality rates of 12.2% and 16.8%, respectively.[44] Largely, long-term outcomes in ICU cancer patients depend on the prognostic properties of the cancer itself, whereas the SIL on ICU admission has little impact.[17,32]

Acute respiratory failure (ARF) remains the most common ICU admission diagnosis in critically ill cancer patients. It usually is associated with poor outcome, especially if mechanical ventilation is needed in the setting of acute respiratory distress syndrome (ARDS).[43,45–47] The mortality risk with invasive mechanical ventilation (IMV) is disproportionately high.[48,49] A multicenter study of 1004 patients with solid or hematological

---

Table 3
Risk factors for short-term mortality of patients with cancer admitted to the intensive care unit

Association with increased mortality rates	No association with mortality
• Age	• Neutropenia
• SIL (scores)	• Recently administered chemotherapy
• Severity and the number	• Autologous stem cell transplantation
of organ failures	Association with lower mortality rates
• ARF	• Positive blood culture
• IMV	• Antibiotic combination in
• Late ICU admissions	neutropenic sepsis (aminoglycosides?)
• Comorbidities,	• Removal of central venous line in
• PS prior to hospitalization,	neutropenic sepsis
(very) advanced tumor stages	
• Acute graft-versus-host disease	
after allogeneic stem cell transplantation	
• Admission after cardiac arrest	
• Invasive pulmonary aspergillosis	

Data from: Schellongowski P, Sperr WR, Wohlfarth P, et al. Critically ill patients with cancer: chances and limitations of intensive care medicine—a narrative review. ESMO Open 2016;1:e000018. https://doi.org/10.1136/esmoopen-2015- 000018 (Does not require permission).

malignancies found that mortality associated with ARDS is high at 52%.[45] One-third of patients received noninvasive ventilation (NIV) but failed, with the highest failure rates occurring in the most severe ARDS category. NIV failure was associated with higher mortality. IMV in cancer patients was associated independently with increased hospital mortality.[50] NIV and high-flow oxygen therapy (HFNC) have emerged as alternatives to avoid intubation with proved effectiveness to reduce intubation in cancer patients with acute hypoxemic respiratory failure.[51–53] Early use of NIV in immunocompromised patients with hypoxemic ARF reported no significant benefits[54] whereas no significant difference in intubation rates were found when treated with HFNC, standard oxygen, or NIV.[55] Although mortality in cancer patients with ARF receiving IMV was invariably high, more recently there has been some improvement, attributed by investigators to advances in oncology and critical care coupled with careful patient selection.[56]

Performance status (PS) is a simple and widely used scale to assess function and guide treatment in patients with cancer. In patients with solid malignancy, a PS greater than 2 was a predictor of hospital mortality, 70% in a univariate analysis and an odds ratio 3.05 in a multivariate analysis.[47] PS is a key and constant outcome predictor in all critically ill patients. Altered PS may be associated with age and comorbidities or the disease aggressiveness. Poor PS translates into increased mortality irrespective of why the PS is altered, with case fatality reaching 85% to 90% in patients who are bedridden.[12,13,17]

Acute kidney injury (AKI) occurs in up to 70% of critically ill cancer patients; half require renal replacement therapy (RRT). AKI requiring RRT is more common in ICU patients with versus without cancer. The major causes of AKI are sepsis, hypoperfusion and nephrotoxic drugs.[57–59] In hematological malignancy patients, major AKI adverse risk factors were older age (>60 years), SIL (nonrenal Sequential Organ Failure Assessment [SOFA]), history of hypertension, tumor lysis syndrome (TLS), exposure to nephrotoxic agents, and myeloma. Hospital mortality was 44.3% in patients with AKI and 25.4% in patients without AKI.[58] Overall, cancer patients requiring RRT have a higher hospital mortality (57.2%) compared with those who did not require RRT (31.2%). Whether they developed AKI or needed RRT, mortality was close to that of general ICU patients. In a large study of 67,986 cancer patients, AKI was an independent risk factor for all-cause mortality.[60] Development of AKI can jeopardize further cancer treatment, increase the toxicity and/or reduce the delivery of chemotherapy, and exclude patients from clinical trials.[57] Early admission to ICU can lead to better renal and overall outcomes, likely due to management of preventable AKI causes, such as TLS or sepsis.[61]

Until recently, it was believed that neutropenia alone in critically ill cancer patients was associated with high mortality; therefore, life-saving therapies were nonbeneficial.[13,18] Neutropenia should not be used as the sole criteria for an ICU admission decision. Likewise, neutropenia should not be the sole factor in a decision to withhold or withdraw life-sustaining therapies.[62]

In the early 1990s, Sculier and Markiewicz[63] reported 5 patients discharged alive among 49 cardiac arrests in nonsurgical cancer patients. Wallace and colleagues[64] evaluated the effectiveness and patient care costs of cardiopulmonary resuscitation (CPR) in cancer patients already on life support in a comprehensive cancer center. Among 5196 ICU admissions over 7 years, 406 (8%) patients received CPR, 256 patients (63%) died at the time of the arrest, and 150 (37%) had return of spontaneous circulation. Only 7 (2%) patients, however, survived to discharge. They concluded that providing CPR to cancer patients receiving life support is costly and does not lead to long-term survival. Similar results were reported by Khasawneh and colleagues[65] and Reisfield and colleagues,[66] with survival to discharge rates of 5.8% and 6.2%, respectively. In contrast, Champigneulle and colleagues[67] showed an 18% hospital survival rate in cancer patients after cardiac arrest with an overall 6-month survival rate of 14%. In cancer cohorts stratified by solid tumor versus hematological malignancy, resuscitation was successful in 7.1% and 2% of patients, respectively. Malignancy, even if metastatic, is not an absolute contraindication to CPR. Cancer stage, the cause of the cardiac arrest, and patient choice should be taken into consideration in order to decide whether to perform CPR.[68] CPR in critically ill cancer patients, as in other types of disease, is indicated and successful mainly when cardiac arrest is the consequence of an acute insult. If CPR is attempted, the decision to terminate resuscitation should be based on clinical judgment. In the final analysis, the determination that a resuscitation attempt is futile is a matter of medical judgment that only a responsible physician can make.[28]

Severity of Illness Scoring Systems

SIL scoring systems can be specific to disease (eg, Pneumonia Severity Index), organ system (eg, Glasgow Coma Scale score), resource utilization (eg, Therapeutic Intervention Scoring System), nursing workload (Nine Equivalents of Nursing Manpower Use Score), or global (eg, general ICU). Within ICU, scoring systems can be classified into those that assess disease severity on admission and predict outcome, such as APACHE, Simplified Acute Physiology Score (SAPS), and Mortality Probability Model (MPM), and scores that use the presence and severity of organ dysfunction on admission and during ICU course, such as Multiple Organ Dysfunction Score (MODS) and SOFA. These various SIL scores have been developed to meet such diverse needs.[69,70] Over time, as patient demographics, disease prevalence, case mix, and scope of ICU care have changed, scoring systems have been undergone multiple revisions or updates.[71] A comparison of general outcomes using the generic and updated models is summarized in (Table 4).

Table 4
Comparison of general outcome prediction models

Characteristics	APACHE	SAPS	APACHE II	MPM	APACHE III	SAPS II	MPM II	SAPS 3	APACHE IV	MPM III
Year	1981	1984	1985	1985	1991	1993	1993	2005	2006	2007
Countries	1	1	1	1	1	12	12	35	1	1
ICUs	2	8	13	1	40	137	140	303	104	135
Patients	705	679	5815	2783	17,440	12,997	19,124	16,784	110,558	124,855
Selection of variables and their weights	Panel of experts	Panel of experts	Panel of experts	Multiple logistic regression	Multiple logistic regression	Multiple logistic regression	Multiple logistic regression	Multiple logistic regression	Multiple logistic regression	Multiple logistic regression
Variables										
Age	No	Yes	Yes	Yes	Yes	Yes	Yes	Yes	Yes	Yes
Origin	No	No	No	No	Yes	No	No	Yes	Yes	No
Surgical status	No	No	Yes	Yes	Yes	Yes	Yes	Yes	Yes	Yes
Chronic	Yes	No	Yes	Yes	Yes	Yes	Yes	Yes	Yes	Yes
Health status										
Physiology	Yes	Yes	Yes	Yes	Yes	Yes	Yes	Yes	Yes	Yes
Acute diagnosis	No	No	Yes	No	Yes	No	Yes	Yes	Yes	Yes
Number of variables	34	14	17	11	26	17	15	20	142	16
Score	Yes	Yes	Yes	No	Yes	Yes	No	Yes	Yes	No
Mortality prediction	No	No	Yes	Yes	Yes	Yes	Yes	Yes	Yes	Yes

Adapted from with permission. Vincent JL, Moreno R. Clinical review: scoring systems in the critically ill. Crit Care. 2010;14(2):207. https://doi.org/10.1186/cc8204.

APACHE originally was developed in 1981 by Knaus and colleagues[72] to categorize patients by SIL according to the degree of acute illness and an assessment of the chronic health status. A simplified APACHE II was developed using just 12 physiologic variables, down from the 34 used in the original version. APACHE II is the most widely used SIL scoring system in the medical literature.[73] It uses age, admission type, chronic health evaluation, and the most abnormal results in 12 physiologic variables during the 24 hours after ICU admission to generate a weighted score (range 0–71) to predict hospital mortality. For each point increase in the score there, is approximately a 1% increase in-hospital mortality. APACHE III is a further refined version of APACHE II that improves calibration and discrimination through the use of a much larger derivation and validation patient sample.[74] As a result of decline in effective prognostic performance, the original APACHE III was recalibrated in 1998.[75] It is not widely used, however, partly because of complexity and proprietary algorithms that are not available in the public domain.

SAPS was developed and validated in 8 French ICUs using 13 weighted physiologic variables and age to predict risk of ICU death. Like APACHE scores, SAPS is calculated from the worst values obtained during the first 24 hours of ICU admission.[76] SAPS II uses a logistic regression analysis that includes 17 variables: 12 physiologic variables, age, type of admission, and 3 variables related to underlying disease.[77] SAPS 3, a completely new model, was created using advanced statistical methods from 20 variables divided into 3 subscores related to patient characteristics prior to admission, the circumstance of the admission, and the degree of physiologic derangement within 1 hour before or after ICU admission (unlike SAPS II with 24-hour time window). SAPS 3 can predict ICU mortality and detect resource utilization variability between ICUs.[78,79]

MPM and MPM II were developed using logistic regression methods from a single ICU and a large database, respectively. MPM II consists of 2 scores taken at admission and at 24 hours. MPM_0, the admission score, has 15 variables and MPM_{24}, the 24-hour score, has 5 of the admission variables and 8 additional variables. It is designed for patients whose ICU stay is greater than 24 hours.

APACHE, SAPS, and MPM scoring systems were developed predominantly from ICU patients with a noncancer diagnosis. This poses a significant challenge because patients with solid versus hematological malignancy (especially HSCT) have different mortality rates. Scoring systems specifically for cancer populations have been developed, such as the ICU Cancer Mortality Model (ICMM), but have had conflicting results.[80] In 1 study of cancer patients (hospital mortality, 44%) admitted to ICU, SAPS II provided a more accurate prognosis than ICMM.[81] But another study showed ICMM to be equivalent to SAPS II (and APACHE II) in patients (hospital mortality, 34%) admitted to an oncological ICU.[82] These findings suggest that the sensitivity of the scoring system varies with regard to differences in factors, such as ICU type and malignancy.[83] In HSCT patients admitted to ICU, 1 study reported APACHE II was no longer predictive of mortality[46] whereas another study found APACHE II superior in predicting mortality compared with other scoring systems.[84] Soares and colleagues[85] evaluated performance of APACHE II, III, SAPS, MPM, and ICMM in critically ill cancer patients and found that none of the scores accurately predicted outcome, with ICMM having no advantage over other general scores. Sinuff and colleagues[86] evaluated 12 observational studies and found that intensivists discriminate between survivors and nonsurvivors more accurately than do scoring systems during the first 24 hours of ICU admission. With a shift in interest to long-term ICU outcomes, scoring systems that quantify the burden of organ failure have emerged. In contrast to prognostic scores that are typically performed once at the beginning of the ICU stay, the organ

Table 5
Comparison of 3 organ dysfunction scores

Characteristics	Logistic Organ Dysfunction Score	Multiple Organ Dysfunction Score	Sequential Organ Dysfunction Score
Year of publication	1996	1995	1996
Selection of variables and their weights	Multiple logistic regression	Literature review and logistic regression	Panel of experts
Variables used to assess organ dysfunction			
Neurologic	Glasgow Coma Scale	Glasgow Coma Scale	Glasgow Coma Scale
Cardiovascular	Heart rate, systolic blood pressure	Pressure-adjusted heart rate	Mean arterial blood pressure, vasopressor use
Renal	Serum urea or urea nitrogen, creatinine, urine output	Serum creatinine	Serum creatinine, urine output
Respiratory	Pao_2/Fio_2 ratio, mechanical ventilation	Pao_2/Fio_2 Ratio	Pao_2/Fio_2 ratio, mechanical ventilation
Hematologic	White blood cell count, platelet count	Platelet count	Platelet count
Hepatic	Serum bilirubin, prothrombin time	Serum bilirubin	Serum bilirubin

Adapted from with permission. Vincent JL, Moreno R. Clinical review: scoring systems in the critically ill. Crit Care. 2010;14(2):207. https://doi.org/10.1186/cc8204.

dysfunction scores may be measured daily. The most commonly used organ failure scoring systems in general ICU patients are the Logistic Organ Dysfunction System, MODS, and SOFA (**Table 5**).

SOFA originally was developed by Vincent and colleagues[87] to evaluate organ failure in patients with sepsis and later adapted by Peres Bota and colleagues[88] to predict mortality in critically ill patients in shock. In a systematic review of 18 studies, Minne and colleagues[89] found that SOFA scores at admission performed slightly worse than APACHE II/III and were competitive with SAPS II models in predicting ICU mortality. The admission SOFA score was not a good mortality predictor, but a SOFA score increase during the first 48 hours of ICU admission predicts a mortality rate of at least 50%, independent of the initial score.[90] Another study evaluated SOFA score performance to predict ICU and in-hospital mortality in medical and surgical cancer patients; there was good discrimination in predicting mortality.[91] SOFA scoring performs well to predict mortality at ICU discharge but not individual outcomes.[92,93]

SUMMARY

Improvements in cancer therapies and survivorship have altered the perception of benefit from ICU admission. In deciding whether a cancer patient should be admitted to ICU, it is favorable to consider acuity and potential reversibility rather than cancer diagnosis and metastases. ICU triage strategies should focus on the potential benefit. A brief trial of ICU care should be considered, if appropriate, to allow for assessment of reversibility and improvement. Interim assessment can inform decisions regarding continuation of ICU care. The use of prognostic scoring systems provides insight into short-term and long-term outcomes. But there still is moderate disagreement between scoring systems applied during ICU admission, and during ICU stay, in cancer patients.

CONFLICTS OF INTEREST

None.

REFERENCES

1. U.S. Cancer Statistics Working Group. U.S. cancer statistics data visualizations tool, based on November 2018 submission data (1999-2016). U.S. Department of Health and Human Services, Centers for Disease Control and Prevention and National Cancer Institute; 2019. Available at: www.cdc.gov/cancer/dataviz https://www.cdc.gov/cancer/dataviz. Accessed February 20, 2020.
2. Guidelines for intensive care unit admission, discharge, and triage. Task Force of the American College of Critical Care Medicine, Society of Critical Care Medicine. Crit Care Med 1999;27(3):633–8.
3. Miller KD, Siegel RL, Lin CC, et al. Cancer treatment and survivorship statistics, 2016. CA Cancer J Clin 2016;66(4):271–89.
4. Shapiro CL. Cancer survivorship. N Engl J Med 2018;379(25):2438–50.
5. Siegel RL, Miller KD, Jemal A. Cancer statistics, 2016. CA Cancer J Clin 2016; 66(1):7–30.
6. Gutierrez C, McEvoy C, Munshi L, et al. Critical care management of toxicities associated with targeted agents and immunotherapies for cancer. Crit Care Med 2020;48(1):10–21.
7. Lee DW, Gardner R, Porter DL, et al. Current concepts in the diagnosis and management of cytokine release syndrome [published correction appears in Blood 2015 Aug 20;126(8):1048. Dosage error in article text] [published correction appears in Blood 2016 Sep 15;128(11):1533]. Blood 2014;124(2):188–95. https://doi.org/10.1182/blood-2014-05-552729.
8. Tanvetyanon T, Leighton JC. Life-sustaining treatments in patients who died of chronic congestive heart failure compared with metastatic cancer. Crit Care Med 2003;31(1):60–4.
9. Benoit DD, Vandewoude KH, Decruyenaere JM, et al. Outcome and early prognostic indicators in patients with a hematologic malignancy admitted to the intensive care unit for a life-threatening complication. Crit Care Med 2003;31(1): 104–12.
10. Lecuyer L, Chevret S, Thiery G, et al. The ICU Trial: a new admission policy for cancer patients requiring mechanical ventilation*. Crit Care Med 2007;35(3): 808–14.
11. Soares M, Azoulay É. Critical care management of lung cancer patients to prolong life without prolonging dying. Intensive Care Med 2009;35(12):2012–4.
12. Azoulay E, Soares M, Darmon M, et al. Intensive care of the cancer patient: recent achievements and remaining challenges. Ann Intensive Care 2011;1(1):5.
13. Azoulay E, Schellongowski P, Darmon M, et al. The Intensive Care Medicine research agenda on critically ill oncology and hematology patients. Intensive Care Med 2017;43(9):1366–82.
14. Peigne V, Rusinová K, Karlin L, et al. Continued survival gains in recent years among critically ill myeloma patients. Intensive Care Med 2008;35(3):512–8.

15. Soares M, Bozza FA, Azevedo LC, et al. Effects of organizational characteristics on outcomes and resource use in patients with cancer admitted to intensive care units. J Clin Oncol 2016;34(27):3315–24.

16. Azoulay E, Mokart D, Pène F, et al. Outcomes of Critically Ill Patients With Hematologic Malignancies: prospective Multicenter Data From France and Belgium—a Groupe de Recherche Respiratoire en Réanimation Onco-Hématologique Study. J Clin Oncol 2013;31(22):2810–8.

17. Schellongowski P, Staudinger T, Kundi M, et al. Prognostic factors for intensive care unit admission, intensive care outcome, and post-intensive care survival in patients with de novo acute myeloid leukemia: a single center experience. Haematologica 2010;96(2):231–7.

18. Azoulay E, Pène F, Darmon M, et al. Managing critically Ill hematology patients: time to think differently. Blood Rev 2015;29(6):359–67.

19. Azoulay É, Mokart D, Lambert J, et al. Diagnostic strategy for hematology and oncology patients with acute respiratory failure: randomized controlled trial. Am J Respir Crit Care Med 2010;182(8):1038–46.

20. Iserson KV, Moskop JC. Triage in medicine, Part I: concept, history, and types. Ann Emerg Med 2007;49(3):275–81.

21. Swan KG, Swan KG. Triage: the past revisited. Mil Med 1996;161(8):448–52.

22. Edwards M. Triage. Lancet 2009;373(9674):1515.

23. Skandalakis PN, Lainas P, Zoras O, et al. "To afford the wounded speedy assistance": dominique Jean Larrey and Napoleon. World J Surg 2006;30(8):1392–9.

24. Chipman M, Hackley BE, Spencer TS. Triage of mass casualties: concepts for coping with mixed battlefield injuries. Mil Med 1980;145(2):99–100.

25. Simchen E, Sprung CL, Galai N, et al. Survival of critically ill patients hospitalized in and out of intensive care units under paucity of intensive care unit beds. Crit Care Med 2004;32(8):1654–61.

26. Chen LM, Render M, Sales AE, et al. Variation in triage practices among Veterans Administration hospitals. In: 34th Annual Meeting of the Society of General Internal Medicine. Vol. 26. Society of General Internal Medicine (Ed). Phoenix (AZ): Society of General Internal Medicine; 2011. p. S51.

27. Azoulay É, Pochard F, Chevret S, et al. Compliance with triage to intensive care recommendations. Crit Care Med 2001;29(11):2132–6.

28. Nates JL, Nunnally M, Kleinpell R, et al. ICU admission, discharge, and triage guidelines: a framework to enhance clinical operations, development of institutional policies, and further research. Crit Care Med 2016;44(8):1553–602.

29. Nates J, Rathi N, Haque S, et al. ICU triage improves patient flow and resource utilization. Chest 2011;140(4):357A.

30. Howell E, Bessman E, Marshall R, et al. Hospitalist bed management effecting throughput from the emergency department to the intensive care unit. J Crit Care 2010;25(2):184–9.

31. Rathi NK, Haque SA, Morales F, et al. Variability in triage practices for critically ill cancer patients: a randomized controlled trial. J Crit Care 2019;53:18–24.

32. Staudinger T, Stoiser B, Müllner M, et al. Outcome and prognostic factors in critically ill cancer patients admitted to the intensive care unit. Crit Care Med 2000;28(5):1322–8.

33. Barfod C, Lauritzen MM, Danker JK, et al. Abnormal vital signs are strong predictors for intensive care unit admission and in-hospital mortality in adults triaged in the emergency department - a prospective cohort study. Scand J Trauma Resusc Emerg Med 2012;20(1):28.

34. Sprung CL, Geber D, Eidelman LA, et al. Evaluation of triage decisions for intensive care admission. Crit Care Med 1999;27(6):1073–9.

35. Orsini J, Butala A, Ahmad N, et al. Factors influencing triage decisions in patients referred for ICU admission. J Clin Med Res 2013;5(5):343–9.

36. Niskanen M, Kari A, Halonen P. Five-year survival after intensive care–comparison of 12,180 patients with the general population. Finnish ICU Study Group. Crit Care Med 1996;24(12):1962–7.

37. Moore EC, Pilcher DV, Bailey MJ, et al. A simple tool for mortality prediction in burns patients: Apache III score and FTSA. Burns 2010;36(7):1086–91.

38. Mariani P, Servois V, De Rycke Y, et al. Liver metastases from breast cancer: surgical resection or not? A case-matched control study in highly selected patients. Eur J Surg Oncol 2013;39(12):1377–83.

39. Tan AC, Jacques SK, Oatley M, et al. Characteristics and outcomes of oncology unit patients requiring admission to an Australian intensive care unit. Intern Med J 2019;49(6):734–9.

40. Pastores SM, Goldman DA, Shaz DJ, et al. Characteristics and outcomes of patients with hematologic malignancies receiving chemotherapy in the intensive care unit. Cancer 2018;124(14):3025–36.

41. Abbas FM, Sert MB, Rosenshein NB, et al. Gynecologic oncology patients in the surgical ICU. Impact on outcome. J Reprod Med 1997;42(3):173–8.

42. Thiéry G, Azoulay É, Darmon M, et al. Outcome of cancer patients considered for intensive care unit admission: a hospital-wide prospective study. J Clin Oncol 2005;23(19):4406–13.

43. Lueck C, Stadler M, Koenecke C, et al. Improved short- and long-term outcome of allogeneic stem cell recipients admitted to the intensive care unit: a retrospective longitudinal analysis of 942 patients. Intensive Care Med 2018;44(9): 1483–92.

44. Puxty K, McLoone P, Quasim T, et al. Characteristics and outcomes of surgical patients with solid cancers admitted to the intensive care unit. JAMA Surg 2018;153(9):834–40.

45. Azoulay E, Lemiale V, Mokart D, et al. Acute respiratory distress syndrome in patients with malignancies. Intensive Care Med 2014;40(8):1106–14.

46. Bird GT, Farquhar-Smith P, Wigmore T, et al. Outcomes and prognostic factors in patients with haematological malignancy admitted to a specialist cancer intensive care unit: a 5 yr study. Br J Anaesth 2012;108(3):452–9.

47. Kingah P, Alzubaidi N, Yafawi JZD, et al. Factors associated with mortality in patients with a solid malignancy admitted to the intensive care unit - a prospective observational study. J Crit Care Med (Targu Mures) 2018;4(4):137–42.

48. Gruson D, Vargas F, Hilbert G, et al. Predictive factors of intensive care unit admission in patients with haematological malignancies and pneumonia. Intensive Care Med 2004;30(5):965–71.

49. Pastores SM, Voigt LP. Acute respiratory failure in the patient with cancer: diagnostic and management strategies. Crit Care Clin 2010;26(1):21–40.

50. Martos-Benítez FD, Soto-García A, Gutiérrez-Noyola A. Clinical characteristics and outcomes of cancer patients requiring intensive care unit admission: a prospective study. J Cancer Res Clin Oncol 2018;144(4):717–23.

51. Azoulay E, Alberti C, Bornstain C, et al. Improved survival in cancer patients requiring mechanical ventilatory support: impact of noninvasive mechanical ventilatory support. Crit Care Med 2001;29(3):519–25.

52. Depuydt PO, Benoit DD, Roosens CD, et al. The impact of the initial ventilatory strategy on survival in hematological patients with acute hypoxemic respiratory failure. J Crit Care 2010;25(1):30–6.
53. Molina R, Bernal T, Borges M, et al. Ventilatory support in critically ill hematology patients with respiratory failure. Crit Care 2012;16(4):R133.
54. Lemiale V, Mokart D, Resche-Rigon M, et al. Effect of noninvasive ventilation vs oxygen therapy on mortality among immunocompromised patients with acute respiratory failure: a randomized clinical trial. JAMA 2015;314(16):1711.
55. Frat J-P, Thille AW, Mercat A, et al. High-flow oxygen through nasal cannula in acute hypoxemic respiratory failure. N Engl J Med 2015;372(23):2185–96.
56. Soares M, Depuydt PO, Salluh JI. Mechanical ventilation in cancer patients: clinical characteristics and outcomes. Crit Care Clin 2010;26(1):41–58.
57. Benoit DD, Hoste EA, Depuydt PO, et al. Outcome in critically ill medical patients treated with renal replacement therapy for acute renal failure: comparison between patients with and those without haematological malignancies. Nephrol Dial Transpl 2005;20(3):552–8.
58. Darmon M, Vincent F, Canet E, et al. Acute kidney injury in critically ill patients with haematological malignancies: results of a multicentre cohort study from the Groupe de Recherche en Réanimation Respiratoire en Onco-Hématologie. Nephrol Dial Transpl 2015;30(12):2006–13.
59. Soares M, Salluh JI, Carvalho MS, et al. Prognosis of critically ill patients with cancer and acute renal dysfunction. J Clin Oncol 2006;24(24):4003–10.
60. Kang E, Park M, Park PG, et al. Acute kidney injury predicts all-cause mortality in patients with cancer. Cancer Med 2019;8(6):2740–50. https://doi.org/10.1002/cam4.2140.
61. Darmon M, Vincent F, Camous L, et al. Tumour lysis syndrome and acute kidney injury in high-risk haematology patients in the rasburicase era. A prospective multicentre study from the Groupe de Recherche en Réanimation Respiratoire et Onco-Hématologique. Br J Haematol 2013;162(4):489–97.
62. Mokart D, Granata A, Crocchiolo R, et al. Allogeneic hematopoietic stem cell transplantation after reduced intensity conditioning regimen: outcomes of patients admitted to intensive care unit. J Crit Care 2015;30(5):1107–13.
63. Sculier JP, Markiewicz E. Cardiopulmonary resuscitation in medical cancer patients: the experience of a medical intensive-care unit of a cancer centre. Support Care Cancer 1993;1(3):135–8.
64. Wallace S, Ewer MS, Price KJ, et al. Outcome and cost implications of cardiopulmonary resuscitation in the medical intensive care unit of a comprehensive cancer center. Support Care Cancer 2002;10(5):425–9.
65. Khasawneh FA, Kamel MT, Abu-Zaid MI. Predictors of cardiopulmonary arrest outcome in a comprehensive cancer center intensive care unit. Scand J Trauma Resusc Emerg Med 2013;21(1):18.
66. Reisfield GM, Wallace SK, Munsell MF, et al. Survival in cancer patients undergoing in-hospital cardiopulmonary resuscitation: a meta-analysis. Resuscitation 2006;71(2):152–60.
67. Champigneulle B, Merceron S, Lemiale V, et al. What is the outcome of cancer patients admitted to the ICU after cardiac arrest? Results from a multicenter study. Resuscitation 2015;92:38–44.
68. Sculier JP. Cardiopulmonary resuscitation in cancer patients: indications and limits. Clin Intensive Care 1995;6(2):72–5.
69. Keegan MT, Gajic O, Afessa B. Severity of illness scoring systems in the intensive care unit. Crit Care Med 2011;39(1):163–9.

70. Vincent J-L, Bruzzi de Carvalho F. Severity of illness. Semin Respir Crit Care Med 2010;31(1):31–8.

71. Higgins TL, Teres D, Nathanson B. Outcome prediction in critical care: the mortality probability models. Curr Opin Crit Care 2008;14(5):498–505.

72. Knaus WA, Zimmerman JE, Wagner DP, et al. APACHE—acute physiology and chronic health evaluation: a physiologically based classification system. Crit Care Med 1981;9(8):591–7.

73. Knaus WA, Draper EA, Wagner DP, et al. APACHE II: a severity of disease classification system. Crit Care Med 1985;13(10):818–29.

74. Knaus WA, Wagner DP, Draper EA, et al. The APACHE III prognostic system. Risk prediction of hospital mortality for critically ill hospitalized adults. Chest 1991; 100(6):1619–36.

75. Zimmerman JE, Wagner DP, Draper EA, et al. Evaluation of acute physiology and chronic health evaluation III predictions of hospital mortality in an independent database. Crit Care Med 1998;26(8):1317–26.

76. Gall J-RL, Loirat P, Alperovitch A, et al. A simplified acute physiology score for ICU patients. Crit Care Med 1984;12(11):975–7.

77. Le Gall JR. A new Simplified Acute Physiology Score (SAPS II) based on a European/North American multicenter study. JAMA 1993;270(24):2957–63.

78. Moreno RP, Metnitz PGH, Almeida E, et al. SAPS 3—From evaluation of the patient to evaluation of the intensive care unit. Part 2: Development of a prognostic model for hospital mortality at ICU admission. Intensive Care Medicine 2006; 32(5):796.

79. Rothen HU, Stricker K, Einfalt J, et al. Variability in outcome and resource use in intensive care units. Intensive Care Medicine 2007;33(8):1329–36.

80. Groeger JS, Lemeshow S, Price K, et al. Multicenter outcome study of cancer patients admitted to the intensive care unit: a probability of mortality model. J Clin Oncol 1998;16(2):761–70.

81. Schellongowski P, Benesch M, Lang T, et al. Comparison of three severity scores for critically ill cancer patients. Intensive Care Med 2004;30(3):430–6.

82. Berghmans T, Paesmans M, Sculier JP. Is a specific oncological scoring system better at predicting the prognosis of cancer patients admitted for an acute medical complication in an intensive care unit than general gravity scores? Support Care Cancer 2004;12(4):234–9.

83. Wigmore T, Farquhar-Smith P. Outcomes for critically ill cancer patients in the ICU: current trends and prediction. Int Anesthesiol Clin 2016;54(4):e62–75.

84. Michel CS, Teschner D, Schmidtmann I, et al. Prognostic factors and outcome of adult allogeneic hematopoietic stem cell transplantation patients admitted to intensive care unit during transplant hospitalization. Sci Rep 2019;9(1):19911.

85. Soares M, Fontes F, Dantas J, et al. Performance of six severity-of-illness scores in cancer patients requiring admission to the intensive care unit: a prospective observational study. Crit Care 2004;8(4):R194–203.

86. Sinuff T, Adhikari NK, Cook DJ, et al. Mortality predictions in the intensive care unit: comparing physicians with scoring systems. Crit Care Med 2006;34(3): 878–85.

87. Vincent JL, Moreno R, Takala J, et al. The SOFA (Sepsis-related organ failure assessment) score to describe organ dysfunction/failure. On behalf of the working group on sepsis-related problems of the European Society of Intensive Care Medicine. Intensive Care Med 1996;22(7):707–10.

88. Peres Bota D, Melot C, Lopes Ferreira F, et al. The multiple organ dysfunction score (MODS) versus the Sequential organ failure assessment (SOFA) score in outcome prediction. Intensive Care Med 2002;28(11):1619–24.
89. Minne L, Abu-Hanna A, de Jonge E. Evaluation of SOFA-based models for predicting mortality in the ICU: a systematic review. Crit Care 2009;12(6):R161.
90. Ferreira FL, Bota DP, Bross A, et al. Serial evaluation of the SOFA score to predict outcome in critically ill patients. JAMA 2001;286(14):1754–8.
91. Cárdenas-Turanzas M, Ensor J, Wakefield C, et al. Cross-validation of a sequential organ failure assessment score–based model to predict mortality in patients with cancer admitted to the intensive care unit. J Crit Care 2012;27(6):673–80.
92. Lamia B, Hellot MF, Girault C, et al. Changes in severity and organ failure scores as prognostic factors in onco-hematological malignancy patients admitted to the ICU. Intensive Care Med 2006;32(10):1560–8.
93. Ñamendys-Silva SA, Texcocano-Becerra J, Herrera-Gómez A. Application of the sequential organ failure assessment (SOFA) score to patients with cancer admitted to the intensive care unit. Am J Hosp Palliat Care 2009;26(5):341–6.

Intensive Care Unit Organization and Interdisciplinary Care for Critically Ill Patients with Cancer

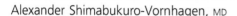

Alexander Shimabukuro-Vornhagen, MD

KEYWORDS

- ICU • Multidisciplinary care • ICU organization • Oncology • Cancer

KEY POINTS

- High-quality critical care for critically ill patients with cancer requires a multidisciplinary care team.
- Critically ill patients with cancer are a highly complex patient population with unique medical needs.
- Effective communication among members of the multidisciplinary care team is critical to achieve the best possible outcomes by avoiding fragmented care, interpersonal conflicts, and delivery of inconsistent information to the patient and the relatives.

BACKGROUND

Critical care is a young medical discipline. Over recent decades there have been substantial medical and technical advances that have resulted in increased chances of survival for critically ill patients. Patients with cancer are a particularly vulnerable patient population. They are at an increased risk of becoming critically ill because of the underlying malignancy, as a consequence of complications of the cancer treatment, or because of an unrelated medical condition.[1] Until recently, patients with cancer have often been considered poor candidates for intensive care unit (ICU) admission. However, the outcomes of patients with cancer requiring critical care has improved substantially over the recent decades.[1]

Novel therapeutic approaches, such as molecularly targeted cancer agents, immune checkpoint blockade, and chimeric antigen receptor (CAR) T-cell therapy, show impressive tumor responses and offer the prospect of long-term disease remission in patients that previously had few or no promising treatment options.[2–4] However, these novel cancer therapies can be associated with severe life-threating

Department I of Internal Medicine, University Hospital of Cologne, Kerpener Str. 62, Cologne 50673, Germany
E-mail address: shima@uk-koeln.de

Crit Care Clin 37 (2021) 19–28
https://doi.org/10.1016/j.ccc.2020.09.003
0749-0704/21/© 2020 Elsevier Inc. All rights reserved.

treatment-related adverse events that necessitate critical care management.[5] As a consequence of these developments, the number of patients with cancer admitted to ICU has been growing over recent decades.[1,6] Patients with cancer account for 15% to 20% of ICU patients.[7] As new effective treatments enter the clinic and the survival of patients with cancer improve, it can be expected that the number of patients with cancer in the ICU will continue to grow. However, the availability of effective cancer therapeutics not only offers novel opportunities but also poses hitherto unknown challenges because it makes decision making in the management of critically ill patients with cancer more complex. As a consequence of the added complexity, treatment has to become more individualized and requires expert knowledge from multiple disciplines.

Patients with cancer are among the most complex patient populations in medicine.[8] Acute critical illness adds additional complexity. ICU patients are a patient population with highly complex care needs. It therefore is no surprise that clinical studies have found that multidisciplinary ICU teams lead to improved outcomes. In critically ill patients with cancer, the already complex medical management of the acute condition leading to ICU admission is further complicated by the underlying malignancy and the additional aspects this entails. State-of-the-art care in this setting can only be ensured by an interdisciplinary care team capable of providing the broad expertise that covers the whole spectrum of care needs of patients with cancer. Every health care worker involved in the care of patients with cancer has to be familiar with the main aspects of interdisciplinary management of patients with malignant diseases. This article therefore summarizes what is currently known about the role of multidisciplinary care for critically ill patients with cancer.

COMPONENTS OF MULTIDISCIPLINARY CARE FOR PATIENTS WITH CANCER

Multidisciplinary care consists of comprehensive care provided by a multiprofessional team that collaboratively manages patients. Multiprofessional team–based care has been shown to improve the management of complex patients and has been adopted in many fields of medicine. In North America and Europe, the multidisciplinary team approach has become the standard in the clinical management of patients with cancer. One of the main strengths of the multidisciplinary team approach is that it can make use of the diverse viewpoints of the team members. Collaborative patient assessment, and treatment planning that involves a broad expertise, ensures that all relevant aspects of patient care are considered and alternative treatment options are discussed. Studies have shown that interdisciplinary team–based cancer care results in better adherence to guidelines and better patient satisfaction.[9–11] Apart from providing optimal care to critically ill patients, multidisciplinary teams offer the ideal platform to perform the type of cross-disciplinary research that is required to achieve significant diagnostic and therapeutic advances in the care of critically ill patients with cancer.[12]

There are several key features that are essential for the practice of multidisciplinary critical care: (1) an organizational structure of ICU services that promotes the multidisciplinary team performance; (2) a diverse team of health care professionals that cover the whole spectrum of expertise required to care for critically ill patients with cancer; (3) frequent, respectful, and effective communication among all team members.

ORGANIZATIONAL INTENSIVE CARE UNIT STRUCTURE

Organizational structure and ICU care processes are key aspects of high-quality critical care delivery and optimal patient outcomes. The ability to identify key organizational features for optimal management of patients with cancer is complicated by the considerable variability in the organization and delivery of critical care. There are large differences both within and between health care systems with regard to how critically ill patients with cancer are cared for.[13–15] Nationally and internationally, there is a wide variety of organizational models for ICUs.[14,16] Furthermore, the number of ICU beds varies widely even among developed countries.[17] However, little is known about how variations in ICU use affect patient outcomes.

The organizational structure of multidisciplinary ICU care therefore has to be tailored to the local infrastructure, resources, and patient population. There are 3 main ICU organizational models: open ICUs, closed ICUs, and semiclosed ICUs. Closed ICUs function as an independent unit that is managed by full-time intensivists. Most of the evidence indicates that the closed ICU concept is associated with improved quality and outcomes. More specialized ICU care does not automatically entail better outcomes.[18] Effective multidisciplinary care teams can likely compensate for most of the advantages that specialty ICUs can offer. ICU staffing and the resulting workload affect the patient outcomes and the well-being of patients, family, and ICU staff. Inadequate staffing can have a negative impact on the job satisfaction of physicians and nurses.[19] Establishing organizational structures that facilitate a positive ICU culture is paramount to promoting the physical and psychological well-being of ICU staff and enabling them to provide patients and families with the best care possible.

The outcome of critically ill patients with cancer is in part determined by the treatment they received before and after their ICU stays. Effective critical care therefore starts before the patients have entered the ICU and extends beyond their discharge from ICU. The multidisciplinary care for patients with cancer should therefore extend beyond the ICU stay. Physicians and nurses that take care of patients with cancer should be proficient at detecting warning signs of clinical deterioration and be familiar with the most important therapeutic measures needed. Medical emergency teams that are staffed by members of the critical care team can support the teams on the ward with identifying and managing deteriorating patients and can facilitate the transition to ICU. Another important issue that has so far received little attention is the long-term outcome of patients with cancer after critical care. For many patients, the challenges are far from over after discharge from ICU. An ICU stay has long-term physical and psychological impacts that can affect the patient's life months and years after receiving treatment in the ICU.[20] Cancer specialists and patients are often not aware of these sequelae of critical care treatment. ICU survivors can have a broad range of physical, mental, and psychological impairments. Post-ICU clinics that see patients after they have been discharged from the ICU can help to address the long-term sequelae of ICU care.

Composition of the Multidisciplinary Intensive Care Unit Team

A multidisciplinary team–based approach that includes health care professionals from various disciplines is most likely to be able to address the diverse needs of critically ill patients with cancer. The multidisciplinary care team should therefore be composed of members from all health care professions that cover the spectrum of expertise required to optimally manage a given patient with cancer.

Hematology/oncology

Common reasons for ICU admission of patients with cancer include complications of the underlying malignancy, adverse events caused by cancer treatment, and critical illness unrelated to the cancer. In the ICU, patients with cancer continue to require specialized cancer care. Therefore, the expertise of cancer specialist is essential for the management of patients with cancer that are admitted to the ICU. Input from the patient's hematologist/oncologist is important to ensure continuity of care. Among all the health care workers taking care of critically ill patients with cancer, the patient's hematologist/oncologist usually is the most well informed with regard to the patient's prior health status, current medical conditions, and goals of care. Critical care physicians rely on cancer specialists to evaluate the prognosis of the patient and the indication for ICU admission. Furthermore, the oncological expertise is often important for the diagnostic work-up and medical management of cancer-related acute medical conditions.[1] In addition, some patients need cancer therapy during the stay in the ICU.[21,22] The oncologist's/hematologist's experience with the selection and dosing of cancer therapies is essential for the safe administration of cancer treatments in the ICU setting. The hematologist/oncologist also plays a crucial role in setting goals of care and transition to palliative care in patients in whom life-prolonging therapies are no longer justified. Importantly, close collaboration of the cancer specialists with the ICU team has been associated with a lower mortality.[23] Oncologists and intensivists should meet on a frequent basis to assess treatment success and discuss the future treatment plan.

Critical care

An ICU is a specially equipped ward that is dedicated to treating patients that are in a life-threatening medical condition. It is staffed with specially trained physicians and nurses that are trained to provide life-supporting medical interventions such as mechanical ventilation and vasopressor support. The core medical ICU team consists of ICU physicians; critical care nurses; and, in some ICUs, advanced practice providers. The main expertise of the core ICU team is the provision of life-sustaining therapies for critically ill patients in order to restore or maintain organ functions.

In most ICUs, besides managing the patients' acute medical conditions, critical care physicians are responsible for assessing the indication for ICU admission and coordination of the multidisciplinary care team. The presence of a board-certified intensivist is associated with improved ICU outcome in patients with cancer.[24] Decision making regarding ICU admission and aggressive life-sustaining treatment of patients with cancer is a highly challenging task because intensivists have to determine the prognosis of the patient's acute condition leading to the request for ICU admission in the context of the prognosis of the underlying malignancy. As mentioned earlier, close collaboration with a cancer clinician is an evidence-based practice that can improve the survival of critically ill patients with cancer. Intensive care physicians should therefore aim to involve an oncologist in crucial decisions whenever possible.

Critical care nurses play a central role in the care of patients with cancer in the ICU. Among all members of the multidisciplinary care team, nurses usually spend the most time with the patients. They are the most likely to detect and respond to acute changes in the patient's condition. Critical care nurses should therefore be familiar with the most common complications that can occur in patients with solid tumor or hematologic malignancies. Furthermore, nurses are an important communication partner for patients and families. They are the ICU team members that are in closest contact with patients and relative and often are asked to reproduce and explain the information provided by physicians. By providing this information in a clear and accessible way, they can enhance understanding of the current treatment concept. Moreover, critical care nurses often act as advocates representing their patients' views and concerns, particularly if no relatives are present.

Clinical pharmacists

The growing number of drugs and the increasing use of drug combinations adds novel therapeutic options but also makes pharmacologic management increasingly complex, particularly in cancer therapy. In critically ill patients, the pharmacologic treatment is further complicated by the frequent presence of impaired organ function, altered volume of distribution, and drug-drug interactions. In many ICUs, clinical pharmacists are important members of the critical care team.[25] Several studies have shown that clinical pharmacists can improve patient outcomes in critical care. Input from a clinical pharmacist during critical care rounds improves the safety and effectiveness of pharmacotherapy. Areas of pharmacologic therapy that have been improved by the availability of a clinical pharmacist in ICUs include adverse drug events,[26] drug-drug interactions,[27] sedation,[28] and antimicrobial treatment.[29] Soares and colleagues[23] showed that the presence of a clinical pharmacist was associated with decreased mortality in critically ill patients with cancer. This finding comes as no surprise considering the large number of drugs that patients with cancer receive either as part of the cancer treatment or for the management of its complications. Clinical pharmacists that are part of a multidisciplinary care team need special knowledge about the pharmacodynamics, pharmacokinetics, and side effect profiles of drugs that are frequently used in patients with cancer.

Palliative care

Palliative care is a key component of comprehensive care for patients with cancer, regardless of diagnosis or prognosis. It therefore should also be part of collaborative ICU care.[30] Even though most intensivists are familiar with the provision of basic palliative care needs for patients in the ICU, optimal palliative care in the ICU requires more expertise and time than intensivists usually have available. Palliative care can be implemented by a member of the ICU team or by a separate external consult team. The care for dying patients benefits from the contribution of palliative care experts. Palliative care can assist in symptom management and supporting the patients and families. The support of a palliative care team can help with transitioning patients that do not benefit from ICU care (eg, because they exhausted all therapeutic options or because they continue to deteriorate despite treatment) to a care setting that is more appropriate and more in line with their needs and wishes.

Spiritual care

For many people, spirituality and religion are an important part of their lives.[31] Spiritual and religious belief can have a strong influence on the treatment of patients with cancer. Spirituality can serve as a valuable resource for patients as well as health care professionals. Most patients with cancer report spiritual and religious needs.[32] Many patients with cancer wish to discuss spiritual issues with their treating physicians, but the spiritual care needs are all too often not adequately met in the ICU.[33] Spiritual well-being of patients and their relatives is important.[34] Studies have shown that provision of spiritual care can have a beneficial impact on the patient and family experience as well as the clinical outcome.[32–34] Therefore, all intensivists should have a basic knowledge to assess and address the spiritual needs of their patients. Ideally, they should be supported by professionally trained spiritual care providers that are experts in attending to the spiritual needs of the patients. Despite the benefits of providing chaplaincy services, only a minority of patients with cancer receive spiritual care.[35] In light of the positive effects of addressing patients' religious and spiritual needs, provision of spiritual care services should be a standard in ICUs caring for patients with cancer and this is a target for further improvement.

Additional team members

Depending on the setting, this core ICU team is typically supported by additional team members, such as social workers, physical therapists, nutritionists, and respiratory therapists. These team members provide important expert services that are needed to obtain optimal treatment outcomes, support patient and family well-being, and facilitate recovery from critical illness. Social workers provide important logistic and psychosocial support for the patients and their families.[36] They provide important psychological support and help to coordinate family meetings.

TEAM COORDINATION AND COMMUNICATION

Despite all its benefits for the patients, multidisciplinary care also has some disadvantages and the potential for harm. More care does not necessarily lead to better care. Because many different specialties are involved in the multidisciplinary care of patients with cancer, there is a risk that care becomes fragmented. If patient care becomes fragmented, multidisciplinary care can paradoxically lead to worse care and decreased satisfaction of patients, their families, and health care providers. Thus, coordination and effective communication are the basis of successful collaborative care.

Multidisciplinary care therefore needs to be well coordinated in order to unfold its full potential. The coordination of the multidisciplinary critical care team is often the responsibility of the ICU physician or a special coordinating nurse. Multidisciplinary critical care rests on the coordinated contribution of multiple health care professionals to the care of an individual patient. By nature, the multiprofessional team approach requires regular communication among the multidisciplinary team members. Communication is the central aspect of successful multidisciplinary care. Effective communication among all members involved in the care of a patient is key to achieving the best outcomes for the patient. In contrast, poor communication is a leading cause of worse ICU team performance and delivery of low-quality health care that can result in patient harm, ICU staff burnout, and increased cost. In order to allow each team member to contribute optimally to care, communication has to be open and respectful. Every team member should have the opportunity to voice concerns.

One aspect of critical care for patients with cancer that is often overlooked is the impact on the health care providers taking care of the patients with cancer. The ICU environment is stressful not only for patients but also for the ICU staff. Caring for patients with cancer often presents critical care teams with unique medical and ethical challenges that can lead to conflict, moral distress, and burnout.[37–39] Perceived inappropriateness of ICU care can cause job dissatisfaction in ICU nurses and physicians.[40]

The quality of communication among the multidisciplinary care team members also affects the communication with patients and their families. The experience of communication with the ICU team has an important impact on the ICU experience and well-being of surrogate decision makers.[41] Patients and their relatives should receive consistent messages from all members of the multidisciplinary care team. This communication requires that the team members develop a common understanding of the goals of care. Poor communication among the multidisciplinary team members and between team members and the patients or relatives can cause distress in patients and their relatives. In contrast, effective team communication reduces conflicts and enhances team spirit and job satisfaction, thereby contributing to high-quality care. Formal and informal team meetings are an opportunity to have an open exchange of ideas and opinions and enable the formulation of a common understanding of the treatment goals. Frequent communication and interprofessional education constitute a considerable investment of time and resources but ultimately pays off by improving the ICU culture and increasing the overall quality of care.

Meeting all the complex demands of critical care for patients with cancer requires constant learning and iterative improvements of processes. Both oncology and critical care are continuously evolving. In order to keep up with new developments in the management of critically ill patients with cancer, the members of the multidisciplinary care team have to update their knowledge in their field of expertise. Beyond this specialty training, additional interprofessional education and training should be offered. At present, there are only few opportunities for cross-disciplinary education and training but the professional societies are increasingly recognizing the need and are starting to establish specialized venues and programs that provide the necessary knowledge.

ECONOMIC ASPECTS

The treatment of cancer is expensive. Modern cancer therapies can often cost more than $100,000. The provision of critical care adds substantial cost to the already highly expensive cancer treatment. In the United States, the mean cost for patients with acute myeloid leukemia who require ICU care is twice the cost of patients who are not admitted to an ICU.[42] CAR T cells are the newest addition to the cancer treatment armamentarium. However, CAR T cells are associated with unique toxicities, namely cytokine release syndrome and immune effector cell–associated neurotoxicity syndrome.[5,43] Critical care contributes substantially to the total cost of CAR T-cell therapy.[44] The added team members that constitute the multidisciplinary care team add to the cost of providing critical care for patients with cancer. However, despite the increased expenses for additional staff, studies suggest that multidisciplinary care could be cost-effective. Multidisciplinary care can help to optimize ICU use and thereby decrease costs.[45]

SUMMARY

Oncology and critical care are becoming increasingly complex. In order to achieve optimal outcomes for critically ill patients with cancer, an interdisciplinary care approach is necessary. Crucial members of a multidisciplinary care team include oncologists/hematologists, intensivists, critical care nurses, social workers, physical therapists, clinical pharmacists, and spiritual care providers. Multidisciplinary ICU management is associated with increased patient and family satisfaction and improved outcomes. Even though the value of multidisciplinary ICU care is generally recognized, there are still many gaps in the knowledge of what is necessary for optimal multidisciplinary care for critically ill patients with cancer. Further research investigating key aspects of the interdisciplinary management of critically ill patients with cancer is needed to further improve the evidence base of multidisciplinary critical care. Better integration of multidisciplinary critical care into the continuum of care for patients with cancer offers the prospect of further improvements in the outcomes of patients with cancer.

CLINICS CARE POINTS

- Multidisciplinary care improves the outcome of critically ill cancer patients.
- Multidisciplinary care rounds should include a board-certified intensivist, a cancer specialist, and a pharmacist.
- A time-limited ICU trial is a valulable ICU admission strategy to address prognostic uncertainty.

DISCLOSURE

The author has nothing to disclose.

REFERENCES

1. Shimabukuro-Vornhagen A, Böll B, Kochanek M, et al. Critical care of patients with cancer. CA Cancer J Clin 2016;66(6):496–517.
2. Tsimberidou A-M. Targeted therapy in cancer. Cancer Chemother Pharmacol 2015;76(6):1113–32.
3. Postow MA, Callahan MK, Wolchok JD. Immune checkpoint blockade in cancer therapy. J Clin Oncol 2015;33(17):1974–82.
4. June CH, Sadelain M. Chimeric antigen receptor therapy. N Engl J Med 2018; 379(1):64–73.
5. Shimabukuro-Vornhagen A, Gödel P, Subklewe M, et al. Cytokine release syndrome. J Immunother Cancer 2018;6(1):56.
6. Sauer CM, Dong J, Celi LA, et al. Improved survival of cancer patients admitted to the intensive care unit between 2002 and 2011 at a U.S. Teaching hospital. Cancer Res Treat 2019;51(3):973–81.
7. Taccone FS, Artigas AA, Sprung CL, et al. Characteristics and outcomes of cancer patients in European ICUs. Crit Care 2009;13(1):R15.
8. Tonelli M, Wiebe N, Manns BJ, et al. Comparison of the complexity of patients seen by different medical subspecialists in a universal health care system. JAMA Netw Open 2018;1(7):e184852.
9. Bjegovich-Weidman M, Haid M, Kumar S, et al. Establishing a community-based lung cancer multidisciplinary clinic as part of a large integrated health care system: aurora health care. J Oncol Pract 2010;6(6):e27–30.
10. Vinod SK, Sidhom MA, Delaney GP. Do multidisciplinary meetings follow guideline-based care? J Oncol Pract 2010;6(6):276–81.
11. Vinod SK, Sidhom MA, Gabriel GS, et al. Why do some lung cancer patients receive no anticancer treatment? J Thorac Oncol 2010;5(7):1025–32.
12. Why interdisciplinary research matters. Nature 2015;525(7569):305.
13. Bekelman JE, Halpern SD, Blankart CR, et al. Comparison of site of death, health care utilization, and hospital expenditures for patients dying with cancer in 7 developed countries. JAMA 2016;315(3):272–83.
14. Wunsch H, Angus DC, Harrison DA, et al. Variation in critical care services across North America and Western Europe. Crit Care Med 2008;36(10):2787–97, e1-9.
15. Chang DW, Shapiro MF. Association between intensive care unit utilization during hospitalization and costs, use of invasive procedures, and mortality. JAMA Intern Med 2016;176(10):1492–9.
16. Vincent JL, Suter P, Bihari D, et al. Organization of intensive care units in Europe: lessons from the EPIC study. Intensive Care Med 1997;23(11):1181–4.
17. Rhodes A, Ferdinande P, Flaatten H, et al. The variability of critical care bed numbers in Europe. Intensive Care Med 2012;38(10):1647–53.
18. Lott JP, Iwashyna TJ, Christie JD, et al. Critical illness outcomes in specialty versus general intensive care units. Am J Respir Crit Care Med 2009;179(8): 676–83.
19. Toh SG, Ang E, Devi MK. Systematic review on the relationship between the nursing shortage and job satisfaction, stress and burnout levels among nurses in oncology/haematology settings. Int J Evid Based Healthc 2012;10(2):126–41.
20. Azoulay E, Vincent J-L, Angus DC, et al. Recovery after critical illness: putting the puzzle together-a consensus of 29. Crit Care 2017;21(1):296.

21. Pastores SM, Goldman DA, Shaz DJ, et al. Characteristics and outcomes of patients with hematologic malignancies receiving chemotherapy in the intensive care unit. Cancer 2018;124(14):3025–36.
22. Wohlfarth P, Staudinger T, Sperr WR, et al. Prognostic factors, long-term survival, and outcome of cancer patients receiving chemotherapy in the intensive care unit. Ann Hematol 2014;93(10):1629–36.
23. Soares M, Bozza FA, Azevedo LCP, et al. Effects of organizational characteristics on outcomes and resource use in patients with cancer admitted to intensive care units. J Clin Oncol 2016;34(27):3315–24.
24. Song JH, Kim S, Lee HW, et al. Effect of intensivist involvement on clinical outcomes in patients with advanced lung cancer admitted to the intensive care unit. PLoS One 2019;14(2):e0210951.
25. Rudis MI, Brandl KM. Position paper on critical care pharmacy services. Society of Critical Care Medicine and American College of Clinical Pharmacy Task Force on critical care pharmacy services. Crit Care Med 2000;28(11):3746–50.
26. Leape LL, Cullen DJ, Clapp MD, et al. Pharmacist participation on physician rounds and adverse drug events in the intensive care unit. JAMA 1999;282(3):267–70.
27. Rivkin A, Yin H. Evaluation of the role of the critical care pharmacist in identifying and avoiding or minimizing significant drug-drug interactions in medical intensive care patients. J Crit Care 2011;26(1):104.e1-6.
28. Marshall J, Finn CA, Theodore AC. Impact of a clinical pharmacist-enforced intensive care unit sedation protocol on duration of mechanical ventilation and hospital stay. Crit Care Med 2008;36(2):427–33.
29. MacLaren R, Bond CA, Martin SJ, et al. Clinical and economic outcomes of involving pharmacists in the direct care of critically ill patients with infections. Crit Care Med 2008;36(12):3184–9.
30. Baggs JG, Norton SA, Schmitt MH, et al. The dying patient in the ICU: role of the interdisciplinary team. Crit Care Clin 2004;20(3):525–40, xi.
31. Peteet JR, Balboni MJ. Spirituality and religion in oncology. CA Cancer J Clin 2013;63(4):280–9.
32. Astrow AB, Kwok G, Sharma RK, et al. Spiritual needs and perception of quality of care and satisfaction with care in hematology/medical oncology patients: a multicultural assessment. J Pain Symptom Manage 2018;55(1):56–64.e1.
33. Astrow AB, Wexler A, Texeira K, et al. Is failure to meet spiritual needs associated with cancer patients' perceptions of quality of care and their satisfaction with care? J Clin Oncol 2007;25(36):5753–7.
34. Ho JQ, Nguyen CD, Lopes R, et al. Spiritual care in the intensive care unit: a narrative review. J Intensive Care Med 2018;33(5):279–87.
35. Epstein-Peterson ZD, Sullivan AJ, Enzinger AC, et al. Examining forms of spiritual care provided in the advanced cancer setting. Am J Hosp Palliat Care 2015;32(7):750–7.
36. Zebrack B, Kayser K, Oktay J, et al. The association of oncology social work's project to assure quality cancer care (APAQCC). J Psychosoc Oncol 2018;36(1):19–30.
37. Poncet MC, Toullic P, Papazian L, et al. Burnout syndrome in critical care nursing staff. Am J Respir Crit Care Med 2007;175(7):698–704.
38. Embriaco N, Azoulay E, Barrau K, et al. High level of burnout in intensivists: prevalence and associated factors. Am J Respir Crit Care Med 2007;175(7):686–92.

39. Mealer ML, Shelton A, Berg B, et al. Increased prevalence of post-traumatic stress disorder symptoms in critical care nurses. Am J Respir Crit Care Med 2007;175(7):693–7.

40. Azoulay E, Timsit J-F, Sprung CL, et al. Prevalence and factors of intensive care unit conflicts: the conflicus study. Am J Respir Crit Care Med 2009;180(9): 853–60.

41. Wendlandt B, Ceppe A, Choudhury S, et al. Modifiable elements of ICU supportive care and communication are associated with surrogates' PTSD symptoms. Intensive Care Med 2019;45(5):619–26.

42. Halpern AB, Culakova E, Walter RB, et al. Association of risk factors, mortality, and care costs of adults with acute myeloid leukemia with admission to the intensive care unit. JAMA Oncol 2017;3(3):374–81.

43. Neelapu SS, Tummala S, Kebriaei P, et al. Chimeric antigen receptor T-cell therapy - assessment and management of toxicities. Nat Rev Clin Oncol 2018;15(1): 47–62.

44. Yang H, Hao Y, Chai X, et al. Estimation of total costs in patients with relapsed or refractory diffuse large B-cell lymphoma receiving tisagenlecleucel from a US hospital's perspective. J Med Econ 2020;23(9):1016–24.

45. MacLaren R, Bond CA. Effects of pharmacist participation in intensive care units on clinical and economic outcomes of critically ill patients with thromboembolic or infarction-related events. Pharmacotherapy 2009;29(7):761–8.

Critical Care of Hematopoietic Stem Cell Transplant Patients

Rachael A. Fornwalt, RN, MSN, ACNP[a], Emily P. Brigham, MD, MHS[b],
R. Scott Stephens, MD[c],*

KEYWORDS

- Hematopoietic stem cell transplant • Bone marrow transplant
- Acute respiratory distress syndrome • Neutropenic sepsis
- Graft-versus-host disease • Cytokine release syndrome • Engraftment syndrome
- Acute renal failure

KEY POINTS

- Approximately 15% of patients require critical care after hematopoietic stem cell transplant (HSCT).
- The immunologic milieu is markedly altered after HSCT.
- Respiratory failure and sepsis are the most common causes of critical illness after HSCT.
- Complications of HSCT can affect any organ system.
- Specialized HSCT intensive care units (ICUs) and ICU providers may improve outcomes.

INTRODUCTION

Hematopoietic stem cell transplant (HSCT) is an essential therapeutic modality in the treatment of malignant and nonmalignant hematologic disease. In 2018, approximately 14,000 autologous HSCTs and more than 9000 allogeneic transplants were performed in the United States.[1] Refinement of transplant techniques over the last 2 decades has dramatically decreased transplant-related mortality, but approximately 15% of HSCT patients still require critical care, with an associated intensive care unit (ICU) mortality of approximately 50%.[2] Respiratory failure and septic shock are the

[a] Oncology Intensive Care Unit, Johns Hopkins Sidney Kimmel Comprehensive Cancer Center, Johns Hopkins Hospital, Harry and Jeanette Weinberg Building, Pod 5C, 401 North Broadway, Baltimore, MD 21231, USA; [b] Oncology Intensive Care Unit, Division of Pulmonary and Critical Care Medicine, Department of Medicine, Johns Hopkins University, 1830 East Monument Street, 5th Floor, Baltimore, MD 21205, USA; [c] Oncology Intensive Care Unit, Division of Pulmonary and Critical Care Medicine, Departments of Medicine and Oncology, Johns Hopkins University, 1800 Orleans Street, Suite 9121 Zayed Tower, Baltimore, MD 21287, USA
* Corresponding author.
E-mail address: rsteph13@jhmi.edu

Crit Care Clin 37 (2021) 29–46
https://doi.org/10.1016/j.ccc.2020.08.002
0749-0704/21/© 2020 Elsevier Inc. All rights reserved.

most common reasons for ICU admission after HSCT, but HSCT complications can affect any organ system.

IMMUNOLOGIC CONSEQUENCES OF HEMATOPOIETIC STEM CELL TRANSPLANT

The immunologic consequences of HSCT are both the primary driver of complications and the key feature differentiating HSCT patients from the general ICU population. In all HSCTs, a cytotoxic conditioning regimen is necessary to suppress the bone marrow and immune system and allow the transplanted cells to engraft. The resulting pancytopenia resolves with engraftment or native marrow recovery. In autologous HSCT, immune dysfunction generally ends with successful engraftment of the autologous stem cells (**Fig. 1**).[3] In contrast, allogeneic transplant introduces a foreign immune system, leading to more complex and more persistent immune dysfunction (see **Fig. 1**). Even after hematopoietic recovery, the immunologic consequences of allogeneic HSCT can cause further life-threatening complications, including graft-versus-host disease (GVHD). Accordingly, allogeneic transplants are associated with significantly more morbidity and mortality than autologous transplants.

Traditional HSCT preparative regiments are myeloablative (MA), and have the dual goal of eliminating residual malignant disease in the marrow and promoting engraftment. More recently developed nonmyeloablative (NMA) regimens seem to decrease transplant-related mortality, but at the possible cost of increased long-term relapse.[4,5] Either related or unrelated donors can be used, with a variety of stem cell sources, including bone marrow, peripheral blood, and umbilical cord blood. Whether related or unrelated, full HLA-matched donors can be difficult to find, especially in minority patients. Effective GVHD prophylaxis with posttransplant cyclophosphamide has facilitated expansion of the donor pool to include related haploidentical donors (each patient shares at least 1 haplotype with each parent, each child, 50% of siblings, and often other relatives).[6–9]

In both MA and NMA transplants, regardless of donor relation and stem cell source, neutropenia, lymphopenia, monocytopenia, and thrombocytopenia persist until donor cell engraftment or bone marrow recovery. This period of aplasia places the HSCT patient at high risk for infectious complications and dramatically changes the immune

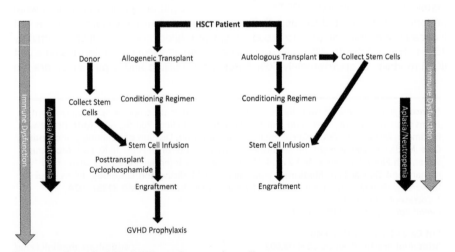

Fig. 1. Outline of HSCT. GVHD, graft-versus-host disease.

response and the resolution of organ injury.[10–13] Immune defenses are also impaired, because conditioning regimens disrupt the intestinal mucosal barrier and cause qualitative and quantitative dysfunction of alveolar macrophages, lymphocytes, and neutrophils.[14–17] The gut and lung microbiomes are also altered, and these changes are associated with post-HSCT complications.[18–21] Combined, these factors contribute to a markedly altered posttransplant immunologic milieu.

ENGRAFTMENT SYNDROME AND CYTOKINE RELEASE SYNDROME

With both autologous and allogeneic HSCT, engraftment syndrome can occur at the time of neutrophil recovery, and is thought to be caused by the earlier recovery of neutrophils than regulatory T cells, leading to uncontrolled neutrophil activation. Engraftment syndrome presents with fever, capillary leak, noncardiogenic pulmonary edema, and organ dysfunction.[22] The incidence of engraftment syndrome seems higher after haploidentical HSCT than in fully matched HSCT.[23] In severe cases, corticosteroids (eg, methylprednisolone 1–1.5 mg/kg/d) may be useful.[22]

Although engraftment syndrome occurs 7 to 14 days after HSCT, the increasing use of peripheral blood stem cells (PBSCs) can cause critical illness immediately after graft infusion.[24] Compared with bone marrow, PBSCs include more mature donor T cells in the transplanted product. This higher T-cell dose can result in a profound cytokine release syndrome (CRS) of fevers, vascular permeability, hemodynamic instability, acute kidney injury, and respiratory failure.[25,26] CRS is particularly common after haploidentical PBSC transplant, and typically resolves when posttransplant cyclophosphamide is given for GVHD prophylaxis.[26] Corticosteroids may also be used, but at the possible expense of graft survival. Emerging data suggest a possible role for anti–interleukin-6 therapy with tocilizumab.[25]

RESPIRATORY FAILURE

Acute respiratory failure is the most common reason for ICU admission after HSCT. At least 15% of patients develop acute respiratory distress syndrome (ARDS), with a mortality of 50% to 70%.[27–29] Infection is the most frequent cause of respiratory failure (**Table 1**).[30,31] Empiric antimicrobial therapy should cover common pneumonic bacteria and account for resistant organisms; this typically requires coverage for *Pseudomonas*, resistant gram positives, and atypical pneumonias. Fungal infections must also be considered.[32] Respiratory viruses are a major problem, and even viruses not thought of as respiratory agents, such as cytomegalovirus and human herpesvirus 6, can also cause significant respiratory injury.[33–39]

Noninvasive ventilation (NIV) is frequently used in HSCT patients based on older reports of mortality reduction with NIV compared with invasive mechanical ventilation (IMV) in immunosuppressed patients.[40–42] More recent data have questioned the benefit of NIV.[43] High tidal volumes during NIV predict NIV failure, which is associated with high mortality.[40,44,45] Heated humidified high-flow nasal cannula oxygen is a promising new option in early respiratory failure.[46–48] If IMV is required, management of ARDS should follow established standards and low tidal volume ventilation should be used[49–51] (**Table 2**). Prone positioning should be strongly considered for Pao_2/Fio_2 (fraction of inspired oxygen) less than 150 mm Hg.[52] Neuromuscular blockade may benefit some patients with moderate to severe ARDS.[53] Although extracorporeal membrane oxygenation (ECMO) is increasingly used in severe ARDS,[54] ECMO outcomes in HSCT patients are extremely poor.[55,56]

Early recognition and treatment of specific infectious causes of respiratory failure may improve outcomes.[57] Chest computed tomography scanning is indicated in all

Table 1
Common pulmonary infections after hematopoietic stem cell transplant

Infection	Common Pathogens	Risk Factors for Occurrence and Severity	Reference
Bacterial	Streptococcus pneumoniae Streptococcus viridans Staphylococcus aureus Pseudomonas aeruginosa Acinetobacter Stenotrophomonas maltophilia Nocardia asteroides	Neutropenia Oral mucositis Aspiration Antecedent viral pneumonia	[31]
Viral	Influenza Adenovirus Respiratory syncytial virus Rhinovirus Parainfluenza Human metapneumovirus Cytomegalovirus	Neutropenia Lymphopenia Allogeneic transplant Bone marrow graft source Steroid therapy Infection before engraftment Presence of copathogens Older age GVHD	[31,33–35]
Fungal	Aspergillus species Pneumocystis jirovecii Mucorales (eg, Rhizopus, Mucor) Fusarium species Histoplasma capsulatum Coccidioides immitis Blastomyces dermatitidis	Prolonged neutropenia Lymphopenia Steroids GVHD Geographic exposure Residential exposure	[31,32]

patients.[58] Although a noninvasive evaluation is generally adequate, bronchoscopy is useful in some patients. Diagnostic yield and clinical utility are highest if bronchoscopy is performed within 24 hours of ICU admission.[42,57,59,60] Bronchoalveolar lavage (BAL) is safe even with profound thrombocytopenia.[61,62] Transbronchial biopsies carry the risk of bleeding and add little utility to BAL alone.[57,63] Progressively bloody BAL aliquots can identify diffuse alveolar hemorrhage (DAH), which occurs in up to 12% of HSCT patients.[64,65] Corticosteroids are the mainstay of DAH treatment, with greatest efficacy at doses less than 250 mg/d of methylprednisolone.[65] Exclusion of infection may suggest idiopathic pneumonia syndrome (IPS), which affects up to 15% of patients after MA allogeneic HSCT (but <2% after NMA HSCT).[66]

Table 2
Management of acute respiratory distress syndrome

ARDS Patient Category	Intervention
All patients (Pao_2/Fio_2 <300 mm Hg)	Low tidal volume ventilation (6–8 mL/kg/PBW) Fluid conservative strategy Treatment of underlying cause
Moderate-severe ARDS (Pao_2/Fio_2 <150 mm Hg)	Prone positioning Neuromuscular blockade in select patients

See text for references.
Abbreviations: Fio_2, fraction of inspired oxygen; PBW, predicted body weight.

Corticosteroids and the anti–tumor necrosis factor-alpha antibody etanercept have been used to treat IPS with mixed results; mortality approaches 100% if IMV is required.[66–68]

NEUTROPENIC SEPSIS

Neutropenic fever and sepsis (**Table 3**) are major problems after HSCT, occurring in approximately 80% and 10% of HSCT patients, respectively.[58,69–72] In patients who progress to septic shock, reported mortality is approximately 50%, with mortality predictors including GVHD, respiratory failure, positive blood cultures, and multiorgan failure.[72–74] Appropriate empiric antibiotics must be started immediately, and attempts at microbiologic diagnosis should not delay antibiotic administration.[58,70] Empiric antimicrobial regimens must cover common sources and organisms and typically include an antipseudomonal penicillin/cephalosporin or carbapenem (**Table 4**).[58,69,70,75] Resistant gram-positive coverage is indicated for hemodynamic instability or if appropriate risk factors exist. Routine addition of an aminoglycoside is not recommended.[70,76,77] Antifungal agents with activity against yeasts and molds are indicated with shock or prolonged neutropenia.[58,69,70] Multidrug-resistant organisms (eg, vancomycin-resistant enterococcus, carbapenem-resistant Enterobacteriaceae) are increasingly common and are associated with high mortalities.[78–81]

Survival in neutropenic sepsis is significantly worse than that of nonneutropenic sepsis.[42,74,82] Although neutropenic sepsis may differ biologically from nonneutropenic sepsis, no data to date support any difference in resuscitation practices, and standard sepsis management strategies apply.[70,76] Fluid resuscitation with balanced crystalloids may be advantageous.[83] Potentially infected intravascular catheters should be removed.[74] Hematopoietic growth factors and granulocyte transfusions should not be routinely used.[69,84,85]

Table 3	
Neutropenic fever, neutropenic sepsis, and neutropenic septic shock	
Neutropenic Fever	ANC<1500 cells/mm³ (<500 cells/mm³ at many centers) And Any temperature >38.3°C Or Sustained temperature >38.0°C for >1 h
Neutropenic Sepsis	ANC<500 cells/mm³ And qSOFA ≥ 2 Respiratory rate ≥22 breaths/min Altered mentation/mental status Systolic blood pressure ≤100 mm Hg Or High suspicion for infection and organ dysfunction
Neutropenic Septic Shock	ANC <500 cells/mm³ And qSOFA ≥ 2 And Vasopressors needed to keep MAP ≥65 mm Hg and lactate >2 mmol/L

Abbreviations: ANC, absolute neutrophil count; MAP, mean arterial pressure; qSOFA, Quick Sequential Organ Failure Assessment score.

Table 4
Typical pathogens, sources, and empiric antibiotics in neutropenic sepsis

Source	Pathogen	Antibiotic Options			
		Anti-pseudomonal beta-lactam	Resistant Gram-positive coverage	Anti-fungal coverage	Aminoglycosides
Unknown, No prior resistant Gram-positives	Coagulase-negative Staphylococci Escherichia coli Enterococcus species	Piperacillin-tazobactam or Cefepime, or Carbapenem (Imipenem, Meropenem)			
Abdomen	Escherichia coli Pseudomonas aeruginosa Enterococcus species Klebsiella species Clostridium species				
Urogenital	Escherichia coli Pseudomonas aeruginosa Klebsiella species				
Lung	Pseudomonas aeruginosa, Streptococcus pneumonia, Viridans streptococci, Acinetobacter species		Vancomycin or Linezolid		
Soft Tissue	Staphylococcus aureus alpha-hemolytic streptococci				
Oral Mucosa	Streptococci species				
Central venous catheter	Coagulase-negative Staphylococci Coryneform bacteria Propionibacterium species Stenotrophomonas maltophilia				
Unknown, Prior resistant Gram-positives	Coagulase-negative Staphylococci Staphylococcus aureus Escherichia coli Enterococcus species				
Unknown, prolonged neutropenia, abdominal pain, pulmonary nodules	Candida albicans, Candida tropicalis, Candida parapsilosis, Aspergillus species			Echinocandins (caspofungin, micafungin) or Voriconazole	
Persistent Hemodynamic Instability Allergy Resistant Organism				or Liposomal Amphotericin	Amikacin, Tobramycin, Gentamicin

Adapted from Penack O, Becker C, Buchheidt D, et al. Management of sepsis in neutropenic patients: 2014 updated guidelines from the Infectious Diseases Working Party of the German Society of Hematology and Medical Oncology (AGIHO). *Ann Hematol.* 2014;93(7):1083-1095; with permission.

ORGAN-SPECIFIC COMPLICATIONS
Cardiac Complications

Traditional cardiac risk factors increase the risk of post-HSCT complications, and recent data show a link between clonal hematopoiesis and cardiovascular disease.[86,87] Cardiac risk may also be increased by many oncologic therapies, including agents (eg, cyclophosphamide) used in HSCT preparative regimens.[86] Infections and peritransplant volume shifts may also precipitate cardiac complications.[88]

Arrhythmias, most commonly atrial fibrillation, affect nearly 30% of HSCT patients.[89,90] New arrhythmia may indicate cardiac failure, and a high index of suspicion for ventricular dysfunction is warranted after HSCT.[91,92] Manifestations of heart failure can range from nonspecific symptoms to fulminant shock. HSCT patients are at increased risk of type I ischemia (plaque rupture) caused by endothelial injury and pre-existing risk factors.[93,94] Management of type I events is complicated by thrombocytopenia and coagulopathy.[95–97] Type II ischemic events secondary to cardiac strain can also occur, as can stress cardiomyopathy and virial myocarditis. Pericardial effusions and tamponade physiology require rapid recognition and emergent intervention.[98,99] Management of cardiac dysfunction is largely identical to that in the general population. Mechanical interventions, including intra-aortic balloon pump, coronary stenting, and ECMO, may be considered on a case-by-case basis.[100]

Neurologic Complications

Neurologic complications are frequent after HSCT.[101] The most worrisome threat is intracerebral hemorrhage, which must be a constant consideration in thrombocytopenic patients. Suspicions of central nervous system (CNS) infection may require modification of antimicrobial regimens to ensure CNS penetration. Seizures and generalized encephalopathy can occur, often with cryptic causes. Posterior reversible encephalopathy syndrome is increasingly recognized, especially in patients receiving tacrolimus-based GVHD prophylaxis. Close collaboration with neurology and neurocritical care specialists may be required.

Acute Kidney Injury

Acute kidney injury (AKI) affects up to 40% of patients after HSCT, with higher incidence after allogeneic transplant than autologous transplant.[102,103] In addition to usual causes of AKI, specific contributors to AKI after HSCT include preparative chemotherapeutic regimens, nephrotoxins (eg, tacrolimus, cyclosporine, antimicrobials), CRS, GVHD, and hepatic sinusoidal obstruction.[102] Hemorrhagic cystitis caused by chemotherapy toxicity or viral infection can cause significant blood loss and obstructive nephropathy because of blood clots. Continuous bladder irrigation may be necessary. The requirement for renal replacement therapy portends a high mortality.[102]

Liver Dysfunction

Liver injury occurs in up to 80% of allogeneic HSCT patients; important causes include drug-induced injury, viral hepatitis, and shock.[104] Hepatic veno-occlusive disease (VOD), or sinusoidal obstruction syndrome (SOS), is a specific form of posttransplant injury primarily seen after MA HSCT.[105,106] VOD/SOS damages the hepatic endothelium, obliterates hepatic sinusoids, and causes hepatocyte necrosis. Diagnosis is based on clinical findings, including hepatomegaly, increased bilirubin level, ascites, and weight gain. Therapeutic options are limited and include ursodeoxycholic acid and defibrotide.

TRANSFUSION SUPPORT, BLEEDING, AND HEMATOLOGIC COMPLICATIONS AFTER HEMATOPOIETIC STEM CELL TRANSPLANT

Transfusion support plays an essential role after HSCT, because effective red blood cell (RBC) and platelet production is precluded until marrow recovery. Red blood cell transfusion should generally target a hemoglobin goal of greater than 7 g/dL (8 g/dL with active cardiac ischemia).[107–110] Bleeding complications are common in thrombocytopenic HSCT patients, with spontaneous intracranial and retroperitoneal hemorrhages of particular concern. Prophylactic platelet transfusion to a goal of 10,000 platelets/µL decreases the risk of spontaneous bleeding.[111–113] Planned invasive procedures or active bleeding warrant higher goals. If bleeding does occur, treatment includes RBC transfusion support, coagulopathy correction, and attempts at procedural hemostasis if indicated. Oral tranexamic acid, intravenous aminocaproic acid, recombinant factor VII, and intravenous prothrombin complex concentrate are potential off-label options for uncontrolled bleeding.

Unexpected thrombocytopenia or thrombocytopenia accompanied by renal or neurologic failure should prompt consideration of HSCT-associated thrombotic microangiopathy (HSCT-TMA). HSCT-TMA resembles thrombotic thrombocytopenic purpura and atypical hemolytic uremic syndrome and occurs in up to 40% of patients after allogeneic HSCT.[114,115] HSCT-TMA is probably caused by endothelial injury and complement activation, and typically occurs in the first 100 days after transplant. Treatment includes stopping possible precipitants and controlling blood pressure. Both rituximab and the anticomplement antibody eculizumab have been used, but without evidence of efficacy.[115]

ACUTE GRAFT-VERSUS-HOST DISEASE

Acute GVHD is a major contributor to peritransplant morbidity and mortality, and is caused by donor-origin T cells recognizing recipient tissues as foreign and instigating an immune response against the transplant recipient.[116] It generally occurs within the first 100 days after transplant and can affect the skin, mucosa, intestinal tract, and liver (**Table 5**).[116–118] Frank epidermal desquamation, massive hematochezia, and fulminant liver failure can result. Severe skin acute GVHD is akin to a burn injury; transfer to a burn center may be required. Corticosteroids are the primary therapy.[116,119] Because GVHD prophylaxis has improved, overall GVHD mortality is decreasing.[7,119]

CRITICAL CARE PROCEDURES IN HEMATOPOIETIC STEM CELL TRANSPLANT PATIENTS
Vascular Access

Vascular access, although essential for medication administration and fluid resuscitation, is often difficult in critically ill patients because of hemodynamic instability and intravascular volume depletion. HCST-associated thrombocytopenia, coagulopathy, and immunosuppression further increase the risk of procedural and infectious complications. Key considerations for vascular access in HSCT patients are listed in **Box 1**.[120–126] The best defense against catheter-related blood stream infection is daily reassessment of vascular catheter need and prompt removal when no longer necessary.

Airway Management

Airway management in critically ill HSCT patients requires specific consideration and the anticipation of possible challenges. Any patient with airway bleeding may be difficult to intubate because of poor visualization. Severe mucositis can cause oral bleeding, mucosal sloughing, and trismus, making intubation challenging. An experienced laryngoscopist is essential, as is immediate availability of video laryngoscopes and airway equipment. Subglottic suction endotracheal tubes may reduce ventilator-associated pneumonias.[127] If bronchoscopy is planned, adequate endotracheal tube size must be balanced against the risk of tracheal stenosis or laryngeal damage with larger tubes.[128]

Table 5
Presentation and grading of acute graft-versus-host disease

Organ Site	Presentation	Grading
Skin	Erythema Maculopapular rash Blisters/ulceration Desquamation	Stage 0: no rash Stage 1: maculopapular rash, <25% BSA Stage 2: maculopapular rash, 25%–50% BSA Stage 3: maculopapular rash, >50% BSA Stage 4: erythredema (>50%) + bullae and desquamation >5% BSA
Gastrointestinal tract	Anorexia Nausea, vomiting Diarrhea Abdominal pain Ileus Bloody diarrhea	Stage 0: no nausea, vomiting, anorexia; diarrhea <500 mL/d Stage 1: persistent nausea, vomiting, anorexia; diarrhea 500–999 mL/d Stage 2: diarrhea 1000–1500 mL/d Stage 3: diarrhea >1500 mL/d Stage 4: severe pain or grossly bloody stool
Liver	Increased bilirubin level Cholestasis	Stage 0: bilirubin<2 mg/dL Stage 1: bilirubin 2–3 mg/dL Stage 2: bilirubin 3.1–6 mg/dL Stage 3: bilirubin 6.1–15 mg/dL Stage 4: bilirubin >15 mg/dL

Abbreviation: BSA, body surface area.
Data from Refs.[116–118]

Point-of-Care Ultrasonography

Point-of-care ultrasonography is a valuable tool for both procedural guidance and rapid clinical assessment to guide patient management. The utility of procedural guidance in thrombocytopenic patients is self-evident. Incorporation of basic lung, cardiac, and abdominal ultrasonography into the assessment of decompensating patients can provide valuable real-time information in undifferentiated cardiac and respiratory failure.[122,129,130] In patients with complex pleural effusions, ultrasonography-guided small-bore pleural catheters (eg, 14 French) are as effective for pleural drainage as larger-bore catheters, and confer less pain and procedural risk.[131]

Box 1
Key considerations for vascular access in hematopoietic stem cell transplant patients

- Choose a compressible site for CVC placement (internal jugular or distal subclavian veins)[121]
- Subclavian sites have lower infection rates[121]
- Avoid femoral CVCs if possible
- Use strict aseptic technique[125]
- Use POCUS for procedural guidance[120,122]
- Consider micropuncture access techniques[123]
- Antibiotic-impregnated catheters may decrease CRBSI[124]
- Adhesive securement devices may decrease bleeding and infection compared with sutures[126]

Abbreviations: CRBSI, catheter-related bloodstream infection; CVC, central venous catheter; POCUS, point-of-care ultrasonography.

ORGANIZATION OF HEMATOPOIETIC STEM CELL TRANSPLANT CRITICAL CARE

HSCT volumes are increasing, and the association of earlier ICU admission with improved survival shows the need for adequate HSCT critical care facilities.[72,82] Many high-volume transplant centers have developed specialty HSCT ICUs. Although specialty HSCT ICUs have several potential benefits, there are few data to support (or dissuade) their development. Development of best practices for HSCT critical care, including optimum ICU organization, is an important area for study,[42] and includes optimum staffing patterns for HSCT ICUs. Nursing shortages are perennial, compounded by the challenge of equipping nurses with the requisite skill set for HSCT critical care. In the face of intensivist shortages, advanced practice providers (nurse practitioners and physician assistants) are increasingly used to provide critical care.[132] The subspecialty nature of HSCT ICUs may be particularly suited to advanced practice providers. In addition, distress and burnout among health care workers caring for HSCT patients is well documented and should be a significant consideration in staffing decisions.[133,134]

SUMMARY

Life-threatening complications are frequent after HSCT, and optimum critical care is essential. HSCT intensivists must understand the process and immunologic consequences of HSCT. Experience leading to pattern recognition can facilitate anticipation and early intervention in critical illness. HSCT critical care is a multidisciplinary endeavor, and the importance of close collaboration with hematologists, oncologists, and infectious disease specialists, as well as nursing, physical and occupational therapists, respiratory therapists, pharmacists, and other specialists, cannot be overstated. Much work remains to maximize outcomes in this unique population of critically ill patients.

DISCLOSURE

Ms R.A. Fornwalt, Dr E.P. Brigham, and Dr R.S. Stephens have no relevant financial disclosures.

REFERENCES

1. D'Souza A, Fretham C. Current uses and outcomes of hematopoietic cell transplantation (HCT): CIBMTR summary slides, 2019 2019. Available at: https://www.cibmtr.org. Accessed February 20, 2020.
2. Saillard C, Darmon M, Bisbal M, et al. Critically ill allogenic HSCT patients in the intensive care unit: a systematic review and meta-analysis of prognostic factors of mortality. Bone Marrow Transplant 2018;53(10):1233–41.
3. Abrahamsson S, Muraro PA. Immune re-education following autologous hematopoietic stem cell transplantation. Autoimmunity 2008;41(8):577–84.
4. Slavin S, Nagler A, Naparstek E, et al. Nonmyeloablative stem cell transplantation and cell therapy as an alternative to conventional bone marrow transplantation with lethal cytoreduction for the treatment of malignant and nonmalignant hematologic diseases. Blood 1998;91(3):756–63.
5. Scott BL, Pasquini MC, Logan BR, et al. Myeloablative versus reduced-intensity hematopoietic cell transplantation for acute myeloid leukemia and myelodysplastic syndromes. J Clin Oncol 2017;35(11):1154–61.
6. Luznik L, O'Donnell PV, Symons HJ, et al. HLA-haploidentical bone marrow transplantation for hematologic malignancies using nonmyeloablative

conditioning and high-dose, posttransplantation cyclophosphamide. Biol Blood Marrow Transplant 2008;14(6):641–50.

7. Luznik L, Bolanos-Meade J, Zahurak M, et al. High-dose cyclophosphamide as single-agent, short-course prophylaxis of graft-versus-host disease. Blood 2010;115(16):3224–30.

8. Dezern AE, Luznik L, Fuchs EJ, et al. Post-transplantation cyclophosphamide for GVHD prophylaxis in severe aplastic anemia. Bone Marrow Transplant 2011;46(7):1012–3.

9. Elmariah H, Kasamon YL, Zahurak M, et al. Haploidentical bone marrow transplantation with post-transplant cyclophosphamide using non-first-degree related donors. Biol Blood Marrow Transplant 2018;24(5):1099–102.

10. Luan YY, Dong N, Xie M, et al. The significance and regulatory mechanisms of innate immune cells in the development of sepsis. J Interferon Cytokine Res 2014;34(1):2–15.

11. McDonald B. Neutrophils in critical illness. Cell Tissue Res 2018;371(3):607–15.

12. Reilly JP, Anderson BJ, Hudock KM, et al. Neutropenic sepsis is associated with distinct clinical and biological characteristics: a cohort study of severe sepsis. Crit Care 2016;20(1):222.

13. Claushuis TA, van Vught LA, Scicluna BP, et al. Thrombocytopenia is associated with a dysregulated host response in critically ill sepsis patients. Blood 2016; 127(24):3062–72.

14. Middleton EA, Weyrich AS, Zimmerman GA. Platelets in pulmonary immune responses and inflammatory lung diseases. Physiol Rev 2016;96(4):1211–59.

15. Mokart D, Guery BP, Bouabdallah R, et al. Deactivation of alveolar macrophages in septic neutropenic ARDS. Chest 2003;124(2):644–52.

16. Cordonnier C, Escudier E, Verra F, et al. Bronchoalveolar lavage during neutropenic episodes: diagnostic yield and cellular pattern. Eur Respir J 1994;7(1): 114–20.

17. van der Velden WJ, Herbers AH, Netea MG, et al. Mucosal barrier injury, fever and infection in neutropenic patients with cancer: introducing the paradigm febrile mucositis. Br J Haematol 2014;167(4):441–52.

18. O'Dwyer DN, Zhou X, Wilke CA, et al. Lung dysbiosis, inflammation, and injury in hematopoietic cell transplantation. Am J Respir Crit Care Med 2018;198(10): 1312–21.

19. Kusakabe S, Fukushima K, Maeda T, et al. Pre- and post-serial metagenomic analysis of gut microbiota as a prognostic factor in patients undergoing haematopoietic stem cell transplantation. Br J Haematol 2020;188(3):438–49.

20. Andermann TM, Peled JU, Ho C, et al. The microbiome and hematopoietic cell transplantation: past, present, and future. Biol Blood Marrow Transplant 2018; 24(7):1322–40.

21. Peled JU, Gomes ALC, Devlin SM, et al. Microbiota as predictor of mortality in allogeneic hematopoietic-cell transplantation. N Engl J Med 2020;382(9): 822–34.

22. Cornell RF, Hari P, Drobyski WR. Engraftment syndrome after autologous stem cell transplantation: an update unifying the definition and management approach. Biol Blood Marrow Transplant 2015;21(12):2061–8.

23. Chen Y, Xu LP, Liu KY, et al. High incidence of engraftment syndrome after haploidentical allogeneic stem cell transplantation. Eur J Haematol 2016;96(5): 517–26.

24. Anasetti C, Logan BR, Lee SJ, et al. Peripheral-blood stem cells versus bone marrow from unrelated donors. N Engl J Med 2012;367(16):1487–96.

25. Abboud R, Keller J, Slade M, et al. Severe cytokine-release syndrome after T cell-replete peripheral blood haploidentical donor transplantation is associated with poor survival and anti-IL-6 therapy is safe and well tolerated. Biol Blood Marrow Transplant 2016;22(10):1851–60.

26. Imus PH, Blackford AL, Bettinotti M, et al. Severe cytokine release syndrome after haploidentical peripheral blood stem cell transplantation. Biol Blood Marrow Transplant 2019;25(12):2431–7.

27. Azoulay E, Lemiale V, Mokart D, et al. Acute respiratory distress syndrome in patients with malignancies. Intensive Care Med 2014;40(8):1106–14.

28. Allareddy V, Roy A, Rampa S, et al. Outcomes of stem cell transplant patients with acute respiratory failure requiring mechanical ventilation in the United States. Bone Marrow Transplant 2014;49(10):1278–86.

29. Yadav H, Nolan ME, Bohman JK, et al. Epidemiology of acute respiratory distress syndrome following hematopoietic stem cell transplantation. Crit Care Med 2016;44(6):1082–90.

30. Azoulay E, Pickkers P, Soares M, et al. Acute hypoxemic respiratory failure in immunocompromised patients: the Efraim multinational prospective cohort study. Intensive Care Med 2017;43(12):1808–19.

31. Girmenia C, Martino P. Pulmonary infections complicating hematological disorders. Semin Respir Crit Care Med 2005;26(5):445–57.

32. Young AY, Leiva Juarez MM, Evans SE. Fungal pneumonia in patients with hematologic malignancy and hematopoietic stem cell transplantation. Clin Chest Med 2017;38(3):479–91.

33. Vakil E, Evans SE. Viral pneumonia in patients with hematologic malignancy or hematopoietic stem cell transplantation. Clin Chest Med 2017;38(1):97–111.

34. Renaud C, Xie H, Seo S, et al. Mortality rates of human metapneumovirus and respiratory syncytial virus lower respiratory tract infections in hematopoietic cell transplantation recipients. Biol Blood Marrow Transplant 2013;19(8):1220–6.

35. Dignan FL, Clark A, Aitken C, et al. BCSH/BSBMT/UK clinical virology network guideline: diagnosis and management of common respiratory viral infections in patients undergoing treatment for haematological malignancies or stem cell transplantation. Br J Haematol 2016;173(3):380–93.

36. Chemaly RF, Shah DP, Boeckh MJ. Management of respiratory viral infections in hematopoietic cell transplant recipients and patients with hematologic malignancies. Clin Infect Dis 2014;59(Suppl 5):S344–51.

37. Legoff J, Zucman N, Lemiale V, et al. Clinical significance of upper airway virus detection in critically ill hematology patients. Am J Respir Crit Care Med 2019; 199(4):518–28.

38. Iglesias L, Perera MM, Torres-Minana L, et al. CMV viral load in bronchoalveolar lavage for diagnosis of pneumonia in allogeneic hematopoietic stem cell transplantation. Bone Marrow Transplant 2017;52(6):895–7.

39. Zhou X, O'Dwyer DN, Xia M, et al. First-onset herpesviral infection and lung injury in allogeneic hematopoietic cell transplantation. Am J Respir Crit Care Med 2019;200(1):63–74.

40. Cortegiani A, Madotto F, Gregoretti C, et al. Immunocompromised patients with acute respiratory distress syndrome: secondary analysis of the LUNG SAFE database. Crit Care 2018;22(1):157.

41. Hilbert G, Gruson D, Vargas F, et al. Noninvasive ventilation in immunosuppressed patients with pulmonary infiltrates, fever, and acute respiratory failure. N Engl J Med 2001;344(7):481–7.

42. Azoulay E, Schellongowski P, Darmon M, et al. The Intensive Care Medicine research agenda on critically ill oncology and hematology patients. Intensive Care Med 2017;43(9):1366–82.
43. Lemiale V, Mokart D, Resche-Rigon M, et al. Effect of noninvasive ventilation vs oxygen therapy on mortality among immunocompromised patients with acute respiratory failure: a randomized clinical trial. JAMA 2015;314(16):1711–9.
44. Carteaux G, Millan-Guilarte T, De Prost N, et al. Failure of noninvasive ventilation for de novo acute hypoxemic respiratory failure: role of tidal volume. Crit Care Med 2016;44(2):282–90.
45. Frat JP, Ragot S, Coudroy R, et al. Predictors of intubation in patients with acute hypoxemic respiratory failure treated with a noninvasive oxygenation strategy. Crit Care Med 2018;46(2):208–15.
46. Azoulay E, Lemiale V, Mokart D, et al. Effect of high-flow nasal oxygen vs standard oxygen on 28-day mortality in immunocompromised patients with acute respiratory failure: the HIGH randomized clinical trial. JAMA 2018;320(20):2099–107.
47. Frat JP, Thille AW, Mercat A, et al. High-flow oxygen through nasal cannula in acute hypoxemic respiratory failure. New Engl J Med 2015;372(23):2185–96.
48. Rochwerg B, Granton D, Wang DX, et al. High flow nasal cannula compared with conventional oxygen therapy for acute hypoxemic respiratory failure: a systematic review and meta-analysis. Intensive Care Med 2019;45(5):563–72.
49. Acute Respiratory Distress Syndrome Network, Brower RG, Matthay MA, et al. Ventilation with lower tidal volumes as compared with traditional tidal volumes for acute lung injury and the acute respiratory distress syndrome. N Engl J Med 2000;342(18):1301–8.
50. Fan E, Del Sorbo L, Goligher EC, et al. An Official American Thoracic Society/European Society of Intensive Care Medicine/Society of Critical Care Medicine clinical practice guideline: mechanical ventilation in adult patients with acute respiratory distress syndrome. Am J Respir Crit Care Med 2017;195(9):1253–63.
51. Wiedemann HP, Wheeler AP, Bernard GR, et al. Comparison of two fluid-management strategies in acute lung injury. N Engl J Med 2006;354(24):2564–75.
52. Guerin C, Reignier J, Richard JC, et al. Prone positioning in severe acute respiratory distress syndrome. N Engl J Med 2013;368(23):2159–68.
53. National Heart, Lung, and Blood Institute PETAL Clinical Trials Network, Moss M, Huang DT, Brower RG, et al. Early neuromuscular blockade in the acute respiratory distress syndrome. N Engl J Med 2019;380(21):1997–2008.
54. Combes A, Hajage D, Capellier G, et al. Extracorporeal membrane oxygenation for severe acute respiratory distress syndrome. N Engl J Med 2018;378(21):1965–75.
55. Schmidt M, Schellongowski P, Patroniti N, et al. Six-month outcome of immunocompromised severe ARDS patients rescued by ECMO. an international multicenter retrospective study. Am J Respir Crit Care Med 2018;197(10):1297–307.
56. Wohlfarth P, Beutel G, Lebiedz P, et al. Characteristics and outcome of patients after allogeneic hematopoietic stem cell transplantation treated with extracorporeal membrane oxygenation for acute respiratory distress syndrome. Crit Care Med 2017;45(5):e500–7.
57. Morton C, Puchalski J. The utility of bronchoscopy in immunocompromised patients: a review. J Thorac Dis 2019;11(12):5603–12.

58. Heinz WJ, Buchheidt D, Christopeit M, et al. Diagnosis and empirical treatment of fever of unknown origin (FUO) in adult neutropenic patients: guidelines of the Infectious Diseases Working Party (AGIHO) of the German Society of Hematology and Medical Oncology (DGHO). Ann Hematol 2017;96(11):1775–92.

59. Lucena CM, Torres A, Rovira M, et al. Pulmonary complications in hematopoietic SCT: a prospective study. Bone Marrow Transplant 2014;49(10):1293–9.

60. Azoulay E, Mokart D, Lambert J, et al. Diagnostic strategy for hematology and oncology patients with acute respiratory failure: randomized controlled trial. Am J Respir Crit Care Med 2010;182(8):1038–46.

61. Cefalo M, Puxeddu E, Sarmati L, et al. Diagnostic performance and safety of bronchoalveolar lavage in thrombocytopenic haematological patients for invasive fungal infections diagnosis: a monocentric, retrospective experience. Mediterr J Hematol Infect Dis 2019;11(1):e2019065.

62. Kim YH, Suh GY, Kim MH, et al. Safety and usefulness of bronchoscopy in ventilator-dependent patients with severe thrombocytopenia. Anaesth Intensive Care 2008;36(3):411–7.

63. O'Dwyer DN, Duvall AS, Xia M, et al. Transbronchial biopsy in the management of pulmonary complications of hematopoietic stem cell transplantation. Bone Marrow Transplant 2018;53(2):193–8.

64. Gupta S, Jain A, Warneke CL, et al. Outcome of alveolar hemorrhage in hematopoietic stem cell transplant recipients. Bone Marrow Transplant 2007;40(1):71–8.

65. Rathi NK, Tanner AR, Dinh A, et al. Low-, medium- and high-dose steroids with or without aminocaproic acid in adult hematopoietic SCT patients with diffuse alveolar hemorrhage. Bone Marrow Transplant 2015;50(3):420–6.

66. Panoskaltsis-Mortari A, Griese M, Madtes DK, et al. An official American Thoracic Society research statement: noninfectious lung injury after hematopoietic stem cell transplantation: idiopathic pneumonia syndrome. Am J Respir Crit Care Med 2011;183(9):1262–79.

67. Thompson J, Yin Z, D'Souza A, et al. Etanercept and corticosteroid therapy for the treatment of late-onset idiopathic pneumonia syndrome. Biol Blood Marrow Transplant 2017;23(11):1955–60.

68. Yanik GA, Horowitz MM, Weisdorf DJ, et al. Randomized, double-blind, placebo-controlled trial of soluble tumor necrosis factor receptor: enbrel (etanercept) for the treatment of idiopathic pneumonia syndrome after allogeneic stem cell transplantation: blood and marrow transplant clinical trials network protocol. Biol Blood Marrow Transplant 2014;20(6):858–64.

69. Freifeld AG, Bow EJ, Sepkowitz KA, et al. Clinical practice guideline for the use of antimicrobial agents in neutropenic patients with cancer: 2010 update by the infectious diseases society of America. Clin Infect Dis 2011;52(4):e56–93.

70. Kochanek M, Schalk E, von Bergwelt-Baildon M, et al. Management of sepsis in neutropenic cancer patients: 2018 guidelines from the infectious diseases working party (AGIHO) and intensive care working party (iCHOP) of the German society of hematology and medical oncology (DGHO). Ann Hematol 2019;98(5):1051–69.

71. Singer M, Deutschman CS, Seymour CW, et al. The third international consensus definitions for sepsis and septic shock (Sepsis-3). JAMA 2016;315(8):801–10.

72. Azoulay E, Mokart D, Pene F, et al. Outcomes of critically ill patients with hematologic malignancies: prospective multicenter data from France and Belgium—a

groupe de recherche respiratoire en reanimation onco-hematologique study. J Clin Oncol 2013;31(22):2810–8.

73. Kumar G, Ahmad S, Taneja A, et al. Severe sepsis in hematopoietic stem cell transplant recipients*. Crit Care Med 2015;43(2):411–21.

74. Legrand M, Max A, Peigne V, et al. Survival in neutropenic patients with severe sepsis or septic shock. Crit Care Med 2012;40(1):43–9.

75. Penack O, Becker C, Buchheidt D, et al. Management of sepsis in neutropenic patients: 2014 updated guidelines from the infectious diseases working party of the German society of hematology and medical oncology (AGIHO). Ann Hematol 2014;93(7):1083–95.

76. Rhodes A, Evans LE, Alhazzani W, et al. Surviving sepsis campaign: international guidelines for management of sepsis and septic shock: 2016. Crit Care Med 2017;45(3):486–552.

77. Paul M, Dickstein Y, Schlesinger A, et al. Beta-lactam versus beta-lactam-aminoglycoside combination therapy in cancer patients with neutropenia. Cochrane Database Syst Rev 2013;(6):CD003038.

78. Montassier E, Batard E, Gastinne T, et al. Recent changes in bacteremia in patients with cancer: a systematic review of epidemiology and antibiotic resistance. Eur J Clin Microbiol Infect Dis 2013;32(7):841–50.

79. Forcina A, Lorentino F, Marasco V, et al. Clinical impact of pretransplant multidrug-resistant gram-negative colonization in autologous and allogeneic hematopoietic stem cell transplantation. Biol Blood Marrow Transplant 2018;24(7): 1476–82.

80. Satlin MJ, Jenkins SG, Walsh TJ. The global challenge of carbapenem-resistant Enterobacteriaceae in transplant recipients and patients with hematologic malignancies. Clin Infect Dis 2014;58(9):1274–83.

81. Weinstock DM, Conlon M, Iovino C, et al. Colonization, bloodstream infection, and mortality caused by vancomycin-resistant enterococcus early after allogeneic hematopoietic stem cell transplant. Biol Blood Marrow Transplant 2007; 13(5):615–21.

82. Azoulay E, Pene F, Darmon M, et al. Managing critically Ill hematology patients: time to think differently. Blood Rev 2015;29(6):359–67.

83. Semler MW, Self WH, Wanderer JP, et al. Balanced crystalloids versus saline in critically ill adults. N Engl J Med 2018;378(9):829–39.

84. Smith TJ, Bohlke K, Lyman GH, et al. Recommendations for the use of WBC growth factors: American Society of Clinical Oncology clinical practice guideline update. J Clin Oncol 2015;33(28):3199–212.

85. Estcourt LJ, Stanworth SJ, Hopewell S, et al. Granulocyte transfusions for treating infections in people with neutropenia or neutrophil dysfunction. Cochrane Database Syst Rev 2016;(4):CD005339.

86. Blaes A, Konety S, Hurley P. Cardiovascular complications of hematopoietic stem cell transplantation. Curr Treat Options Cardiovasc Med 2016;18(4):25.

87. Jaiswal S, Natarajan P, Silver AJ, et al. Clonal hematopoiesis and risk of atherosclerotic cardiovascular disease. N Engl J Med 2017;377(2):111–21.

88. Armenian SH, Sun CL, Shannon T, et al. Incidence and predictors of congestive heart failure after autologous hematopoietic cell transplantation. Blood 2011; 118(23):6023–9.

89. Tonorezos ES, Stillwell EE, Calloway JJ, et al. Arrhythmias in the setting of hematopoietic cell transplants. Bone Marrow Transplant 2015;50(9):1212–6.

90. Peres E, Levine JE, Khaled YA, et al. Cardiac complications in patients undergoing a reduced-intensity conditioning hematopoietic stem cell transplantation. Bone Marrow Transplant 2010;45(1):149–52.

91. Rotz SJ, Ryan TD, Jodele S, et al. The injured heart: early cardiac effects of hematopoietic stem cell transplantation in children and young adults. Bone Marrow Transplant 2017;52(8):1171–9.

92. Armenian SH, Horak D, Scott JM, et al. Cardiovascular function in long-term hematopoietic cell transplantation survivors. Biol Blood Marrow Transplant 2017; 23(4):700–5.

93. Chow EJ, Mueller BA, Baker KS, et al. Cardiovascular hospitalizations and mortality among recipients of hematopoietic stem cell transplantation. Ann Intern Med 2011;155(1):21–32.

94. Almici C, Skert C, Bruno B, et al. Circulating endothelial cell count: a reliable marker of endothelial damage in patients undergoing hematopoietic stem cell transplantation. Bone Marrow Transplant 2017;52(12):1637–42.

95. Chang HM, Moudgil R, Scarabelli T, et al. Cardiovascular complications of cancer therapy: best practices in diagnosis, prevention, and management: part 1. J Am Coll Cardiol 2017;70(20):2536–51.

96. Chang HM, Okwuosa TM, Scarabelli T, et al. Cardiovascular complications of cancer therapy: best practices in diagnosis, prevention, and management: part 2. J Am Coll Cardiol 2017;70(20):2552–65.

97. Jacobs JA, Pickworth K, Boudoulas KD, et al. Outcomes for cancer patients with acute ST-segment elevation myocardial infarction undergoing primary percutaneous coronary intervention. Cardiovasc Revasc Med 2019;20(8):711–5.

98. Norkin M, Ratanatharathorn V, Ayash L, et al. Large pericardial effusion as a complication in adults undergoing SCT. Bone Marrow Transplant 2011;46(10): 1353–6.

99. Liu YC, Chien SH, Fan NW, et al. Risk factors for pericardial effusion in adult patients receiving allogeneic haematopoietic stem cell transplantation. Br J Haematol 2015;169(5):737–45.

100. Moslehi JJ. Cardiovascular toxic effects of targeted cancer therapies. N Engl J Med 2016;375(15):1457–67.

101. Benz R, Schanz U, Maggiorini M, et al. Risk factors for ICU admission and ICU survival after allogeneic hematopoietic SCT. Bone Marrow Transplant 2014; 49(1):62–5.

102. Sedhom R, Sedhom D, Jaimes E. Mini-review of kidney disease following hematopoietic stem cell transplant. Clin Nephrol 2018;89(6):389–402.

103. Liu H, Li YF, Liu BC, et al. A multicenter, retrospective study of acute kidney injury in adult patients with nonmyeloablative hematopoietic SCT. Bone Marrow Transplant 2010;45(1):153–8.

104. Norvell JP. Liver disease after hematopoietic cell transplantation in adults. Transplant Rev (Orlando) 2015;29(1):8–15.

105. Dalle JH, Giralt SA. Hepatic veno-occlusive disease after hematopoietic stem cell transplantation: risk factors and stratification, prophylaxis, and treatment. Biol Blood Marrow Transplant 2016;22(3):400–9.

106. Lewis C, Kim HT, Roeker LE, et al. Incidence, predictors, and outcomes of veno-occlusive disease/sinusoidal obstruction syndrome after reduced-intensity allogeneic hematopoietic cell transplantation. Biol Blood Marrow Transplant 2020; 26(3):529–39.

107. Hebert PC, Wells G, Blajchman MA, et al. A multicenter, randomized, controlled clinical trial of transfusion requirements in critical care. Transfusion

Requirements in Critical Care Investigators, Canadian Critical Care Trials Group. N Engl J Med 1999;340(6):409–17.

108. Tay J, Allan DS, Chatelain E, et al. Liberal versus restrictive red blood cell transfusion thresholds in hematopoietic cell transplantation: a randomized, open label, phase III, noninferiority trial. J Clin Oncol 2020;38(13):1463–73.

109. Carson JL, Guyatt G, Heddle NM, et al. Clinical practice guidelines from the AABB: red blood cell transfusion thresholds and storage. JAMA 2016;316(19): 2025–35.

110. Carson JL, Stanworth SJ, Alexander JH, et al. Clinical trials evaluating red blood cell transfusion thresholds: an updated systematic review and with additional focus on patients with cardiovascular disease. Am Heart J 2018;200:96–101.

111. Wandt H, Schaefer-Eckart K, Wendelin K, et al. Therapeutic platelet transfusion versus routine prophylactic transfusion in patients with haematological malignancies: an open-label, multicentre, randomised study. Lancet 2012; 380(9850):1309–16.

112. Stanworth SJ, Estcourt LJ, Powter G, et al. A no-prophylaxis platelet-transfusion strategy for hematologic cancers. N Engl J Med 2013;368(19):1771–80.

113. Kumar A, Mhaskar R, Grossman BJ, et al. Platelet transfusion: a systematic review of the clinical evidence. Transfusion 2015;55(5):1116–27 [quiz: 1115].

114. Wanchoo R, Bayer RL, Bassil C, et al. Emerging concepts in hematopoietic stem cell transplantation-associated renal thrombotic microangiopathy and prospects for new treatments. Am J Kidney Dis 2018;72(6):857–65.

115. Elsallabi O, Bhatt VR, Dhakal P, et al. Hematopoietic stem cell transplant-associated thrombotic microangiopathy. Clin Appl Thromb Hemost 2016; 22(1):12–20.

116. Zeiser R, Blazar BR. Acute graft-versus-host disease - biologic process, prevention, and therapy. N Engl J Med 2017;377(22):2167–79.

117. Harris AC, Young R, Devine S, et al. International, multicenter standardization of acute graft-versus-host disease clinical data collection: a report from the Mount Sinai Acute GVHD International Consortium. Biol Blood Marrow Transplant 2016; 22(1):4–10.

118. Ferrara JL, Levine JE, Reddy P, et al. Graft-versus-host disease. Lancet 2009; 373(9674):1550–61.

119. Khoury HJ, Wang T, Hemmer MT, et al. Improved survival after acute graft-versus-host disease diagnosis in the modern era. Haematologica 2017; 102(5):958–66.

120. Saugel B, Scheeren TWL, Teboul JL. Ultrasound-guided central venous catheter placement: a structured review and recommendations for clinical practice. Crit Care 2017;21(1):225.

121. Malek AI, Raad I. Catheter- and device-related infections in critically ill cancer patients. In: Nates JL, Price KJ, editors. Oncologic Critical Care. 1st edition. Springer Nature; 2019. p. 1401–17.

122. Campbell SJ, Bechara R, Islam S. Point-of-care ultrasound in the intensive care unit. Clin Chest Med 2018;39(1):79–97.

123. Murarka S, Movahed MR. The use of micropuncture technique for vascular or body cavity access. Rev Cardiovasc Med 2014;15(3):245–51.

124. Lorente L, Lecuona M, Jimenez A, et al. Chlorhexidine-silver sulfadiazine- or rifampicin-miconazole-impregnated venous catheters decrease the risk of catheter-related bloodstream infection similarly. Am J Infect Control 2016; 44(1):50–3.

125. Wolf HH, Leithauser M, Maschmeyer G, et al. Central venous catheter-related infections in hematology and oncology: guidelines of the infectious diseases working party (AGIHO) of the German society of hematology and oncology (DGHO). Ann Hematol 2008;87(11):863–76.

126. Luo X, Guo Y, Yu H, et al. Effectiveness, safety and comfort of StatLock securement for peripherally-inserted central catheters: a systematic review and meta-analysis. Nurs Health Sci 2017;19(4):403–13.

127. Caroff DA, Li L, Muscedere J, et al. Subglottic secretion drainage and objective outcomes: a systematic review and meta-analysis. Crit Care Med 2016;44(4): 830–40.

128. Shinn JR, Kimura KS, Campbell BR, et al. Incidence and outcomes of acute laryngeal injury after prolonged mechanical ventilation. Crit Care Med 2019; 47(12):1699–706.

129. Lichtenstein DA. BLUE-protocol and FALLS-protocol: two applications of lung ultrasound in the critically ill. Chest 2015;147(6):1659–70.

130. Raffaella G, Lorenzo L, Elisabetta X, et al. Lung ultrasound to evaluate invasive fungal diseases after allogeneic hematopoietic stem cell transplantation. Infect Chemother 2019;51(4):386–92.

131. Rahman NM, Maskell NA, Davies CW, et al. The relationship between chest tube size and clinical outcome in pleural infection. Chest 2010;137(3):536–43.

132. Kreeftenberg HG, Pouwels S, Bindels A, et al. Impact of the advanced practice provider in adult critical care: a systematic review and meta-analysis. Crit Care Med 2019;47(5):722–30.

133. Grulke N, Larbig W, Kachele H, et al. Distress in patients undergoing allogeneic haematopoietic stem cell transplantation is correlated with distress in nurses. Eur J Oncol Nurs 2009;13(5):361–7.

134. Neumann JL, Mau LW, Virani S, et al. Burnout, moral distress, work-life balance, and career satisfaction among hematopoietic cell transplantation professionals. Biol Blood Marrow Transplant 2018;24(4):849–60.

Toxicities Associated with Immunotherapy and Approach to Cardiotoxicity with Novel Cancer Therapies

Cristina Gutierrez, MD[a], Prabalini Rajendram, MD[b],
Stephen M. Pastores, MD, MACP, FCCP, FCCM[c],*

KEYWORDS

- Checkpoint inhibitors • Chimeric antigen receptor T-cell therapy
- Cytokine release syndrome • Neurotoxicity • Cardiotoxicity • Pneumonitis
- Oncology • Critical illness

KEY POINTS

- Immune checkpoint inhibitors (ICIs), although highly successful in treating various malignancies, can be associated with uncommon but life-threatening organ toxicities, including pneumonitis, myocarditis, hepatic and renal failure, endocrinopathies, and central and peripheral nervous system syndromes.
- Treatment of ICI-related toxicities include immunosuppression with corticosteroids. For corticosteroid-refractory cases, further immunosuppressive therapy with mycophenolate, infliximab, and intravenous immunoglobulin may be required.
- The 2 most common toxicities associated with chimeric antigen receptor (CAR) T-cell therapy are cytokine release syndrome (CRS) and immune effector cell–associated neurotoxicity syndrome (ICANS).
- In addition to standard guidelines for managing circulatory shock, respiratory failure, encephalopathy, cerebral edema, and seizures, the treatment of CRS and ICANS relies on cytokine (interleukin-6) blockade and corticosteroids.
- Early detection and prophylactic management of patients at high risk for cardiotoxicity from novel oncologic therapy is key in reducing cardiovascular morbidity and mortality.

[a] Department of Critical Care Medicine, University of Texas MD Anderson Cancer Center, 1515 Holcombe Boulevard, Houston, TX 77030, USA; [b] Department of Critical Care, Respiratory Institute, Cleveland Clinic, 9500 Euclid Avenue, Cleveland, OH 44195, USA; [c] Department of Anesthesiology and Critical Care Medicine, Memorial Sloan Kettering Cancer Center, Weill Cornell Medical College, 1275 York Avenue C-1179, New York, NY 10065, USA
* Corresponding author.
E-mail address: pastores@mskcc.org

Crit Care Clin 37 (2021) 47–67
https://doi.org/10.1016/j.ccc.2020.08.003
0749-0704/21/© 2020 Elsevier Inc. All rights reserved.

INTRODUCTION

In recent years, major advances in oncology especially the advent of targeted agents and immunotherapies (immune checkpoint inhibitors [ICIs] and chimeric antigen receptor [CAR] T-cell therapy) have led to improved quality of life and survival rates in patients with cancer. However, an increasing number of adverse effects and unique toxicities caused by these novel anticancer therapies are reported. This article focuses on the clinical features, and grading and management of toxicities associated with ICIs and CAR T-cell therapy. In addition, because cardiotoxicity is one of the most harmful effects of anticancer therapeutics, we describe the risk factors and mechanisms of cardiovascular injury associated with newer agents, screening technologies for at-risk patients, and preventive and treatment strategies.

IMMUNE CHECKPOINT INHIBITOR TOXICITIES

The first immune checkpoint inhibitor (ICI) approved for the treatment of cancer was ipilimumab, for metastatic melanoma, in 2011.[1] To date, a total of 7 ICIs have been approved by the Food and Drug Administration (FDA) for various malignancies including renal cell carcinoma, non–small cell and small cell lung cancer, hepatocellular, cervical and urothelial cancer[2,3](**Table 1**). T-cell activation is downregulated by the cytotoxic T lymphocyte–associated antigen 4 (CTLA-4), programmed cell death protein 1 (PD-1), and programmed death ligand-1 (PD-L1) pathways. ICIs act by enhancing the immune system to fight against cancer cells by blocking these pathways.[4] Although this mechanism of action is effective in disturbing the tumoral milieu, the resulting enhanced inflammatory response can lead to toxic effects, or what are collectively called "immune-related adverse events" (irAEs).

General Features

Toxicities mediated by ICIs can affect multiple organs, including the skin, gastrointestinal tract, lungs, and cardiovascular, neurologic, endocrine, renal, hepatic, hematological, musculoskeletal, and ocular systems. Although each one of these presentations carries its own specific features, some generalizations can be made of irAEs.

- Time of onset and dosing: The time of onset of irAEs can vary from as early as 1 week to as late as 12 months after treatment initiation. Cumulative doses of ICIs have not been associated with increased risk of developing irAEs.[4] Patients who develop mild irAEs can receive a repeat ICI "challenge" but this is not recommended in severe toxicities.
- Incidence of severe toxicities: The severity of irAEs caused by ICIs is measured with the Common Terminology Criteria for Adverse Events grading system. CTLA-4 inhibitors have a higher incidence (27% vs 16%) and greater severity of irAEs than PD-1/PD-L1 inhibitors, and their incidence can rise to 50% when using combination therapy.[2,5,6] A recent meta-analysis showed that mortality from irAEs ranged from 0.63% to 1.2% and was higher with CTLA-4 inhibitor therapy and those patients with myocarditis, myositis, pneumonitis, and hepatitis.[7]
- Risk factors and predictors of toxicity: Precise data to predict which patients will develop irAEs are not available. The use of specific targets (CTLA-4 vs PD-1/PD-L1) are associated with a higher incidence of specific organ toxicities (see **Table 1**).[4] At the same time, some malignancies seem to have a higher incidence of certain toxicities.[8] Genetic evaluation of patients who have developed irAEs

Table 1
Food and Drug Administration–approved immune checkpoint inhibitors, targets, toxicity features, and indications

Target	Toxicity Features	Checkpoint Inhibitor	Indications
CTLA-4	Higher rates of toxicity (including G3-G4) when compared to PD-1/PDL-1 blockade Most common: Dermatologic - rash Colitis Hepatotoxicity Hypophysitis Transverse myelitis	Ipilimumab	Melanoma, renal cell carcinoma, colorectal carcinoma
PD-1	Grade 3 and 4 toxicities vary from disease site Most common: Dermatologic - vitiligo Pneumonitis Cardiotoxicity Thyroid dysfunction	Pembro-lizumab	Melanoma, cervical, endometrial, esophageal and gastric, head and neck SCC, renal cell carcinoma, urothelial, hepatocellular carcinoma. NSCLC, SCLC, diffuse large-cell lymphoma
		Nivolumab	Melanoma, NSCLC, SCLC, colorectal, head and neck SCC, Hodgkin lymphoma, hepatocellular and renal cell carcinoma, urothelial carcinoma
		Cemiplimab	Cutaneous SCC
PDL-1	Toxicity is lower when compared to PD-1 blockade	Atezolizumab	Urothelial, NSCLC, SCLC, breast carcinoma
	Most common: Pneumonitis Cardiotoxicity	Avelumab	Merkel cell carcinoma, renal cell carcinoma, urothelial carcinoma
		Durvalumab	Urothelial carcinoma, NSCLC

Abbreviations: NSCLC, non–small cell lung carcinoma; SCC, squamous cell carcinoma; SCLC, small cell lung carcinoma.

have not determined significant correlations.[9] On the contrary, specific in vivo changes of T-cell, B-cell, and natural killer (NK) cell activity have been described in association to specific toxicities.[10–12]

- Treatment of toxicities: Discontinuation of the ICI and use of immunosuppressive therapy are the cornerstones of treating severe irAEs. Clinical practice guidelines from the American Society of Clinical Oncology, National Comprehensive Cancer Network, and European Society for Medical Oncology are available.[13–15] Twenty-five percent of patients can be refractory to corticosteroids and recommendations for treating these cases vary.[16] A "targeted" treatment approach based on the patient's inflammatory profile (T-cell, B-cell, or NK-cell mediated) has recently been suggested but further evidence is needed to support this strategy.[17]

The main complications observed in the critical care setting include pulmonary, cardiac, and neurologic irAEs (see **Table 1**).

Pulmonary Toxicity

ICI-related pneumonitis is more common with PD-1/PDL-1 inhibitors than with CTLA-4 inhibitors (10% vs <1%).[15] A higher incidence is observed with combination therapy and among patients with lung cancer, and those receiving concomitant radiation therapy or epidermal growth factor receptor tyrosine kinase inhibitors (TKIs).[18–22] The incidence of pneumonitis has recently been reported to be as high as 20%, most likely due to the increased use of ICIs for other malignancies.[8,19,21] In most cases, pneumonitis presents with mild symptoms (dyspnea, dry cough, fever, and chest pain), which usually resolve with discontinuation of therapy and low-dose corticosteroids.[19,22] Rarely, the clinical presentation can be rapidly progressive and fulminant, leading to respiratory failure, with reported mortality of approximately 15%.[7,19] Pneumonitis in patients with lung cancer is associated with worse outcomes when compared with patients with other malignancies.[3,23] The median time of onset is usually 3 months; however, cases have been described as late as 19 months after treatment initiation.[19]

Diagnosis of pneumonitis should include ruling out other causes of lung injury and respiratory failure; most importantly infections, diffuse alveolar hemorrhage, progression of disease, and other drug toxicities. Concomitant findings on examination of other irAEs should help guide the diagnosis, because as many as 58% of cases of pneumonitis have other toxicities associated with ICIs.[19] Although bronchoscopy can be helpful to rule out infectious complications, there are no specific findings described for ICI-related pneumonitis. Radiological findings include ground-glass opacities or patchy nodular infiltrates predominantly in the lower lobes, cryptogenic organizing pneumonia, and interstitial and hypersensitivity-like infiltrates.[19,24,25] Sarcoid-like patterns manifested as hilar lymphadenopathy associated with or without micronodules, ground-glass opacities, and peribronchial interstitial thickening have also been described.[3,14] Lung biopsies are not performed routinely but can be helpful to rule out lymphangitic spread or infection.[13] The 2 most common histologic findings are organizing pneumonia and cellular interstitial pneumonitis.[19,26]

Treatment of ICI-related pneumonitis includes corticosteroids, although as many as 40% of patients require additional immunosuppressive therapy.[19] Guidelines recommend using methylprednisolone and to consider other immunosuppressive agents such as infliximab (anti–tumor necrosis factor [TNF]-alpha antibody), mycophenolate mofetil, cyclophosphamide and intravenous immune globulin (IVIg) if no improvement is observed within 48 hours of corticosteroid treatment[3,14,15] (**Table 2**). A slow taper (over 4–6 weeks) is recommended as worsening of symptoms has been described when corticosteroids are discontinued before 4 weeks.[13,14]

Cardiac Toxicities

Cardiac toxicities secondary to ICIs are considered rare (<1%), more common with PD-1/PDL-1 inhibitors and have a mortality rate of 50%.[27,28] Patients who received combination therapy, and those with refractory arrhythmias or cardiogenic shock are at increased risk of death.[27–30] T-cell regulation and expression of CTLA-4, PD-1 and PD-L1 play an important role in myocardial injury, thus their blockade with ICIs can have an impact on cardiac toxicity.[31–34] The median onset of cardiovascular irAEs is 10 weeks after initiation of ICIs, with reports as early as 2 days and as late as 8 months.[27,29,35] The use of other cardiotoxic agents such as TKIs, can increase the incidence of ICI-related cardiotoxicity.[36,37] Data to support that risk factors for coronary artery disease increase the risk of cardiovascular irAEs remains unclear.[27,35,38]

Clinical presentations of cardiovascular irAEs include myocarditis, pericarditis, heart failure, and arrhythmias.[28–30] The most common arrhythmias include atrial fibrillation (30%), ventricular tachycardia/fibrillation (27%), and conduction abnormalities such as heart block (17%).[30,38] Reports of myocardial infarction are described in the literature but it is unclear if these ischemic events are due to plaque rupture versus coronary vasculitis or vasospasm triggered by the ICI.[29] Decreased ventricular

Table 2
Treatment of immune checkpoint inhibitor–related toxicity

Type of Toxicity	First-Line Therapy[a]	Second-Line Therapy[a]
Pneumonitis (grade 3–4)	• Methylprednisolone 1–4 mg/kg/ d (slow taper)	• Infliximab 5 mg/kg • MMF 1 g q 12 h • IVIg for 5 d • Cyclophosphamide
Cardiotoxicity-myocarditis (grade 3–4)	• Methylprednisolone 1–2 mg/kg/ d or 1 g/d	• MMF • Infliximab • Anti-thymocyte globulin • Tacrolimus • IVIg
Neurotoxicities: (Grade 3–4)		
Guillain-Barre syndrome/ Myasthenia gravis	• IVIg (0.4 mg/kg/d) or plasmapheresis • Pyridostigmine	• Consider Methylprednisolone 1– 4 mg/kg/d[b] • Azathioprine • Cyclosporine • MMF
Aseptic meningitis/ encephalitis	• Methylprednisolone 1–2 mg/kg/ d	• Methylprednisolone (1 g/d) • + IVIg if no improvement • Rituximab
Transverse myelitis	• Methylprednisolone 2 mg/kg/ day-1 g/d • IVIg	• Plasmapheresis • IVIg

Abbreviations: IVIg, intravenous immune globulin; MMF, mycophenolate mofetil.
[a] Recommendations based on guidelines from American Society of Clinical Oncology, European Society for Medical Oncology, National Comprehensive Cancer Network (NCCN).[13–15]
[b] Guidelines vary on whether if corticosteroids should be first-line or second-line therapy for myasthenia gravis and Guillain-Barre syndrome (GBS). NCCN recommends dosing for GBS to be 1 g/d of methylprednisolone intravenous.

ejection fraction (EF) can occur in patients with myocarditis and in those without evidence of myocardial injury with Takotsubo-like physiology.[32,38] Most patients with left ventricular (LV) dysfunction improve with corticosteroids.[27]

As with other irAEs, it is important to rule out other causes for cardiac dysfunction such as acute coronary syndrome, electrolyte imbalances, other medication toxicities, and infection (eg, viral myocarditis).[34] So far, a validated risk assessment tool has not been developed therefore some institutions recommend the creation of algorithms to expedite the workup and treatment for suspected ICI-related cardiovascular irAEs.[34,35,39,40]

Myocarditis is more common with anti-PD-1/PD-L1 therapy, and while extremely rare (incidence of <0.5%), it is usually fulminant if the diagnosis and treatment are delayed.[28,29] Myocarditis has been known to be associated with myositis and neurologic complications such as myasthenia gravis; thus, close cardiac monitoring is recommended for patients presenting with myalgias and muscle weakness.[27] Half of the patients with ICI-related myocarditis have a higher rate of major cardiovascular events, compared with the general population with myocarditis.[35] Most patients will have abnormal troponins and pro-brain natriuretic peptide (BNP); however abnormal electrocardiograms (ECGs) and echocardiogram are only described in 50% of patients.[30,35,38,39] ECG findings include prolongation of the PR interval, AV block, ventricular arrhythmias, frequent premature contractions, ST depression or diffuse T-wave inversion.[34,39] Elevated troponins (>1.5 ng/mL) are associated with increased mortality.[34,35] Echocardiogram may show decreased LV or right ventricular EF with global or regional abnormalities.[35] The gold standard for diagnosis of myocarditis is an endomyocardial biopsy revealing lymphocytic infiltration of the myocardium and cardiac conduction system.[34] Cardiac MRI can be helpful; however, it can be normal in almost 50% of patients (compared with 20% of cases in non–ICI-related myocarditis).[37,41]

Treatment recommendations for cardiovascular irAEs include holding ICI therapy and initiation of corticosteroids (see **Table 2**). In patients who do not promptly respond, higher doses of corticosteroids may be administered along with IVIg, infliximab, mycophenolate and anti-thymocyte globulin.[13,15,29,30,41,42] Caution is recommended when administering infliximab as this agent has been associated with increased risk of decompensated heart failure.[34]

Neurotoxicity

ICI-related neurologic irAEs usually present within 3 months (2–12 weeks) of treatment initiation, although neuromuscular disorders present earlier.[43] Although uncommon, they have significant morbidity and mortality especially when associated with other toxicities such as myocarditis.[5,7,43] Clinical presentation may include encephalopathy, aseptic meningitis, encephalitis, seizures, transverse myelitis, posterior reversible encephalopathy syndrome (PRES), Guillain-Barre syndrome (GBS), and myasthenia gravis (MG).[5,43] Reactivation of underlying neurologic syndromes, such as multiple sclerosis, MG, and neurosarcoidosis, have also been described.[43–45] Central nervous system (CNS) progression of cancer, infection, seizure disorder, and metabolic causes as causes of neurologic symptoms should be ruled out. GBS and MG are thought to occur due to activation of the immune system against the host after the inhibition of either CTLA-4 or PD-1/PD-L1.[43,46,47] Although the clinical presentation can be classical, variability can be observed due to concomitant presentation of other polyradiculoneuropathies and myositis.[44]

Diagnostic workup should include a thorough clinical examination, cerebrospinal fluid (CSF) analysis, neuroimaging studies (brain and/or spine MRI), electroencephalography (EEG) and electromyography (EMG).[3] Lymphocytic pleocytosis and elevated protein is commonly found on CSF analysis in patients with GBS. Acetylcholine receptor (AChR) and antistriated antibodies are helpful in cases of suspected MG, although they are not always positive in these patients.[44]

Treatment for both MG and GBS include corticosteroids, plasmapheresis, and IVIg; although the role of IVIg is less clear (see **Table 2**).[5,14,15,45,48] Pyridostigmine may be useful for MG in addition to corticosteroids. Because many cases present with concurrent myositis, corticosteroid-sparing treatments can be considered to avoid worsening the myositis. Medications that can exacerbate MG should be avoided.[15] Rituximab, mycophenolate, and infliximab have been used in some cases.[4,5,15,45]

In patients presenting with aseptic meningitis, encephalitis and encephalopathy, infectious causes should be ruled out and treated concomitantly until a definite diagnosis is made.[4,5,43,44,49] Brain MRI and CSF studies can be helpful; however, there are no specific findings related to ICI toxicity.[3,50] Treatments include corticosteroids, IVIg, and rituximab in refractory cases (see **Table 2**).[14,15,45,50,51] Responses to treatment vary significantly and relapses can be observed when tapering corticosteroids.[45] Seizures should be treated with antiepileptic agents and discontinuation of the ICI.[5,47] PRES presents with similar clinical and radiological findings as in the general population.[5,43,45] Transverse myelitis has been reported with ipilimumab and reversed after high-dose corticosteroids.[5,45]

Other Considerations for the Intensive Care Unit

Other irAEs can present in critically ill patients with cancer treated with ICIs, although may not be the leading cause of intensive care unit (ICU) admission. Hypophysitis, occurs in 10% of patients treated with anti-CTLA-4 therapy; therefore, adrenal insufficiency and hypothyroidism should be considered if there is clinical suspicion.[3] Hyperthyroidism, diabetes insipidus, and diabetes (causing hyperglycemic emergencies) are described.[3,15,16] Endocrinopathies caused by ICIs do not reverse when the agents are discontinued, therefore hormonal therapy is required long term.[13]

Renal toxicities are also described with ICIs and permanent renal dysfunction is associated with increased mortality.[52] Although risk factors have not been described, concerns of activation of an underlying autoimmune disease (eg, vasculitis) or confounding with other nephrotoxic agents, such as proton pump inhibitors and sepsis, can lead to further nephrotoxicity.[52]

Elevation of liver function tests are more common with anti-CTLA-4 therapy, and although severe toxicity is rare, cases of refractory liver failure have been described.[3,15] Although the use of ICIs alone is not associated to an increased risk of infections, the use of immunosuppressive therapy for the management of irAEs can cause significant immunosuppression.[22] Therefore, institutional guidelines on initiation of prophylactic therapy for opportunistic infections, should be followed. Last, it is important for the intensivist be aware that flares of known or undiagnosed, autoimmune diseases are observed with the initiation of ICIs.[53] Although they are reported as mild in most cases, considering autoimmune pathologies and vasculitis as part of the differential diagnosis in a patient with multiorgan failure is crucial.

CHIMERIC ANTIGEN RECEPTOR T-CELL-THERAPY–ASSOCIATED TOXICITIES

CAR T-cell therapy, is a form of adoptive cell therapy that uses genetically engineered autologous or allogeneic T-cells expressing an artificial receptor to redirect the specificity of the T cells against a tumoral antigen.[54] The most studied CAR T-cell therapy products target CD19 antigen expressed in B-cell leukemia and lymphoma and have revolutionized the treatment of patients with relapsed/refractory B-cell hematologic malignancies. The median survival for patients who are refractory to second-line chemotherapy or relapse after autologous stem cell transplantation is approximately 6 months.[55–57] However, clinical trials proved the efficacy of CAR T-cell therapy in refractory diffuse large B-cell lymphoma (DLBCL), with reported high clinical response rates of 50% to 90%.[58–61]

As a consequence of these unprecedented response rates, in 2017 the US FDA approved 2 anti-CD19 CAR T-cell therapy products; axicabtagene ciloleucel (YES-CARTA) for DLBCL and tisagenlecleucel (KYMRIAH) for acute lymphoblastic leukemia (ALL),[62] and relapsed/refractory DLBCL in 2017.[63,64] The promise of CAR T-cell therapy for the treatment of B-cell hematologic malignancies has laid the foundation for ongoing clinical trials to evaluate extending this treatment strategy to other malignancies.

Despite the high rates of complete remission, this treatment is often associated with specific toxicities; B-cell aplasia, graft versus host disease, cytokine release syndrome (CRS), and immune effector cell–associated neurotoxicity syndrome (ICANS) (also referred to as neurotoxicity). CRS and ICANS, the 2 most common toxicities that have the potential to lead to multiorgan failure and death, are reversible, therefore prompt recognition and management of these complications is important to mitigate adverse outcomes.

Pathophysiology and Clinical Features of Cytokine Release Syndrome and Immune Effector Cell-Associated Neurotoxicity Syndrome

CRS can occur within hours to days of CAR T-cell infusion and is mediated by release of cytokines by activated T cells.[60,61] CRS occurs when antigen recognition by CAR T-cells leads to activation, proliferation and cytokine release, precipitating a cascade reaction leading to activation of T cells, B cells, NK cells, and macrophages.[65] Increased levels of cytokines such as interleukin-6 (IL-6), IL-2, IL-2 receptor-a, IL-8, IL-10, interferon (IFN)-γ, and tumor necrosis factor (TNF)-γ have been associated in patients with CRS.[66–70] In addition to cytokines, nonspecific biomarkers such as ferritin and C-reactive protein (CRP) levels have been linked to increased severity of CAR T-cell-therapy–associated toxicities. Although elevated levels of CRP ≥20 mg/dL correlate with severe CRS with a 100% specificity, the predictive value of this biomarker is still unknown.[71,72]

Clinical symptomology of CRS can be challenging to identify, as the presentation is broad and can mimic sepsis. CRS commonly presents with high fevers, tachycardia, hypotension, and/or hypoxemia. Cardiovascular toxicities can manifest as arrhythmias, cardiomyopathy with decreased EF, vasodilatory shock and/or cardiogenic shock. CRS can also cause noncardiogenic pulmonary edema secondary to pulmonary capillary leak syndrome leading to acute respiratory failure and progression to acute respiratory distress syndrome. Other organ systems may be involved leading to acute kidney injury, hepatic and gastrointestinal dysfunction, cytopenias, and dissemination intravascular coagulation. Grading of CRS is based on the severity of these symptoms.[73,74]

The presentation of symptoms with ICANS are variable, and not necessarily associated with CRS and therefore suggest a different pathophysiology and mechanism of injury than CRS. Two pathophysiological mechanisms have been proposed to explain ICANS. One suggested mechanism is a cytokine-mediated CNS injury due to high levels of serum and CSF IL-2, IL-6, IFN-γ, and TNF-α.[73–75] The alternative explanation is that neurotoxicity is secondary to an active diffusion of CAR T-cells across the blood brain barrier (BBB) as indicated by the detection of the cells in CSF. Endothelial activation and injury, disseminated intravascular coagulation, capillary leak, and increased BBB permeability also play an important roles.[76]

Several risk factors such as tumor characteristics, patient characteristics and therapy regimen have been related to severity of CRS and neurotoxicity. Higher activation and proliferation of CAR T-cells is observed in patients with higher tumor burden predicting more toxicity.[73] Cell dosing, chemotherapy regimens before cell infusion, and cell construct also have an effect on cell proliferation and activity.[73–75] Last, a patient's age and comorbidities have been linked to increased risk and severity of CAR T-cell-therapy–associated toxicity.[77]

ICANS associated with anti-CD19 CAR T-cell therapy has been reported in 40% to 60% of patients. Symptoms present in biphasic pattern with the first phase occurring simultaneously with CRS and within 5 days of CAR T-cell infusion, and the second phase occurring after CRS resolution. Common symptoms of mild neurotoxicity include diminished attention, confusion, agitation and mild aphasia, tremors and dysgraphia. Neurotoxicity is classified as severe when the symptoms progress to global aphasia, agitation, obtundation, seizures, status epilepticus, and cerebral edema.[76–79] A neurologic assessment score, CAR T-cell-therapy–associated TOXicity (CARTOX)-10, had been developed to recognize early signs of encephalopathy and assist in grading severity.[79] A modified version of CARTOX-10 now termed Immune Effector Cell-Associated Encephalopathy (ICE) score (**Table 3**) was developed to create a

Table 3		
Immune effector cell–associated encephalopathy (ICE) score		
Test[a]	**Task**	**Points[b]**
Orientation	Orientation to year, month, city, hospital	4
Naming	Ability to name objects	3
Following commands	Ability to follow 1 or 2 step commands (simple commands)	1
Writing	Ability to write a standard sentence	1
Attention	Ability to count backward from 100 by 10	1

[a] Test used to assess cognitive function.
[b] Maximum number of points for each cognitive function for a maximum total of 10.
Adapted from Lee DW, Santomasso BD, Locke FL et al. ASTCT consensus grading for cytokine release syndrome neurologic toxicity associated with immune effector cells. Biol Blood Marrow Transplant 2019; 25: 625-638; with permission.

simplified and unified method to assess encephalopathy and is used to grade ICANS.[74]

Diagnostic workup and treatment of cytokine release syndrome (CRS)

Patients with grade 1 toxicity can be managed with monitoring and supportive care of fever (acetaminophen, cooling blankets), malaise, and myalgias. However, grade 2 or higher toxicities require ICU admission for monitoring and support of hemodynamic instability, respiratory compromise, and multiple organ failure. Initial management of hypotension and circulatory shock with fluid resuscitation and vasopressor support should mirror standard ICU practices.

Cardiac dysfunction is severe and rapid but typically reverse, resembling stress cardiomyopathy or cardiomyopathy related to sepsis and is associated with high mortality.[80] Expert consensus suggests obtaining an echocardiogram to determine LVEF, troponins, and ECG, as these may be indicators of severe CRS. It is essential to monitor serum lactate levels as surrogate of end-organ perfusion and administer intravenous fluids, vasopressor, and/or inotropic agents to optimize cardiac output.[73,74] It is prudent to consider other etiologies of shock and perform blood cultures, urine cultures and start antibiotics if index of suspicion for septic shock is high.[81] Arrhythmias (atrial fibrillation, QT prolongation), including fatal arrhythmias, have also been reported.[71] Acute hypoxemic respiratory failure should be managed with supplemental oxygen (preferably using high-flow nasal cannula) or noninvasive ventilation with bilevel positive airway pressure as first-line approach for mild to moderate acute hypoxemic respiratory failure.[82,83] Mechanical ventilation needs to be considered for higher grade (grade 4) CRS; and lung protective (low tidal volumes and judicious application of positive end-expiratory pressure) strategies should be implemented in the care of these patients with consideration for adjunctive therapies such as prone positioning.[84] Other supportive therapies such as extracorporeal membrane oxygenation, should be considered on a case by case basis in consultation with a multidisciplinary team of clinicians. Treatment of acute renal failure, and consideration for renal replacement therapies should be considered according to standard guidelines.[73,79]

In addition to organ supportive measures, the mainstay of therapy for CRS-related toxicities is the use of monoclonal antibodies (mAbs) with activity against circulating IL-6 (tocilizumab or siltuximab). Both agents have different mechanism of action; tocilizumab binds to membrane IL-6 receptors (IL-6R) whereas siltuximab binds to circulating IL-6. Tocilizumab (8 mg/kg for adults) is recommended for grade 2 or higher

CRS; for patients with hypotension unresponsive to fluid resuscitation and in persistent hypoxia with fraction of inspired oxygen requirement of greater than 40% or 6L nasal cannula/minute. The dose of tocilizumab can be repeated if CRS does not improve with the initial dose. In some cases, serum IL-6 levels can be elevated after tocilizumab administration suggesting there is persistent inflammatory response associated with CRS.[85] For this reason, it has been theorized that siltuximab (11 mg/kg administered as a single dose) can be used in refractory cases; however, there are insufficient data to support this theory. Similarly, anecdotal use of other cytokine-directed treatment, including TNF-α (etanercept, infliximab) and IL-1R blockade (anakinra), in refractory cases have been reported.[86–88]

Current guidelines suggest there is a role for use of corticosteroids for grade 3 or higher CRS toxicity or grade 2 CRS refractory to tocilizumab or siltuximab. **Table 4** summarizes the clinical presentation, grading and management of CRS. Because there is a lack of randomized controlled trials of the choice of agent, dose, and duration of treatment with tocilizumab and corticosteroids, managing severe toxicities of CAR T-cell therapy requires careful deliberation and frequent monitoring of patient's response to therapy.

Diagnostic workup and treatment of immune effector cell-associated neurotoxicity syndrome (ICANS)

Brain imaging studies (computed tomography [CT] or MRI), EEG, lumbar puncture (if no contraindications are present), and an expert neurologic examination with fundoscopy is recommended for the appropriate diagnosis and gradation of neurotoxicity. The 2 commonly encountered presentations of severe neurotoxicity are seizures (convulsive or nonconvulsive) and cerebral edema, which can lead to neurologic devastation if not recognized and managed in a timely manner.

Nonconvulsive seizures that are associated with CAR T-cell therapy can progress to status epilepticus in 10% of patients.[79] Thus, prophylactic antiepileptics or for those with grade 1 or 2 neurotoxicity, can be considered. Benzodiazepines and levetiracetam are the most common agents used in nonconvulsive and convulsive seizures.

In addition to monitoring in the ICU, administration of antiepileptics for seizures, corticosteroids are recommended for patients with grade 3 and 4 neurotoxicity. Corticosteroids can be considered in grade 2 toxicity if the CAR T-cell construct has been linked with severe neurotoxicity. Dexamethasone has excellent CNS penetration and may be preferred over methylprednisolone. The optimal duration of corticosteroids is unknown, therefore tapering of corticosteroids is suggested after resolution of clinical symptoms.[77,79] Because tocilizumab and siltuximab are too large molecules to enter the BBB, the use of these agents for neurotoxicity after CRS resolution is not recommended. However, tocilizumab and siltuximab are recommended for patients with concurrent CRS and grade 1 or higher neurotoxicity.

Monitoring for signs of elevated intracranial pressure (ICP) with fundoscopy, transcranial Doppler, or measurement of optic nerve sheath diameter should be performed when corticosteroid use is being considered. Brain MRI or CT scan is used to rule out other intracranial pathologies such as hemorrhagic or ischemic stroke. The clinical presentation, grading and management of ICANS is described in **Table 5**. Standard guidelines should be followed to manage these conditions paying special attention to controlling elevated ICP and intubation strategies for airway protection.[77] Assessment and careful consideration of alternate causes of encephalopathy should be entertained and diagnostic strategies used according to standard of care.

Table 4
Grading of cytokine release syndrome

CRS Parameter	Grade 1	Grade 2	Grade 3	Grade 4
Constitutional (fever)	Temperature ≥38ₒC Malaise, myalgia, arthralgia	Temperature ≥38ₒC Malaise, myalgia, arthralgia	Temperature ≥38ₒC Malaise, myalgia, arthralgia	Temperature ≥38ₒC Malaise, myalgia, arthralgia
	With	With	With	With
Cardiac (hypotension)	None	Hypotension/Shock: responsive to IV fluids <24 hr Cardiomyopathy: EF>40% or 10% decrease in EF Arrythmia: Stable dysrhythmias	Hypotension/Shock: requiring one vasopressor (±vasopressin) Cardiomyopathy: EF 20%–39% or 10% decrease in EF Arrythmia: Unstable dysrhythmias	Hypotension/Shock: Refractory requiring multiple vasopressors Cardiomyopathy: EF<20% Arrythmia: Life-threatening
	And/or	And/or	And/or	And/or
Respiratory (hypoxia)	None	Hypoxemia requiring low flow nasal cannula≤6 L/min	Hypoxemia requiring high-flow nasal cannula ≥6 L/min Venturi mask or Nonrebreather mask	Hypoxemia requiring noninvasive positive pressure or mechanical ventilation
Treatment	Supportive care	Admission to ICU Tocilizumab (or consider siltuximab) Consider Corticosteroids if symptoms prevail	Tocilizumab or siltuximab in cases refractory to tocilizumab Corticosteroids: Dexamethasone 10 mg IV q6hrs (or equivalent dosing of methylprednisolone)[a]	Tocilizumab or siltuximab in cases refractory to tocilizumab Corticosteroids: Methylprednisolone 1 g/d[a]

Abbreviations: EF, ejection fraction; ICU, intensive care unit; IV, intravenous.
[a] Recommend tapering dose and duration based on patient's response to therapy.

Data from Lee DW, Santomasso BD, Locke FL, et al. ASTCT Consensus Grading for Cytokine Release Syndrome and Neurologic Toxicity Associated with Immune Effector Cells. *Biol Blood Marrow Transplant.* 2019;25(4):625-638. https://doi.org/10.1016/j.bbmt.2018.12.758; and Gutierrez C, McEvoy C, Mead E et al. Management of the critically ill adult chimeric antigen receptor-T cell therapy patient: A critical care perspective. Critical Care Med 2018; 46 (9) 1402-1410

Table 5
Immune effector cell–associated neurotoxicity syndrome (ICANS) consensus grading

Neurotoxicity Domain	Grade 1	Grade 2	Grade 3	Grade 4
ICE Score	7–9	3–6	0–2	0
Consciousness	Awakens spontaneously	Awakens to voice	Awakens only to tactile stimulus	Unarousable, stupor, coma
Seizure	None	None	Partial seizure, or convulsive seizures resolving spontaneously; or nonconvulsive seizure that responds with antiepileptics	Status epilepticus (repetitive clinical or electrical seizures without return to baseline)
Cerebral edema/ICP	None	None	Focal/local edema on imaging	Diffuse cerebral edema; clinical signs of herniation such as Cushing's triad; posturing; cranial nerve VI palsy; papilledema
Motor findings	None	None	None	Severe focal motor deficits; hemiparesis; or paraparesis
Supportive care and diagnostic imaging	CT or MRI brain and EEG Frequent neurologic assessment Consider seizure prophylaxis Lumbar puncture (if no contraindications)	CT or MRI brain and EEG Frequent neurologic assessment Consider seizure prophylaxis Lumbar puncture (if no contraindications)	CT or MRI brain and EEG Frequent neurologic assessment Treat seizures with benzodiazepines, levetiracetam or other antiepileptic agents as necessary Lumbar puncture (if no contraindications)	CT or MRI brain and continuous EEG Frequent neurologic assessment Treatment of status epilepticus as per institutional guidelines

Treatment	Supportive care and monitoring		
	Supportive care and monitoring for progression Consider corticosteroids if symptoms are persistent or if CAR construct has been associated with severe neurotoxicity	Corticosteroids: Dexamethasone 10 mg IV every 6 h (or equivalent dosing of methylprednisolone) Tocilizumab or siltuximab if concomitant CRS symptoms are present	Corticosteroids: Methylprednisolone 1 g/d Tocilizumab or siltuximab if concomitant CRS symptoms are present

Abbreviations: CAR, chimeric antigen receptor; CRS, cytokine release syndrome; CT, computed tomography; EEG, encephalography; ICE, Immune Effector Cell-Associated Encephalopathy; IV, intravenous.

Data from Lee DW, Santomasso BD, Locke FL, et al. ASTCT Consensus Grading for Cytokine Release Syndrome and Neurologic Toxicity Associated with Immune Effector Cells. *Biol Blood Marrow Transplant.* 2019;25(4):625-638. https://doi.org/10.1016/j.bbmt.2018.12.758; and Gutierrez C, McEvoy C, Mead E et al. Management of the critically ill adult chimeric antigen receptor-T cell therapy patient: A critical care perspective. *Critical Care Med* 2018; 46 (9) 1402-1410.

NOVEL ONCOLOGIC THERAPY AND CARDIOTOXICITY

Many of the new anticancer therapeutics can be associated with cardiovascular (CV) toxicities including heart failure, cardiac conduction abnormalities, arrhythmias, pulmonary hypertension, pericardial disease, and arterial and venous thrombosis, resulting in significant morbidity and mortality. Cardio-oncology has become a distinct interdisciplinary specialty consisting of cardiologists and oncologists dedicated to minimizing CV risk and preventing CV disease in patients with cancer and survivors.[89]

Much of the published literature on the cardiotoxicities associated with traditional chemotherapeutic agents focused on the risk of developing LV dysfunction with anthracyclines (eg, doxorubicin) and of heart failure and ischemia, bradycardia, and QT prolongation with cyclophosphamide, 5-flurouracil, cisplatin, and arsenic. In the case of doxorubicin, cardiotoxicity is dose dependent; at doses of ≥ 400 mg/m^2, the risk of developing LV dysfunction is greater than 5%.[90]

In the case of trastuzumab (anti-HER2), high rates of myocardial contractile dysfunction (27%) due to HER2 inhibition of cell repair have been observed since the pivotal trial.[91] Unlike the anthracyclines, cardiac toxicity from trastuzumab does not show the typical structural changes, is not cumulative-dose dependent and more likely to be reversible. It is notable that the incidence of cardiac events such as congestive heart failure is highest when trastuzumab and anthracyclines are given together.

Various cardiotoxicities can occur in patients receiving TKIs including hypertension (nilotinib, cabozantinib, dabrafenib, bosutinib), fluid retention (imatinib), atrial and ventricular arrhythmias (ibrutinib, sunitinib, sorafenib), QT prolongation (dasatinib, nilotinib), and pulmonary hypertension with dasatinib.[92]

Vascular endothelial growth factor (VEGF) inhibitors (sunitinib, ponatinib, bevacizumab) have been associated with hypertension, cardiomyopathy, proteinuria, and vascular toxic events.[93] Hypertension can occur in 25% to 80% of treated patients, mainly due to direct inhibition of VEGF signaling resulting in an imbalance between the production of vasodilators (nitric oxide, prostacyclin) and vasoconstrictors (endothelin-1), loss of capillary circulation, and alteration in glomerular function, which all contribute to causing hypertension.[92] Angiotensin-converting enzyme inhibitors are considered first-line therapy for hypertension in these patients. Verapamil and diltiazem, both CYP3A4 inhibitors, should probably be avoided to treat hypertension in patients receiving sunitinib, sorafenib, and other VEGFR-TKIs, but may be considered in patients receiving bevacizumab. High-risk subjects who are to be initiated on VEGF inhibitors should have aggressive hypertension management. The cardiomyopathy associated with VEGF inhibitors is characterized by systolic dysfunction in at least 10% of patients, although many patients do not have heart failure symptoms.

The use of carfilzomib, a proteasome inhibitor, has been associated with hypertension, arrhythmias, and heart failure. Immunomodulatory agents (thalidomide, lenalidomide, and pomalidomide) used for the treatment of multiple myeloma and light chain (AL) amyloidosis are associated with arterial and venous thromboembolism. Similarly, histone deacetylase inhibitors (eg, romidepsin) and CDK 4/6 inhibitors (eg, ribociclib) can cause QT prolongation.[94]

The cardiotoxicities associated with ICIs and CAR T-cell therapy were described earlier.

STRATEGIES TO MITIGATE RISK OF CARDIOTOXICITY

Early detection and prophylactic management of patients at high risk for cardiotoxicity from anticancer therapies is key in reducing morbidity and mortality. Correction of modifiable CV risk factors (smoking, alcohol, obesity) and serum electrolytes and reduction of psychological distress should be undertaken. Measurement of cardiac biomarkers such as troponins and natriuretic peptides (BNP and N-terminal BNP) as markers of myocardial cell injury, may be helpful in identifying subclinical cardiotoxicity and predicting the likelihood of developing LV dysfunction particularly in patients treated with anthracyclines, taxanes, and trastuzumab.[95] However, elevated levels of BNP and N-terminal BNP have not consistently correlated with echocardiographic evidence of LV dysfunction. Novel biomarkers for risk stratification of heart failure with preserved EF such as protein biomarker of cardiac stress (ST2), matrix metalloproteinase-2, and growth differentiation factor-15 have recently been identified.[96]

Current guidelines for monitoring cardiac function in these patients still involves evaluating for signs for heart failure and serial assessment of LVEF with 2-dimensional (2D) echocardiography.[97,98] Cardiotoxicity is defined on echocardiography as a reduction in LVEF greater than 10% with a cutoff value of less than 50%. Given the limitations of standard 2D echocardiography in detecting LV dysfunction, new imaging techniques such as 3D echocardiography and speckle-tracking echocardiography and cardiac MRI, if available, are increasingly being used although further studies are needed to confirm their benefits.[99–101]

Dexrazoxane is a cardioprotective agent that is used clinically to decrease doxorubicin cardiotoxicity and anthracycline-induced extravasation injury. Although originally thought to act solely as an iron chelator that reduces iron-dependent doxorubicin-induced oxidative damage, it is now believed that its cardioprotective effect may be due largely to its ability to inhibit and reduce topoisomerase IIβ protein levels in the heart.[102]

Several cardiovascular agents have been demonstrated to be cardioprotective against anthracyclines including beta-blockers (carvedilol, nebivolol), angiotensin-converting enzyme (ACE) inhibitors (enalapril), angiotensin receptor blockers (valsartan, telmisartan), aldosterone antagonists (spironolactone) ,and statins (atorvastatin).[89,103] With carvedilol, the mechanism for the cardioprotective effect appears to be related to its antioxidant properties. However, serial echocardiography and use of beta-blockers and ACE inhibitors have not been shown to confer long-term cardioprotection. Future strategies could include the use of autologous progenitor cardiac cells.[104]

SUMMARY

The use of ICIs and CAR T-cell therapy have significantly improved the prognosis of many patients with solid and hematologic malignancies. Despite their important clinical benefits, these therapies can be associated with diverse and complex immune-related adverse events, including fatal toxicities. General and organ-specific guidelines for the management of toxicities due to ICIs and CAR T-cell therapy are available. Cardiovascular toxicities from novel agents including heart failure, myocarditis, cardiac conduction abnormalities, arrhythmias, and pulmonary hypertension can result in significant morbidity and mortality. Multidisciplinary teams working collaboratively with ICU clinicians are essential to effectively manage serious toxicities.

DISCLOSURE

The authors have no commercial or financial conflicts of interest related to this article.

REFERENCES

1. Hodi FS, O'Day SJ, McDermott DF, et al. Improved survival with ipilimumab in patients with metastatic melanoma. N Engl J Med 2010;363(8):711–23.
2. Marin-Acevedo JA, Chirila RM, Dronca RS. Immune checkpoint inhibitor toxicities. Mayo Clin Proc 2019;94(7):1321–9.
3. Friedman CF, Proverbs-Singh TA, Postow MA. Treatment of the immune-related adverse effects of immune checkpoint inhibitors: a review. JAMA Oncol 2016; 2(10):1346–53.
4. Postow MA, Sidlow R, Hellmann MD. Immune-related adverse events associated with immune checkpoint blockade. N Engl J Med 2018;378(2):158–68.
5. Neagu MR, Jenkins RW, Reardon D. Neurological complications of immune-based therapies. Cham (Switzerland): Springer; 2018.
6. Larkin J, Chiarion-Sileni V, Gonzalez R, et al. Combined nivolumab and ipilimumab or monotherapy in untreated melanoma. N Engl J Med 2015;373(1):23–34.
7. Wang DY, Salem JE, Cohen JV, et al. Fatal toxic effects associated with immune checkpoint inhibitors: a systematic review and meta-analysis. JAMA Oncol 2018;4(12):1721–8.
8. Nishino M, Giobbie-Hurder A, Hatabu H, et al. Incidence of programmed cell death 1 inhibitor-related pneumonitis in patients with advanced cancer: a systematic review and meta-analysis. JAMA Oncol 2016;2(12):1607–16.
9. Wolchok JD, Weber JS, Hamid O, et al. Ipilimumab efficacy and safety in patients with advanced melanoma: a retrospective analysis of HLA subtype from four trials. Cancer Immune 2010;10:9.
10. Das R, Bar N, Ferreira M, et al. Early B cell changes predict autoimmunity following combination immune checkpoint blockade. J Clin Invest 2018; 128(2):715–20.
11. Hopkins AM, Rowland A, Kichenadasse G, et al. Predicting response and toxicity to immune checkpoint inhibitors using routinely available blood and clinical markers. Br J Cancer 2017;117(7):913–20.
12. Patil PD, Burotto M, Velcheti V. Biomarkers for immune-related toxicities of checkpoint inhibitors: current progress and the road ahead. Expert Rev Mol Diagn 2018;18(3):297–305.
13. Haanen J, Carbonnel F, Robert C, et al. Management of toxicities from immunotherapy: ESMO Clinical Practice Guidelines for diagnosis, treatment and follow-up. Ann Oncol 2017;28(suppl_4):iv119–42.
14. Puzanov I, Diab A, Abdallah K, et al. Managing toxicities associated with immune checkpoint inhibitors: consensus recommendations from the Society for Immunotherapy of Cancer (SITC) toxicity management working group. J Immunother Cancer 2017;5(1):95.
15. Thompson JA, Schneider BJ, Brahmer J, et al. Management of immunotherapy-related toxicities, version 1.2019. J Natl Compr Canc Netw 2019;17(3):255–89.
16. Shoushtari AN, Friedman CF, Navid-Azarbaijani P, et al. Measuring toxic effects and time to treatment failure for nivolumab plus ipilimumab in melanoma. JAMA Oncol 2018;4(1):98–101.
17. Martins F, Sykiotis GP, Maillard M, et al. New therapeutic perspectives to manage refractory immune checkpoint-related toxicities. Lancet Oncol 2019; 20(1):e54–64.
18. Antonia SJ, Villegas A, Daniel D, et al. Durvalumab after chemoradiotherapy in stage III non-small-cell lung cancer. N Engl J Med 2017;377(20):1919–29.

19. Naidoo J, Wang X, Woo KM, et al. Pneumonitis in patients treated with anti-programmed death-1/programmed death ligand 1 therapy. J Clin Oncol 2017; 35(7):709–17.

20. Rashdan S, Minna JD, Gerber DE. Diagnosis and management of pulmonary toxicity associated with cancer immunotherapy. Lancet Respir Med 2018;6(6): 472–8.

21. Suresh K, Psoter KJ, Voong KR, et al. Impact of checkpoint inhibitor pneumonitis on survival in NSCLC patients receiving immune checkpoint immunotherapy. J Thorac Oncol 2019;14(3):494–502.

22. Sears CR, Peikert T, Possick JD, et al. Knowledge gaps and research priorities in immune checkpoint inhibitor-related pneumonitis. An official American Thoracic Society research statement. Am J Respir Crit Care Med 2019;200(6): e31–43.

23. Gettinger SN, Horn L, Gandhi L, et al. Overall survival and long-term safety of nivolumab (anti-programmed death 1 antibody, BMS-936558, ONO-4538) in patients with previously treated advanced non-small-cell lung cancer. J Clin Oncol 2015;33(18):2004–12.

24. Nishino M, Sholl LM, Hodi FS, et al. Anti-PD-1-related pneumonitis during cancer immunotherapy. N Engl J Med 2015;373(3):288–90.

25. Tirumani SH, Ramaiya NH, Keraliya A, et al. Radiographic profiling of immune-related adverse events in advanced melanoma patients treated with ipilimumab. Cancer Immunol Res 2015;3(10):1185–92.

26. Larsen BT, Chae JM, Dixit AS, et al. Clinical and histopathologic features of immune checkpoint inhibitor-related pneumonitis. Am J Surg Pathol 2019;43(10): 1331–40.

27. Moslehi JJ, Salem JE, Sosman JA, et al. Increased reporting of fatal immune checkpoint inhibitor-associated myocarditis. Lancet 2018;391(10124):933.

28. Salem JE, Manouchehri A, Moey M, et al. Cardiovascular toxicities associated with immune checkpoint inhibitors: an observational, retrospective, pharmacovigilance study. Lancet Oncol 2018;19(12):1579–89.

29. Lyon AR, Yousaf N, Battisti NML, et al. Immune checkpoint inhibitors and cardiovascular toxicity. Lancet Oncol 2018;19(9):e447–58.

30. Mir H, Alhussein M, Alrashidi S, et al. Cardiac complications associated with checkpoint inhibition: a systematic review of the literature in an important emerging area. Can J Cardiol 2018;34(8):1059–68.

31. Varricchi G, Galdiero MR, Marone G, et al. Cardiotoxicity of immune checkpoint inhibitors. ESMO Open 2017;2(4):e000247.

32. Tarrio ML, Grabie N, Bu DX, et al. PD-1 protects against inflammation and myocyte damage in T cell-mediated myocarditis. J Immunol 2012;188(10): 4876–84.

33. Nishimura H, Okazaki T, Tanaka Y, et al. Autoimmune dilated cardiomyopathy in PD-1 receptor-deficient mice. Science 2001;291(5502):319–22.

34. Palaskas N, Lopez-Mattei J, Durand JB, et al. Immune checkpoint inhibitor myocarditis: pathophysiological characteristics, diagnosis, and treatment. J Am Heart Assoc 2020;9(2):e013757.

35. Mahmood SS, Fradley MG, Cohen JV, et al. Myocarditis in patients treated with immune checkpoint inhibitors. J Am Coll Cardiol 2018;71(16):1755–64.

36. Choueiri TK, Larkin J, Oya M, et al. Preliminary results for avelumab plus axitinib as first-line therapy in patients with advanced clear-cell renal-cell carcinoma (JAVELIN Renal 100): an open-label, dose-finding and dose-expansion, phase 1b trial. Lancet Oncol 2018;19(4):451–60.

37. Guo CW, Alexander M, Dib Y, et al. A closer look at immune-mediated myocarditis in the era of combined checkpoint blockade and targeted therapies. Eur J Cancer 2020;124:15–24.

38. Escudier M, Cautela J, Malissen N, et al. Clinical features, management, and outcomes of immune checkpoint inhibitor-related cardiotoxicity. Circulation 2017;136(21):2085–7.

39. Bonaca MP, Olenchock BA, Salem JE, et al. Myocarditis in the setting of cancer therapeutics: proposed case definitions for emerging clinical syndromes in cardio-oncology. Circulation 2019;140(2):80–91.

40. Lee Chuy K, Oikonomou EK, Postow MA, et al. Myocarditis surveillance in patients with advanced melanoma on combination immune checkpoint inhibitor therapy: the memorial sloan Kettering Cancer Center experience. Oncologist 2019;24(5):e196–7.

41. Zhang L, Jones-O'Connor M, Awadalla M, et al. Cardiotoxicity of immune checkpoint inhibitors. Curr Treat Options Cardiovasc Med 2019;21(7):32.

42. Johnson DB, Balko JM, Compton ML, et al. Fulminant myocarditis with combination immune checkpoint blockade. N Engl J Med 2016;375(18):1749–55.

43. Johnson DB, Manouchehri A, Haugh AM, et al. Neurologic toxicity associated with immune checkpoint inhibitors: a pharmacovigilance study. J Immunother Cancer 2019;7(1):134.

44. Zimmer L, Goldinger SM, Hofmann L, et al. Neurological, respiratory, musculoskeletal, cardiac and ocular side-effects of anti-PD-1 therapy. Eur J Cancer 2016;60:210–25.

45. Gill C, Rouse S, Jacobson RD. Neurological complications of therapeutic monoclonal antibodies: trends from oncology to rheumatology. Curr Neurol Neurosci Rep 2017;17(10):75.

46. Johnson DB, Chandra S, Sosman JA. Immune checkpoint inhibitor toxicity in 2018. JAMA 2018;320(16):1702–3.

47. Zukas AM, Schiff D. Neurological complications of new chemotherapy agents. Neuro Oncol 2018;20(1):24–36.

48. Liao B, Shroff S, Kamiya-Matsuoka C, et al. Atypical neurological complications of ipilimumab therapy in patients with metastatic melanoma. Neuro Oncol 2014;16(4):589–93.

49. Spain L, Walls G, Julve M, et al. Neurotoxicity from immune-checkpoint inhibition in the treatment of melanoma: a single centre experience and review of the literature. Ann Oncol 2017;28(2):377–85.

50. Laserna A, Tummala S, Patel N, et al. Atezolizumab-related encephalitis in the intensive care unit: case report and review of the literature. SAGE Open Med Case Rep 2018;6. 2050313X18792422.

51. Harrison RA, Tummala S, de Groot J. Neurologic toxicities of cancer immunotherapies: a review. Curr Neurol Neurosci Rep 2020;20(7):27.

52. Cortazar FB, Kibbelaar ZA, Glezerman IG, et al. Clinical features and outcomes of immune checkpoint inhibitor-associated AKI: a multicenter study. J Am Soc Nephrol 2020;31(2):435–46.

53. Menzies AM, Johnson DB, Ramanujam S, et al. Anti-PD-1 therapy in patients with advanced melanoma and preexisting autoimmune disorders or major toxicity with ipilimumab. Ann Oncol 2017;28(2):368–76.

54. June CH, Riddell SR, Schumacher TN. Adoptive cellular therapy: a race to the finish line. Sci Transl Med 2015;7:280.

55. Coiffier B, Thieblemont C, Van Den Neste E, et al. Long-term outcome of patients in the LNH-98.5 trial, the first randomized study comparing rituximab-

CHOP to standard CHOP chemotherapy in DLBCL patients: a study by the Groupe d'Etudes des Lymphomes de l'Adulte. Blood 2010;116:2040–5.

56. Van Den Neste E, Schmitz N, Mounier N, et al. Outcomes of diffuse large B-cell lymphoma patients relapsing after autologous stem cell transplantation: an analysis of patients included in the CORAL study. Bone Marrow Transplant 2017; 52(2):216–21.

57. Nagle SJ, Woo K, Schuster SJ, et al. Outcomes of patients with relapsed/refractory diffuse large B-cell lymphoma with progression of lymphoma after autologous stem cell transplantation in the rituximab era. Am J Hematol 2013;88: 890–4.

58. Locke FL, Neelapu SS, Bartlett, et al. Phase 1 results of ZUMA-1: a multicenter study of KTE-C19 anti-CD19 CAR T cell therapy in refractory aggressive lymphoma. Mol Ther 2017;25:285–95.

59. Locke FL, Neelapu SS, Bartlett NL, et al. Clinical and biologic covariates of outcomes in ZUMA-1: a pivotal trial of axicabtagene ciloleucel (axi-cel; KTE-C19) in patients with refractory aggressive non-Hodgkin lymphoma (r-NHL). J Clin Oncol 2017;35(15_suppl):7512.

60. Schuster SJ, Svoboda J, Chong EA, et al. Chimeric antigen receptor T cells in refractory large B-cell lymphomas. N Engl J Med 2017;377:2545–54.

61. Neelapu SS, Locke FL, Bartlett NL, et al. Axicabtagene ciloleucel CAR T-cell therapy in refractory large B-cell lymphoma. N Engl J Med 2017;377:2531–44.

62. Study of efficacy and safety of CTL019 in pediatric ALL patient (ELIANA) NCT02228096. Available at: https://clinicaltrials.gov/ct2/show/NCT02228096. Accessed February 10, 2020.

63. Safety and efficacy of KTE-C19 in adults with refractory aggressive non-hodgkin lymphoma (ZUMA-1) NCT02445248. Available at: https://clinicaltrials.gov/ct2/show/NCT02348216. Accessed February 10, 2020.

64. Study of efficacy and safety of CTL019 in adult DLBCL patients (JULIET) NCT02445248. Available at: https://clinicaltrials.gov/ct2/show/NCT02445248. Accessed February 10, 2020.

65. Xu XJ, Tang YM. Cytokine release syndrome in cancer immunotherapy with chimeric antigen receptor engineered T cells. Cancer Lett 2014;343:172–8.

66. Teachey DT, Lacey SF, Shaw PA, et al. Identification of predictive biomarkers for cytokine release syndrome after chimeric antigen receptor T- cell therapy for acute lymphoblastic leukemia. Cancer Discov 2016;6(6):664–79.

67. Davila ML, Riviere I, Wang X, et al. Efficacy and toxicity management of 19-29z CAR T cell therapy in B cell acute lymphoblastic leukemia. Sci Transl Med 2014; 6(224):224–5.

68. Santomasso BD, Park JH, Salloum D, et al. Clinical and biological correlates of neurotoxicity associated with CAR T-cell therapy in patients with B-cell acute lymphoblastic leukemia. Cancer Discov 2018;8(8):958–71.

69. Hay KA, Hanafi LA, Li D, et al. Kinetics and biomarkers of severe cytokine release syndrome after CD19 chimeric antigen receptor-modified T-cell therapy. Blood 2017;130(21):2295–306.

70. Maude SL, Frey N, Shaw PA, et al. Chimeric antigen receptor T cell for sustained remissions in leukemia. N Engl J Med 2014;371:1507–17.

71. Lee DW, Kochenderfer JN, Stetler-Stevenson M, et al. T cells expressing CD19 chimeric antigen receptors for acute lymphoblastic leukemia in children and young adults. A phase 1 dose-escalation trial. Lancet 2015;385:517–28.

72. Riegler LL, Jones GP, Lee DW. Current approaches in grading and management of cytokine release syndrome after chimeric antigen receptor T-cell therapy. Ther Clin Risk Manag 2019;15:323–35.

73. Lee DW, Gardner R, Porter DL, et al. Current concepts in the diagnosis and management of cytokine release syndrome. Blood 2014;124(2):188–95.

74. Lee DW, Santomasso BD, Locke FL, et al. ASTCT consensus grading for cytokine release syndrome neurologic toxicity associated with immune effector cells. Biol Blood Marrow Transplant 2019;25:625–38.

75. Brudno JN, Kochenderfer. Toxicities of chimeric antigen receptor T cells: recognition and management. Blood 2016;127(26):3321–30.

76. Gust J, Hay KA, Hanafi LA, et al. Endothelial activation and blood brain barrier disruption in neurotoxicity after adoptive immunotherapy with CD19 CAR-T cells. Cancer Discov 2017;7:1404–19.

77. Gutierrez C, McEvoy C, Mead E, et al. Management of the critically ill adult chimeric antigen receptor-T cell therapy patient: a critical care perspective. Crit Care Med 2018;46(9):1402–10.

78. Park JH, Riviere I, Gonen M, et al. Long-term follow up of CD19 CAR therapy in acute lymphoblastic leukemia. N Engl J Med 2018;378:449–59.

79. Neelapu SS, Tummala S, Kebriaei P, et al. Chimeric antigen receptor T-cell therapy – assessment and management of toxicities. Nat Rev Clin Oncol 2018;15:47–61.

80. Kochenderfer JN, Dudley ME, Feldman SA, et al. B-cell depletion and remission of malignancy along with cytokine-associated toxicity in a clinical trial of anti-CD19 chimeric-antigen-receptor-transduced T cells. Blood 2012;119:2709–20.

81. Rhodes A, Evans LE, Alhazzani W, et al. Surviving sepsis campaign: International guidelines for management of sepsis and septic shock:2016. Intensive Care Med 2017;43:304–77.

82. Rochwerg B, Brochard L, Elliott MW, et al. Official ERS/ATS clinical practice guidelines: noninvasive ventilation for acute respiratory failure. Eur Respir J 2017;50:1602426.

83. Adda M, Coquet I, Darmon M, et al. Predictors of noninvasive ventilation failure in patients with hematologic malignancy and acute respiratory failure. Crit Care Med 2008;36:2766–72.

84. Fan E, Del Sorbo L, Goligher EC, et al. American Thoracic Society, European Society of intensive care medicine, and Society of Critical Care Medicine: an official American Thoracic Society/European Society of Intensive Care Medicine/Society of Critical Care Medicine clinical practice guideline: mechanical ventilation in adult patients with acute respiratory distress syndrome. Am J Respir Crit Care Med 2017;195:1253–63.

85. Nishimoto N, Mima TK, Nakahara H, et al. Mechanisms and pathologic significances in increase in serum interleukin-6 (IL-6), and soluble IL-6 receptor antibody, tocilizumab, in patients with rheumatoid arthritis and castleman disease. Blood 2008;112(10):3959–64.

86. Giavridis T, Van der Stegen SJC, Eyquem J, et al. CAR T cell-induced cytokine release syndrome is mediated by macrophages and abated by IL-1 blockade. Nat Med 2018;24:731–8.

87. Norelli M, Camisa B, Barbiera G, et al. Monocyte-derived IL-1 and IL-6 are differentially required for cytokine-release syndrome and neurotoxicity due to CAR T cells. Nat Med 2018;24:739–48.

88. Grupp SA, Kalos M, Barrett D, et al. Chimeric antigen receptor-modified T cells for acute lymphoid leukemia. N Engl J Med 2013;368(16):1509–18.

89. Cardinale D, Stivala F, Cipolla CM. Oncologic therapies associated with cardiac toxicities: how to minimize risks. Expert Rev Anticancer Ther 2019;19(5):359–74.

90. Cardinale D, Colombo A, Lamantia G, et al. Anthracycline-induced cardiomyopathy: clinical relevance and response to pharmacologic therapy. J Am Coll Cardiol 2010;55(3):213–20.

91. Slamon DJ, Leyland-Jones B, Shak S, et al. Use of chemotherapy plus a monoclonal antibody against HER2 for metastatic breast cancer that overexpresses HER2. N Engl J Med 2001;344(11):783–92.

92. Yeh ETH, Ewer MS, Moslehi J, et al. Mechanisms and clinical course of cardiovascular toxicity of cancer treatment. Oncology. Semin Oncol 2019;46(6): 397–402.

93. Bair SM, Choueiri TK, Moslehi J. Cardiovascular complications associated with novel angiogenesis inhibitors: emerging evidence and evolving perspectives. Trends Cardiovasc Med 2013;23(4):104–13.

94. Guha A, Armanious M, Fradley MG. Update on cardio-oncology: novel cancer therapeutics and associated cardiotoxicities. Trends Cardiovasc Med 2019; 29(1):29–39.

95. Christenson ES, James T, Agrawal V, et al. Use of biomarkers for the assessment of chemotherapy-induced cardiac toxicity. Clin Biochem 2015;48(4–5):223–35.

96. Cypen J, Ahmad T, Testani JM, et al. Novel biomarkers for the risk stratification of heart failure with preserved ejection fraction. Curr Heart Fail Rep 2017;14(5): 434–43.

97. Zamorano JL, Lancellotti P, Rodriguez Munoz D, et al. 2016 ESC Position Paper on cancer treatments and cardiovascular toxicity developed under the auspices of the ESC Committee for Practice Guidelines: The Task Force for cancer treatments and cardiovascular toxicity of the European Society of Cardiology (ESC). Eur Heart J 2016;37(36):2768–801.

98. Plana JC, Galderisi M, Barac A, et al. Expert consensus for multimodality imaging evaluation of adult patients during and after cancer therapy: a report from the American Society of Echocardiography and the European Association of Cardiovascular Imaging. Am Soc Echocardiogr 2014;27(9):911–39.

99. Thavendiranathan P, Poulin F, Lim KD, et al. Use of myocardial strain imaging by echocardiography for the early detection of cardiotoxicity in patients during and after cancer chemotherapy: a systematic review. J Am Coll Cardiol 2014;63(25 Pt A):2751–68.

100. Bloom MW, Hamo CE, Cardinale D, et al. Cancer therapy-related cardiac dysfunction and heart failure: Part 1: definitions, pathophysiology, risk factors, and imaging. Circ Heart Fail 2016;9(1):e002661.

101. Agha A, Zarifa A, Kim P, et al. The role of cardiovascular imaging and serum biomarkers in identifying cardiotoxicity related to cancer therapeutics. Methodist Debakey Cardiovasc J 2019;15(4):258–66.

102. Hasinoff BB, Patel D, Wu X. The role of topoisomerase IIβ in the mechanisms of action of the doxorubicin cardioprotective agent dexrazoxane. Cardiovasc Toxicol 2019;20(3):312–20.

103. Chang HM, Moudgil R, Scarabelli T, et al. Cardiovascular complications of cancer therapy: best practices in diagnosis, prevention, and management: Part 1. J Am Coll Cardiol 2017;70(20):2536–51.

104. Hamo CE, Bloom MW, Cardinale D, et al. Cancer therapy-related cardiac dysfunction and heart failure: Part 2: prevention, treatment, guidelines, and future directions. Circ Heart Fail 2016;9(2):e002843.

Infectious Disease Complications in Patients with Cancer

Susan K. Seo, MD[a,b,*], Catherine Liu, MD[c,d],
Sanjeet S. Dadwal, MD[e]

KEYWORDS

• Infection • Cancer • Immunocompromised • Neutropenia • Sepsis • Critical care

KEY POINTS

• Infection remains a significant cause of morbidity and mortality in critically ill patients with cancer.
• Neutropenia is an important risk factor for infection in patients with cancer.
• Respiratory infections are the leading cause of infection in patients with cancer admitted to the intensive care unit.

Critically ill patients with cancer requiring intensive care unit (ICU) stay are vulnerable to infection because of a variety of factors, including local tumor effects, complex cancer treatments, disruption of physical barriers, neutropenia, humoral and/or cellular dysfunction, asplenia, and presence of foreign devices. Recognizing that patients with cancer can have multiple immune defects concurrently is critical because it affects diagnostic and therapeutic decision making. This article describes common infectious complications that critical care teams may encounter while caring for patients with cancer.

FEVER AND NEUTROPENIA

Febrile, neutropenic patients, particularly those with severe neutropenia for more than 7 days, are at risk for progression to sepsis.[1] The model that is widely used to identify

Funding: This work was funded in part by the National Institute of Health/National Cancer Institute (NIH/NCI) Cancer Center Support Grant P30 CA008748 (SKS) and the NIH/NCI Cancer Center Support Grant P30 CA15704 (CL).
[a] Infectious Disease Service, Department of Medicine, Memorial Sloan Kettering Cancer Center, 1275 York Avenue, New York, NY 10065, USA; [b] Department of Medicine, Weill Cornell Medical College, New York, NY, USA; [c] Vaccine and Infectious Disease Division, Fred Hutchison Cancer Research Center, 1100 Fairview Avenue North, Seattle, WA 98109, USA; [d] Department of Medicine, University of Washington, Seattle, WA, USA; [e] Division of Infectious Diseases, Department of Medicine, City of Hope National Medical Center, 1500 East Duarte Road, Duarte, CA 91010, USA
* Corresponding author. 1275 York Avenue, New York, NY 10065.
E-mail address: seos@mskcc.org

neutropenic patients at low versus high risk for complications is the Multinational Association for Supportive Care in Cancer risk score. The rate of septic shock associated with fever and neutropenia (FN) ranges between 3.2% and 13.4% across centers.[2] With heightened recognition and improved supportive care, survival of neutropenic patients with severe sepsis or septic shock may be improving over time.[3] One challenge is distinguishing noninfectious mimics such as adrenal insufficiency and the cytokine release storm associated with receipt of chimeric antigen receptor T cells.[4]

Diagnosis and Management

It is important to remember that neutropenic patients have attenuated signs and symptoms of infection. A thorough history and physical examination, including inspection of catheter sites, perirectal region, and the skin, are the bedrock of diagnostic evaluation. Initial evaluation also includes chest imaging for patients with respiratory symptoms, at least 2 sets of blood cultures (peripheral and catheter), and cultures of other sites as defined by the clinical presentation.[1] Prompt institution of empiric broad-spectrum antimicrobials (eg, cefepime, piperacillin/tazobactam, carbapenem) is merited to prevent progression to sepsis. Upfront vancomycin use is not necessary unless there is suspected central venous catheter (CVC) infection, skin and soft tissue infection (SSTI), severe pneumonia, or hemodynamic instability. Modifications to the initial antibiotic regimen should be guided by clinical and microbiological data. Patients who remain hemodynamically unstable despite standard FN therapy should have their antimicrobial regimens broadened to include coverage for possible resistant bacteria and/or fungi.

CATHETER-RELATED BLOODSTREAM INFECTIONS

CVCs currently account for ~25% of all bloodstream infections (BSIs) among oncology patients.[5] The most common causes include gram-positive (GP) organisms such as coagulase-negative staphylococci (CoNS), *Staphylococcus aureus*, and *Enterococcus faecium*, but with gram-negative (GN) bacteria such as *Escherichia coli*, *Klebsiella* spp, and *Pseudomonas aeruginosa* also playing an important role. Recently, data suggested an epidemiologic shift among oncology patients toward a GN predominance, which may be attributable to infection prevention strategies primarily targeting GP organisms, including chlorhexidine for insertion site cleaning and use of antimicrobial-impregnated CVCs.[5]

Pathogenesis

The most common source of catheter-related bloodstream infections (CRBSIs) is colonization of the catheter by the patient's own skin flora or contamination of the catheter hub during line insertion or manipulation. Less commonly, CRBSIs are caused by hematogenous seeding of the device from another site or, rarely, by contamination of the infusate. Because colonizing organisms can establish themselves in the catheter's biofilm within 48 to 72 hours after insertion, they can be difficult to eradicate and can cause recurrent infection.

Diagnosis and Management

CRBSIs are defined when simultaneously drawn blood cultures reveal a 3-fold greater number of colonies of the same organism from the CVC than the peripherally drawn culture, or when the CVC-drawn culture turns positive for the same organism at least 2 hours earlier than the peripherally drawn culture, or when the same organism is cultured from blood and the catheter tip.[6] Once the CVC is determined to be the source, management varies by pathogen. Vancomycin is typically used as empiric therapy for GP bacteria.

Empiric therapy for GN pathogens relies on the local antibiogram and severity of disease and should include antipseudomonal coverage for neutropenic patients.

For CoNS BSI, CVC removal and antibiotic treatment for 5 to 7 days are recommended for patients with short-term CVCs.[6] For those with long-term CVCs, catheter retention may be appropriate if clinically stable and without evidence of persistent or relapsed bacteremia. Although the usual antibiotic course is 10 to 14 days, some experts suggest that 5 to 7 days is adequate for uncomplicated cases.[7]

In contrast with CoNS, *S aureus* BSI is often associated with complications (eg, septic phlebitis, endocarditis).[8] Diagnostic work-up includes echocardiography. A minimum 14-day treatment course is recommended for patients with *S aureus* CRBSI, with a longer duration (4–6 weeks) if there is evidence for metastatic sites of infection.[6] Because of high relapse rates, early CVC removal is strongly recommended for patients with both short-term and long-term CVCs.

For candidemia, initial empiric therapy is an echinocandin, and the minimum duration of treatment without metastatic complications is 2 weeks after blood culture clearance.[9] For nonneutropenic patients, early CVC removal is recommended because the source is usually catheter related. For neutropenic patients and those with mucosal barrier injury, it is more difficult to determine the role of the gastrointestinal (GI) tract versus the CVC as the primary source of candidemia. An individualized approach is suggested when considering CVC removal in these patients. One exception is *Candida parapsilosis*, for which CVC removal should always be performed.

In patients with GN CRBSIs associated with persistent bacteremia or severe sepsis, the CVC should be removed.[6] In a study of 300 patients with cancer, CVC removal within 2 days of onset of GN CRBSI was associated with improved microbiological response and decreased mortality.[10] Notably, these findings were not observed for GN BSIs that did not meet criteria for CRBSI or for CRBSI associated with mucosal barrier injury. Antibiotic de-escalation is recommended once culture and susceptibility results are available, and treatment duration is usually 7 to 14 days.[6]

RESPIRATORY INFECTIONS

Pneumonia remains a major cause of morbidity and mortality in critically ill patients with cancer. The challenge for clinicians is that the differential diagnosis for pulmonary infiltrates in oncologic patients includes not just lower respiratory tract infections but also noninfectious causes (eg, cancer progression, diffuse alveolar hemorrhage, drug or radiation toxicity, malignant airway obstruction, pulmonary edema, venous thromboembolic disease), with presenting signs and symptoms ranging from mild dyspnea to rapidly progressive respiratory failure.[11] In many instances, there can be more than 1 lung-related problem at the same time.

Pathogenesis and Host Factors

The pathogenesis of cancer-associated pneumonia has been well described.[12] Host susceptibility factors for pneumonia include general debility, malignancy-related catabolism, preexisting lung disease, functional or anatomic defects, epithelial barrier disruption, and immune system derangements.[12] Neutropenia is the most significant risk factor.[13] Other immune system derangements are associated with infections by specific pathogens (**Table 1**).

Diagnosis and Management

Computed tomography (CT) chest imaging is more sensitive than plain radiography in the detection and characterization of pneumonia, and the description of the radiologic

Table 1
Respiratory pathogens causing pulmonary infiltrates in critically ill patients with cancer

Organism	Epidemiologic Clues	Immune Defect Predisposing to Infection
GP Bacteria		
Nocardia spp	Prolonged corticosteroids	Cell mediated
Rhodococcus equi	Zoonotic exposure (horse farms, race tracks)	Cell mediated
S aureus, including methicillin-resistant strains	Agent of CAP and HAP/VAP	—
Streptococcus pneumoniae	Most common bacterial agent of CAP	Humoral
Streptococcus pyogenes	Agent of CAP	—
Enterococcus spp, including vancomycin-resistant strains	Agent of HAP/VAP	—
GN Bacteria		
Acinetobacter baumannii complex[a]	Agent of HAP/VAP	—
Citrobacter spp	Agent of HAP/VAP	—
Enterobacter spp	Agent of HAP/VAP	—
Escherichia coli[a]	Agent of CAP and HAP/VAP	—
Haemophilus influenzae	Agent of CAP	Humoral
Klebsiella spp[a]	Agent of CAP and HAP/VAP	—
Moraxella catarrhalis	Agent of CAP	—
Proteus spp	Agent of HAP/VAP	—
P aeruginosa[a]	Agent of HAP/VAP; structural lung disease (bronchiectasis)	Neutropenia
Serratia marcescens	Agent of HAP/VAP	—
Stenotrophomonas maltophilia[a]	Agent of HAP/VAP	—
Atypical Bacteria		
Chlamydia pneumoniae	Agent of CAP	—
Chlamydia psittaci	Zoonotic exposure (birds)	—
Coxiella burnetii	Zoonotic exposure (abattoir workers, farm animals)	—
Legionella spp	Agent of CAP and HAP (contaminated hospital water supply)	Cell mediated
Mycoplasma pneumoniae	Agent of CAP	—
Anaerobes	Alcoholism; aspiration; endobronchial obstruction; poor dental hygiene	—

(continued on next page)

Table 1
(continued)

Organism	Epidemiologic Clues	Immune Defect Predisposing to Infection
Mycobacteria		
Atypical mycobacteria	Receipt of tumor necrosis factor inhibitors (infliximab)	Cell mediated; intrinsic/ acquired defects of the Th1 cell and macrophage pathway
Mycobacterium tuberculosis	Alcoholism; hematologic malignancy or head and neck cancer; HIV infection; malnutrition; receipt of Bruton tyrosine kinase inhibitor (ibrutinib), corticosteroids, or tumor necrosis factor inhibitors	—
Fungi		
Aspergillus spp	GVHD; prolonged neutropenia; receipt of Bruton tyrosine kinase inhibitor or corticosteroids	Neutropenia; cell mediated
Blastomyces dermatitidis	Endemic mycosis (exposure to moist soils and in wooded areas along waterways and swamps in North America)	Cell mediated
Coccidioides immitis	Endemic mycosis (southwestern United States)	Cell mediated
Cryptococcus spp	Exposure to pigeon or chicken droppings	Cell mediated
Dematiaceous molds	Exposure to soil and decaying vegetation	—
Fusarium spp	GVHD; prolonged neutropenia; receipt of Bruton tyrosine kinase inhibitor	Neutropenia; cell mediated
Histoplasma capsulatum	Endemic mycosis (Ohio and Mississippi River valleys or Central America); exposure to bird or bat droppings; receipt of Bruton tyrosine kinase inhibitor	Cell mediated
Mucor spp (and other agents of mucormycosis)	Diabetes; GVHD; iron overload; receipt of Bruton tyrosine kinase inhibitor or corticosteroids	Neutropenia; cell mediated
Pneumocystis jiroveci	HSCT recipient; receipt of anti-CD52 monoclonal antibody (alemtuzumab), anti-CD20 antibody (rituximab), Bruton tyrosine kinase inhibitor, corticosteroids, oral alkylating agents (temozolomide), purine analogues (fludarabine), or tumor necrosis factor inhibitors	Cell mediated

(continued on next page)

		Immune Defect Predisposing to
Table 1 *(continued)*		
Organism	**Epidemiologic Clues**	**Infection**
Parasites		
Strongyloides stercoralis	Exposure to soil contaminated with human feces (coal miners); previous residence in tropical or subtropical regions (immigrants, military personnel, travelers); residence in southeastern United States	Cell mediated
Respiratory viruses	Frequent agents of CAP; seasonal variation	—
Adenovirus	—	—
Bocavirus	—	—
Coronavirus	—	—
SARS-CoV-2	Cause of pandemic in 2020	—
Human metapneumovirus	—	—
Influenza A and B	—	—
Parainfluenza Respiratory syncytial virus	Association with postinfectious complications (eg, air-flow obstruction or bronchiolitis obliterans) in HSCT recipients	— Humoral, cell-mediated
Rhinovirus	—	—
Other Viruses		
Cytomegalovirus	GVHD; HSCT recipient; receipt of corticosteroids	Cell mediated

Abbreviations: CAP, community-acquired pneumonia; GVHD, graft-versus-host disease; HAP, hospital-acquired pneumonia; HIV, human immunodeficiency virus; HSCT, hematopoietic stem cell transplant; MDR, multidrug resistant; SARS-CoV-2, severe acute respiratory syndrome coronavirus 2; Th1, T-helper 1; VAP, ventilator-associated pneumonia.
   [a] Includes MDR strains.

pattern of lung infiltration may focus the differential diagnosis to likely causal agents.[12–14] However, CT patterns are nonspecific, particularly in neutropenic patients, and cannot be solely relied on for diagnosis.[12]

In patients from whom high-quality sputum samples cannot be obtained, flexible bronchoscopy with bronchoalveolar lavage is the diagnostic procedure of choice.[12] The pace and severity of pneumonia may determine whether there is time to wait for response to initial therapy or whether to pursue a diagnostic procedure immediately. Molecular diagnostics for the rapid identification of respiratory pathogens, including not only bacteria but also mycobacteria, fungi, and viruses, have been a major advance in recent years.[15] The evidence for using procalcitonin-guided algorithms for critically ill patients with cancer with bacterial pneumonia is limited. The selection of appropriate therapy, dose, duration, and monitoring should be personalized to the patient with cancer based on cause, risk for multidrug-resistant (MDR) pathogens, and other factors.

Microbiological Spectrum

Bacterial pneumonias

Bacteria remain the most common causal agents for pneumonia in patients with cancer. The type of bacterial pneumonia depends on the underlying immune deficit and its duration, as well as whether the infection is community acquired or nosocomial.[14]

Recent studies suggest that community-acquired pneumonia (CAP) in immunocompromised patients generally involves the same pathogens seen in immunocompetent hosts.[16,17] Certain epidemiologic exposures or risk factors increase the likelihood of infection with a particular pathogen (see **Table 1**). *P aeruginosa* deserves special mention because it is known to cause serious infections in neutropenic patients.[13] In addition, secondary bacterial pneumonias following influenza or other respiratory viral infections occur frequently, with *S aureus* and *Streptococcus pneumoniae* being the most commonly isolated organisms, followed by *Haemophilus influenzae* and *Streptococcus pyogenes*.

Causal agents for hospital-acquired pneumonia (HAP)/ventilator-associated pneumonia (VAP) include the ESKAPE pathogens (ie, *E faecium*, *S aureus*, *Klebsiella* spp, *Acinetobacter* spp, *P aeruginosa*, and *Enterobacter* spp) and are frequently MDR (see **Table 1**).[18] Additional pathogens to be considered are *Citrobacter* spp, *E coli*, *Proteus* spp, *Serratia marcescens*, and *Stenotrophomonas maltophilia*. Because MDR rates vary by hospital, ICU, and other factors, the need for routine surveillance is emphasized.

A spotlight on some notable pathogens follows. *S maltophilia* colonization and infection in patients with cancer has been increasingly reported. HAP/VAP caused by this organism tends to occur in patients with extended ICU stay, tracheostomy, prolonged (>7 days) mechanical ventilation, or exposure to broad-spectrum antibiotics.[19] In general, the clinical and radiographic presentations are similar to those seen with other infectious causes of HAP/VAP, but a syndrome of rapidly progressive and fatal hemorrhagic pneumonia caused by *S maltophilia* has been described in patients with hematologic malignancies (HM) and hematopoietic stem cell transplant (HSCT) recipients.[20] Trimethoprim-sulfamethoxazole is the most reliable in vitro agent, but emerging resistance has been reported.[19]

HAP caused by *Legionella* spp can occur at centers where the organism is present in the hospital water supply or where there is ongoing construction.[18] Although *L pneumophila* serotype 1 is the most commonly recognized species, several non-*pneumophila Legionella* types (*Legionella jordanis*, *Legionella micdadei*) can cause pulmonary infections in severely immunocompromised hosts.[21,22]

Nocardia spp is well recognized to cause focal or systemic infection in patients with impaired cell-mediated immunity. Common infecting species include *Nocardia abscessus*, *Nocardia cyriacigeorgica*, *Nocardia farcinica*, and *Nocardia nova*.[23] The lung is the primary site of infection in most cases, but a search for sites of dissemination, including the brain, should be pursued because it affects treatment duration.[24] Because *Nocardia* spp can have markedly different susceptibility patterns, it is important to send the recovered isolate for formal identification and sensitivity testing to guide therapy.

Mycobacterial infections

Pulmonary tuberculosis (TB) usually represents reactivation of latent infection. Patients with HM, particularly foreign-born individuals, and patients with head and neck cancer have disproportionately higher TB rates compared with the general US population.[25] Thus, TB should be considered in these patients with pulmonary infiltrates. Atypical mycobacterial pulmonary infections have also been described in patients with cancer, who are typically older, have solid tumors, and have underlying lung disease.[26]

Fungal infections

Pneumocystis jiroveci has long been recognized to be an important opportunistic and potentially life-threatening pulmonary pathogen in patients with cancer.[27] Risk factors include prolonged corticosteroid use, receipt of immunosuppressive therapy affecting cell-mediated immunity, and HSCT. High suspicion is needed in patients presenting with fever; dry cough; hypoxemia at rest or exertion; and diffuse, bilateral interstitial infiltrates. Bronchoscopy should be pursued for diagnosis. The serum (1,3)-β-D-glucan (BDG) is an adjunctive diagnostic test and cannot be used solely to diagnose *P jiroveci* pneumonitis (PJP) because it is nonspecific, but a negative BDG result essentially rules out PJP because of its excellent negative predictive value.[28]

Prolonged and severe neutropenia is a risk factor for invasive pulmonary aspergillosis, which is mitigated by mold-active azole prophylaxis in the highest-risk patient groups (eg, acute leukemia, allogeneic HSCT).[29,30] Breakthrough mucormycosis infections in patients already taking voriconazole and with new pulmonary findings should be entertained.[31] The differential diagnosis for lung nodules should also include *Cryptococcus* spp, endemic fungi (*Blastomyces*, *Coccidioides*, *Histoplasma*), *Fusarium* spp, and *Geotrichum* spp; epidemiologic clues may provide guidance as to their likelihood (see **Table 1**).[14] Dematiaceous molds, such as *Alternaria* spp and *Cladosporium* spp are increasingly implicated as causes of lung infections in leukemic and transplant patients and pose therapeutic challenges because of variable susceptibilities to the available antifungal agents.

Viral infections

Respiratory viruses are frequent agents of CAP and have seasonal variation (see **Table 1**).[32] Clinical presentations can range from asymptomatic shedding to acute respiratory distress, and providers should be vigilant for signs and symptoms of pulmonary bacterial superinfection.

Cytomegalovirus (CMV) pneumonitis, usually with concomitant viremia, can occur in allogeneic HSCT recipients and patients with HM who have received chemotherapeutic drugs such as alemtuzumab, rituximab, and fludarabine.[33] To a far lesser extent, patients with solid tumors can also reactivate CMV if exposed to T cell–suppressing therapy such as high-dose corticosteroids.[34] Definitive diagnosis requires the presence of CMV inclusion bodies and/or CMV viral antigens in lung tissue.

Severe acute respiratory syndrome coronavirus 2 (SARS-CoV-2) is a novel coronavirus that has resulted in a worldwide pandemic in 2020, with pneumonia being the most frequent serious manifestation of infection. Patients with cancer with SARS-CoV-2 have a higher risk for severe events, including ICU admission, invasive ventilation, and death, compared with patients infected with SARS-CoV-2 but without cancer.[35]

Parasitic infections

Strongyloides stercoralis is an intestinal nematode that can cause hyperinfection and disseminated disease in highly immunocompromised patients.[36] Suspicion should be increased in individuals who have previously resided in tropical and subtropical endemic regions (eg, immigrants, military personnel). The migration of filariform larvae during autoinfection can facilitate bacterial translocation from the GI tract, leading to pneumonia, meningitis, or sepsis. Acute respiratory distress syndrome can occur during severe disease along with multiorgan failure. Mortality is high even with treatment.

GASTROINTESTINAL INFECTIONS
Infections in Solid Tumors

Patients with solid tumors usually present with infections that result as a sequela of tumor obstruction (eg, cholangitis, intra-abdominal abscesses) or, in some cases, complications from GI surgery. Management of these infections often requires antibiotic therapy in combination with source control (eg, percutaneous drainage, surgical washout).

Neutropenic Enterocolitis

Neutropenic enterocolitis (NEC) or typhlitis is a life-threatening chemotherapy-associated complication that occurs most commonly among patients with acute leukemia but has also been observed among other HM patients and those receiving high-dose chemotherapy for solid tumors.[37] The pathogenesis is thought to involve a combination of mucosal injury from cytotoxic drugs, profound neutropenia, and impaired host defenses leading to inflammatory, hemorrhagic, and/or necrotizing involvement of the lower intestinal tract. The incidence ranges from 0.8% to 26%. A recent study of critically ill patients with NEC reports ICU and hospital mortalities of 32% and 39%, respectively.[38]

Common features include fever, diarrhea, abdominal pain, mucositis, nausea, and vomiting, but GI bleeding or obstruction can also be seen.[37] The diagnostic criteria include neutropenia, bowel wall thickening on CT imaging, and exclusion of other diagnoses such as *Clostridioides difficile*. Management of NEC includes bowel rest, nasogastric suction, intravenous (IV) fluids, nutritional and blood product support, as well as broad-spectrum antimicrobial therapy. Surgical intervention is reserved for patients with bowel perforation, persistent GI bleeding despite correction of coagulopathies and thrombocytopenia, or clinical deterioration despite optimal medical management.

Hepatosplenic Candidiasis

Hepatosplenic candidiasis (HC) is primarily observed among patients with acute leukemia, but it is seen less frequently now in the era of antifungal prophylaxis. This condition is thought to result from bloodstream invasion of *Candida* from the GI tract, with the portal system receiving the largest inoculum.[39] The clinical presentation includes high persistent fevers accompanied by right upper quadrant pain, nausea, and vomiting in a previously neutropenic patient who has recently experienced count recovery. An elevated serum alkaline phosphatase can be seen, and abdominal CT or magnetic resonance imaging (MRI) typically shows multiple hypodense lesions in the liver, spleen, and sometimes the kidneys. Because of emerging fluconazole resistance, initial therapy should include an echinocandin for several weeks followed by stepdown therapy to an oral azole after evidence of clinical improvement.[9] Treatment continues until there is radiographic resolution.

Infectious Diarrhea

Patients with cancer are at increased risk for *C difficile* infection (CDI) because of frequent and prolonged hospitalizations, immunosuppression, and exposure to factors that alter the gut microbiota. At the same time, the diagnosis of CDI is challenging because diarrhea is a frequent complication of chemotherapy, transplant-related GI complications, and novel immunotherapies. In addition, the nucleic acid amplification tests (NAATs) that are commonly used for CDI diagnosis do not distinguish between colonization and true infection. Hospital-onset CDI rates have been reported to be higher at cancer centers and may in part be driven by the increased frequency of testing in the context of a high prevalence of diarrhea.[40,41] First-line treatment is oral vancomycin or fidaxomicin.[42] Among patients with fulminant CDI, oral vancomycin combined with IV metronidazole is recommended. If ileus is present, vancomycin can also be administered per rectum. Surgical indications include bowel perforation, septic shock, and associated organ failure.

Community-acquired diarrhea caused by *Salmonella*, *Shigella*, *Yersinia*, and *Campylobacter* is uncommon in patients with cancer. In contrast, norovirus is an important cause of viral gastroenteritis and has been associated with outbreaks in hematology/transplant units and with reported mortality up to 25% in allogeneic HSCT recipients.[43] Supportive care is the mainstay of treatment. Colitis caused by adenovirus can be life threatening among patients with impaired cellular immunity. Cidofovir is the only antiviral option and may be considered in severely ill patients, although close monitoring is needed because of the risk of nephrotoxicity.[44] CMV colitis has been described in allogeneic HSCT recipients and is managed with IV ganciclovir with transition to oral valganciclovir as the colitis resolves.[45] Foscarnet is an alternative if there is concern for ganciclovir-related myelosuppression, but careful monitoring of renal function and electrolytes is needed.

CENTRAL NERVOUS SYSTEM INFECTIONS

A small subset of patients with cancer is at risk for central nervous system (CNS) infections. Patients with primary or secondary brain tumors who have had neurosurgical procedures, including placement of shunts or Ommaya reservoirs, are at risk because of barrier disruption, decreased cellular immunity from corticosteroids, and poor wound healing following corticosteroid and radiation therapy.[46] Patients with deficient humoral immunity or with functional or anatomic asplenia are at risk for meningitis caused by encapsulated bacteria (eg, *S pneumoniae*, *H influenzae*), and those with T-cell defects are vulnerable to opportunistic infections encompassing a wide variety of bacterial, fungal, viral, and parasitic pathogens. For patients anticipating receipt of cytotoxic chemotherapy or HSCT, the risk for CNS infections in the current era is probably lessened by screening and/or antimicrobial prophylaxis.

Diagnostic Approach

Although CT is faster, MRI of the brain can better distinguish among tumor, infection, and radiation effects.[46] After ruling out increased intracranial pressure, lumbar puncture should ideally be performed. Although limitations exist, rapid diagnostics can improve the ability to identify the causal agent. One example is the US Food and Drug Administration (FDA)–approved multiplex NAAT that detects 14 bacterial, viral, and fungal pathogens of community-acquired meningitis and encephalitis.[47]

Clinical Presentation

Meningitis/encephalitis

Meningitis is classically associated with the sudden onset of fever, headache, and nuchal rigidity, whereas encephalitis is distinguished by abnormalities of brain function.[46] The distinction between the two can be frequently blurred because patients can have features of both (meningoencephalitis). Seizures are common with encephalitis and can be detected by electroencephalography.

The cerebrospinal fluid inflammatory response can be muted in patients with cancer.[48] One study showed that most infections occurred in patients with prior neurosurgery and, not surprisingly, bacteria typically associated with device-related infections, including CoNS, *S aureus*, *Propionibacterium acnes*, and *Corynebacterium jeikeium*, were well represented in this series.[48] In contrast, agents usually associated with community-acquired meningitis were uncommon. Nevertheless, the data do not negate the fact that meningitis is a medical emergency and warrants timely empiric antibiotics in patients with cancer suspected to have this diagnosis. Empiric antibacterial regimens for community-associated and health care–associated meningitis are extensively reviewed elsewhere.[49,50] One key consideration is to include an antibiotic with activity against *Listeria* as part of the empiric regimen for meningitis in immunosuppressed patients. For recent neurosurgical patients, IV vancomycin should be combined with a third-generation or fourth-generation cephalosporin (eg, ceftazidime, cefepime) or a carbapenem.

Viruses are common agents of infectious encephalitis. In 1 recent study, causes of viral encephalitis in allogeneic HSCT recipients included human herpesvirus 6 (HHV6), Epstein-Barr virus, herpes simplex virus (HSV), JC virus, varicella zoster virus (VZV), CMV, and adenovirus.[51] Certain examination or imaging features may point to a diagnosis. Flaccid paralysis during the summer may suggest the possibility of West Nile virus infection; temporal lobe involvement is strongly suggestive of HSV; and grouped vesicles in a dermatomal pattern may suggest VZV, although the absence of a rash does not rule out VZV from consideration. VZV can also be associated with isolated facial palsy, other cranial neuropathies, vasculopathy, and myelitis; imaging may show enhancement of affected nerve roots.[46] There are no specific therapies for most CNS viral infections, with the exceptions being high-dose acyclovir for HSV and VZV and ganciclovir or foscarnet for CMV and HHV6.

Focal brain lesions

Focal mass lesions include polymicrobial bacterial abscess, nocardiosis, toxoplasmosis, and invasive fungal infections.[46] In 1 study of autologous and allogeneic HSCT recipients at a tertiary cancer center, the incidence of CNS infections was 4.2% (15 out of 361), with cerebral toxoplasmosis and fungal infections being the leading causes.[52] Toxoplasmosis, which has also been described in patients with Hodgkin lymphoma and other HM, represents reactivation of latent disease and can be fatal if untreated. The most commonly used regimen is the combination of pyrimethamine with sulfadiazine and folinic acid.

Fungal brain abscesses can present with a focal neurologic abnormality, headache, and/or seizure caused by the local destruction or compression of adjacent brain tissue with or without angioinvasion.[53] Clinically relevant pathogens include yeasts (eg, *Candida*, *Cryptococcus*), molds (eg, *Aspergillus*, *Rhizopus*, *Mucor*, *Pseudallescheria*, *Fusarium*), and dimorphic fungi (eg, *Histoplasma*, *Coccidioides*). Definitive diagnosis requires tissue biopsy for histopathologic examination and culture. Amphotericin B and its lipid formulations as well as the azoles (eg, fluconazole, voriconazole, posaconazole) are the 2 primary antifungal classes used to treat CNS fungal infections, but their attendant toxicities can make therapy challenging, particularly when treatment lasts months.[46,53]

URINARY TRACT INFECTIONS
Infections Associated with Urinary Diversion

Radical cystectomy (RC) with urinary diversion (eg, continent cutaneous diversion, ileal conduit, orthotopic neobladder) is an important urologic procedure, but urinary tract infections (UTIs) can occur when there is incomplete voluntary voiding or when bacteria are introduced into the reservoir via suboptimal catheterization practices.[54]

Approximately 20% of these infections are associated with sepsis. Diabetes, perioperative blood transfusion, continent diversion, and urine leak correlate with UTI risk following RC.[55] E coli, Enterococcus spp, Klebsiella spp, and S aureus are the most frequently recovered bacteria.[54,55]

Infections Associated with Ureteral Stents or Percutaneous Nephrostomy Tubes

Obstructive uropathy is frequent in patients with advanced solid tumors, primarily prostate, retroperitoneal, or pelvic tumors, and is managed by placing ureteral stents or percutaneous nephrostomy tubes (PNTs).[11] However, complicated UTIs are common. At 1 tertiary cancer center, the rate of PNT-associated pyelonephritis was 19% (38 out of 200), with risk factors being prior UTI and neutropenia.[56]

Pathogenesis

The pathogenesis of implant-associated UTIs starts with bacterial adhesion onto the indwelling implant surfaces and subsequent biofilm formation.[57] Many uropathogens are capable of making biofilms, and these include E coli, Enterococcus faecalis, P aeruginosa, P mirabilis, S aureus, and Candida spp. The likelihood of bacterial colonization is higher as the duration of implant retention increases. Because indwelling stents can be associated with vesicoureteral reflux of urine, this facilitates retrograde ascension of bacteria into the kidney, leading to pyelonephritis. The entry of bacteria from the renal parenchyma into the renal circulatory system can lead to bacteremia, sepsis, septic shock, and/or renal failure.

Clinical presentation and management

Pyelonephritis is defined by the presence of greater than or equal to 10^5 colony-forming units per milliliter of a uropathogen in the urine accompanied by symptoms (eg, fever, chills, nausea, vomiting, costovertebral angle tenderness, flank pain).[57] Patients with cancer who also have diabetes may be at risk for emphysematous pyelonephritis and papillary necrosis. CT of the abdomen and pelvis is generally reserved for patients who are severely ill, have persistent symptoms despite greater than or equal to 48 hours of appropriate antimicrobial therapy, or have suspected urinary tract obstruction. The approach to empiric antibiotic therapy for hospitalized patients depends in part on the risk for infection with MDR bacteria. For septic patients requiring ICU care, a conservative approach is to combine a carbapenem for coverage of extended-spectrum beta-lactamase–producing organisms and P aeruginosa, as well as IV vancomycin for methicillin-resistant S aureus coverage, until urine and blood culture results are available.[58]

SKIN AND SOFT TISSUE INFECTIONS

SSTIs range from mild (eg, impetigo) to life threatening (eg, necrotizing fasciitis). For immunocompromised patients, the broad differential diagnosis includes drug eruptions, tumor infiltration of the skin and soft tissue, reaction to chemotherapy or radiation therapy, graft-versus-host disease, Sweet syndrome, erythema multiforme, and leukocytoclastic vasculitis.[59] Dermatologic evaluation, including biopsy of skin lesions, is usually warranted. The principal portal of entry is a breach in skin integrity, with S aureus and streptococci largely responsible for SSTI in general. Careful history should be obtained to consider unusual organisms potentially associated with specific exposures (eg, shellfish ingestion and Vibrio vulnificus). In patients with impaired cellular immunity, HSV or VZV reactivation with possible secondary bacterial infection can occur. SSTI may also be a manifestation of disseminated infection, such as that seen with ecthyma gangrenosum in neutropenic patients.[59] This condition results from perivascular invasion of small vessels with secondary ischemic necrosis and is classically associated with *P aeruginosa*, *S aureus*, *Aeromonas* spp, atypical mycobacteria, *Candida* spp, and *Fusarium*. Severe infections such as necrotizing fasciitis and clostridial myonecrosis require urgent surgical debridement in addition to antibiotic therapy.

ANTIMICROBIAL STEWARDSHIP

Antimicrobial stewardship (AS) refers to a systematic effort to educate and persuade health care providers to follow evidence-based prescribing in order to reduce antibiotic overuse or misuse with the goals of stemming further antimicrobial resistance, improving patient outcomes, and reducing unnecessary health care costs.[60] AS is particularly pertinent to the ICU, and specific interventions, such as development of clinical guidelines, prospective audit and feedback, antibiotic time-outs, incorporation of rapid diagnostics, and computerized decision support, have been studied for feasibility in the critical care setting.[61] Timely and appropriate empiric antibiotic therapy has been shown in a variety of infections to reduce mortality, but antibiotic de-escalation, even in critically ill patients with cancer, is also important once microbiological results are available to decrease unnecessary broad-spectrum exposure.[62]

SUMMARY

The gamut of infectious complications in critically ill patients with cancer is broad and can affect single or multiple organ systems. Neutropenia remains an important risk factor for infection, although the degree and severity depend on the type of malignancy and subsequent cancer treatment. Astute clinicians should maintain a high index of suspicion to properly diagnose and manage infections, recognizing also that noninfectious mimics add complexity to the care of these patients.

DISCLOSURE

The authors have nothing to disclose.

REFERENCES

1. Freifeld AG, Bow EJ, Sepkowitz KA, et al. Clinical practice guideline for the use of antimicrobial agents in neutropenic patients with cancer: 2010 update by the infectious diseases society of America. Clin Infect Dis 2011;52:e56–93.
2. Guarana M, Nucci M, Nouer SA. Shock and early death in hematologic patients with febrile neutropenia. Antimicrob Agents Chemother 2019;63: e01250-19.
3. Legrand M, Max A, Peigne V, et al. Survival in neutropenic patients with severe sepsis or septic shock. Crit Care Med 2012;40:43–9.
4. Park JH, Romero FA, Taur Y, et al. Cytokine release syndrome grade as a predictive marker for infections in patients with relapsed or refractory B-cell acute lymphoblastic leukemia treated with chimeric antigen receptor T cells. Clin Infect Dis 2018;67:533–40.
5. Chaftari AM, Hachem R, Jiang Y, et al. Changing epidemiology of catheter-related bloodstream infections in cancer patients. Infect Control Hosp Epidemiol 2018;39:727–9.
6. Mermel LA, Allon M, Bouza E, et al. Clinical practice guidelines for the diagnosis and management of intravascular catheter-related infection: 2009 Update by the Infectious Diseases Society of America. Clin Infect Dis 2009;49:1–45.

7. Raad I, Chaftari AM. Advances in prevention and management of central line-associated bloodstream infections in patients with cancer. Clin Infect Dis 2014; 59(Suppl 5):S340–3.

8. El Zakhem A, Chaftari AM, Bahu R, et al. Central line-associated bloodstream infections caused by Staphylococcus aureus in cancer patients: clinical outcome and management. Ann Med 2014;46:163–8.

9. Pappas PG, Kauffman CA, Andes DR, et al. Clinical practice guideline for the management of candidiasis: 2016 update by the infectious diseases Society of America. Clin Infect Dis 2016;62:e1–50.

10. Fares J, Khalil M, Chaftari AM, et al. Impact of catheter management on clinical outcome in adult cancer patients with gram-negative bacteremia. Open Forum Infect Dis 2019;6:ofz357.

11. Battaglia CC, Hale K. Hospital-acquired infections in critically ill patients with cancer. J Intensive Care Med 2019;34:523–36.

12. Wong JL, Evans SE. Bacterial pneumonia in patients with cancer: novel risk factors and management. Clin Chest Med 2017;38:263–77.

13. Evans SE, Ost DE. Pneumonia in the neutropenic cancer patient. Curr Opin Pulm Med 2015;21:260–71.

14. Stover DE, Kaner RJ. Pulmonary complications in cancer patients. CA Cancer J Clin 1996;46:303–20.

15. Torres A, Lee N, Cilloniz C, et al. Laboratory diagnosis of pneumonia in the molecular age. Eur Respir J 2016;48:1764–78.

16. Rabello LS, Silva JR, Azevedo LC, et al. Clinical outcomes and microbiological characteristics of severe pneumonia in cancer patients: a prospective cohort study. PLoS One 2015;10:e0120544.

17. Di Pasquale MF, Sotgiu G, Gramegna A, et al. Prevalence and etiology of community-acquired pneumonia in immunocompromised patients. Clin Infect Dis 2019;68:1482–93.

18. American Thoracic Society, Infectious Diseases Society of America. Guidelines for the management of adults with hospital-acquired, ventilator-associated, and healthcare-associated pneumonia. Am J Respir Crit Care Med 2005;171: 388–416.

19. Safdar A, Rolston KV. Stenotrophomonas maltophilia: changing spectrum of a serious bacterial pathogen in patients with cancer. Clin Infect Dis 2007;45: 1602–9.

20. Tada K, Kurosawa S, Hiramoto N, et al. Stenotrophomonas maltophilia infection in hematopoietic SCT recipients: high mortality due to pulmonary hemorrhage. Bone Marrow Transplant 2013;48:74–9.

21. Meyer R, Rappo U, Glickman M, et al. Legionella jordanis in hematopoietic SCT patients radiographically mimicking invasive mold infection. Bone Marrow Transplant 2011;46:1099–103.

22. del Castillo M, Lucca A, Plodkowski A, et al. Atypical presentation of Legionella pneumonia among patients with underlying cancer: a fifteen-year review. J Infect 2016;72:45–51.

23. Wang HL, Seo YH, LaSala PR, et al. Nocardiosis in 132 patients with cancer: microbiological and clinical analyses. Am J Clin Pathol 2014;142:513–23.

24. Torres HA, Reddy BT, Raad II, et al. Nocardiosis in cancer patients. Medicine (Baltimore) 2002;81:388–97.

25. Kamboj M, Sepkowitz KA. The risk of tuberculosis in patients with cancer. Clin Infect Dis 2006;42:1592–5.

26. Redelman-Sidi G, Sepkowitz KA. Rapidly growing mycobacteria infection in patients with cancer. Clin Infect Dis 2010;51:422–34.

27. Sepkowitz KA, Brown AE, Telzak EE, et al. Pneumocystis carinii pneumonia among patients without AIDS at a cancer hospital. JAMA 1992;267:832–7.

28. Morjaria S, Frame J, Franco-Garcia A, et al. Clinical performance of (1,3) beta-D glucan for the diagnosis of pneumocystis pneumonia (PCP) in cancer patients tested with PCP polymerase chain reaction. Clin Infect Dis 2019;69:1303–9.

29. Cornely OA, Maertens J, Winston DJ, et al. Posaconazole vs. fluconazole or itraconazole prophylaxis in patients with neutropenia. N Engl J Med 2007;356:348–59.

30. Wingard JR, Carter SL, Walsh TJ, et al. Randomized, double-blind trial of fluconazole versus voriconazole for prevention of invasive fungal infection after allogeneic hematopoietic cell transplantation. Blood 2010;116:5111–8.

31. Trifilio SM, Bennett CL, Yarnold PR, et al. Breakthrough zygomycosis after voriconazole administration among patients with hematologic malignancies who receive hematopoietic stem-cell transplants or intensive chemotherapy. Bone Marrow Transplant 2007;39:425–9.

32. Hijano DR, Maron G, Hayden RT. Respiratory viral infections in patients with cancer or undergoing hematopoietic cell transplant. Front Microbiol 2018;9:3097.

33. Chemaly RF, Torres HA, Hachem RY, et al. Cytomegalovirus pneumonia in patients with lymphoma. Cancer 2005;104:1213–20.

34. Schlick K, Grundbichler M, Auberger J, et al. Cytomegalovirus reactivation and its clinical impact in patients with solid tumors. Infect Agent Cancer 2015;10:45.

35. Liang W, Guan W, Chen R, et al. Cancer patients in SARS-CoV-2 infection: a nationwide analysis in China. Lancet Oncol 2020;21:335–7.

36. Safdar A, Malathum K, Rodriguez SJ, et al. Strongyloidiasis in patients at a comprehensive cancer center in the United States. Cancer 2004;100:1531–6.

37. Nesher L, Rolston KV. Neutropenic enterocolitis, a growing concern in the era of widespread use of aggressive chemotherapy. Clin Infect Dis 2013;56:711–7.

38. Duceau B, Picard M, Pirracchio R, et al. Neutropenic enterocolitis in critically ill patients: spectrum of the disease and risk of invasive fungal disease. Crit Care Med 2019;47:668–76.

39. Cornely OA, Bangard C, Jaspers NI. Hepatosplenic candidiasis. Clin Liver Dis (Hoboken) 2015;6:47–50.

40. Kamboj M, Son C, Cantu S, et al. Hospital-onset Clostridium difficile infection rates in persons with cancer or hematopoietic stem cell transplant: a C3IC network report. Infect Control Hosp Epidemiol 2012;33:1162–5.

41. Kamboj M, Brite J, Aslam A, et al. Artificial differences in Clostridium difficile infection rates associated with disparity in testing. Emerg Infect Dis 2018;24:584–7.

42. McDonald LC, Gerding DN, Johnson S, et al. Clinical practice guidelines for Clostridium difficile infection in adults and children: 2017 update by the infectious diseases Society of America (IDSA) and Society for Healthcare Epidemiology of America (SHEA). Clin Infect Dis 2018;66:e1–48.

43. Schwartz S, Vergoulidou M, Schreier E, et al. Norovirus gastroenteritis causes severe and lethal complications after chemotherapy and hematopoietic stem cell transplantation. Blood 2011;117:5850–6.

44. Matthes-Martin S, Feuchtinger T, Shaw PJ, et al. European guidelines for diagnosis and treatment of adenovirus infection in leukemia and stem cell transplantation: summary of ECIL-4 (2011). Transpl Infect Dis 2012;14:555–63.

45. Ljungman P, de la Camara R, Robin C, et al. Guidelines for the management of cytomegalovirus infection in patients with haematological malignancies and after stem cell transplantation from the 2017 European Conference on Infections in Leukaemia (ECIL 7). Lancet Infect Dis 2019;19:e260–72.

46. Pruitt AA. Central nervous system infections in cancer patients. Semin Neurol 2010;30:296–310.

47. Leber AL, Everhart K, Balada-Llasat JM, et al. Multicenter evaluation of BioFire FilmArray meningitis/encephalitis panel for detection of bacteria, viruses, and yeast in cerebrospinal fluid specimens. J Clin Microbiol 2016;54:2251–61.

48. Safdieh JE, Mead PA, Sepkowitz KA, et al. Bacterial and fungal meningitis in patients with cancer. Neurology 2008;70:943–7.

49. Tunkel AR, Hartman BJ, Kaplan SL, et al. Practice guidelines for the management of bacterial meningitis. Clin Infect Dis 2004;39:1267–84.

50. Tunkel AR, Hasbun R, Bhimraj A, et al. 2017 infectious diseases Society of America's clinical practice guidelines for healthcare-associated ventriculitis and meningitis. Clin Infect Dis 2017;64:e34–65.

51. Schmidt-Hieber M, Schwender J, Heinz WJ, et al. Viral encephalitis after allogeneic stem cell transplantation: a rare complication with distinct characteristics of different causative agents. Haematologica 2011;96:142–9.

52. Denier C, Bourhis JH, Lacroix C, et al. Spectrum and prognosis of neurologic complications after hematopoietic transplantation. Neurology 2006;67:1990–7.

53. Scully EP, Baden LR, Katz JT. Fungal brain infections. Curr Opin Neurol 2008;21:347–52.

54. Clifford TG, Katebian B, Van Horn CM, et al. Urinary tract infections following radical cystectomy and urinary diversion: a review of 1133 patients. World J Urol 2018;36:775–81.

55. Parker WP, Toussi A, Tollefson MK, et al. Risk factors and microbial distribution of urinary tract infections following radical cystectomy. Urology 2016;94:96–101.

56. Bahu R, Chaftari AM, Hachem RY, et al. Nephrostomy tube related pyelonephritis in patients with cancer: epidemiology, infection rate and risk factors. J Urol 2013;189:130–5.

57. Scotland KB, Lo J, Grgic T, et al. Ureteral stent-associated infection and sepsis: pathogenesis and prevention: a review. Biofouling 2019;35:117–27.

58. Golan Y. Empiric therapy for hospital-acquired, Gram-negative complicated intra-abdominal infection and complicated urinary tract infections: a systematic literature review of current and emerging treatment options. BMC Infect Dis 2015;15:313.

59. Moffarah AS, Al Mohajer M, Hurwitz BL, et al. Skin and soft tissue infections. Microbiol Spectr 2016;4:1–16.

60. Barlam TF, Cosgrove SE, Abbo LM, et al. Implementing an antibiotic stewardship program: guidelines by the infectious diseases Society of America and the Society for Healthcare Epidemiology of America. Clin Infect Dis 2016;62:e51–77.

61. Pickens CI, Wunderink RG. Principles and practice of antibiotic stewardship in the ICU. Chest 2019;156:163–71.

62. Paskovaty A, Pastores SM, Gedrimaite Z, et al. Antimicrobial de-escalation in septic cancer patients: is it safe to back down? Intensive Care Med 2015;41:2022–3.

Oncologic Emergencies
Traditional and Contemporary

Jenna Spring, MD[a,b], Laveena Munshi, MD, MSc[a,c,*]

KEYWORDS

- Hyperleukocytosis and leukostasis • Tumor lysis syndrome
- Superior vena cava syndrome • Malignant pericardial effusion
- Metastatic spinal cord compression
- Syndrome of inappropriate antidiuretic hormone • Cytokine release syndrome
- Immune-related adverse events

KEY POINTS

- As the number of intensive care unit (ICU) patients with cancer increases, intensivists must have the ability to recognize and manage oncologic emergencies.
- Clinical decision making around disease- or treatment-related emergencies can be complex, and multidisciplinary input is critical to provide optimal care.
- Novel immune therapies are changing the landscape of cancer-related complications. Side effects of immune-effector cells are particularly important because many of these patients require ICU-level care.

INTRODUCTION

It is becoming increasingly important for intensivists to rapidly identify and treat cancer-related complications. Currently, up to 20% of intensive care unit (ICU) admissions will have an underlying cancer diagnosis.[1] The volume of oncology patients admitted to the ICU may continue to grow as cancer prevalence increases; ICU oncologic admission policies evolve; and novel treatments are introduced with unique toxicities. A multidisciplinary approach, including close collaboration with the patient's oncologist, is essential to ensuring the best possible outcome. In this

[a] Interdepartmental Division of Critical Care Medicine, Department of Medicine, University of Toronto, Sinai Health System and University Health Network, Toronto, Ontario, Canada; [b] Interdepartmental Division of Critical Care Medicine, Department of Medicine, University of Toronto, Sunnybrook Health Sciences Centre, 2075 Bayview Avenue, Room D108, Toronto, Ontario M4N 3M5, USA; [c] Mount Sinai Hospital, 600 University Avenue, Suite 18-206, Toronto, Ontario M5G 1X5, Canada
* Corresponding author. Mount Sinai Hospital, 600 University Avenue, Suite 18-206, Toronto, Ontario M5G 1X5, Canada.
E-mail address: laveena.munshi@sinaihealth.ca
Twitter: @jennaspring (J.S.); @laveenamunshi (L.M.)

Crit Care Clin 37 (2021) 85–103
https://doi.org/10.1016/j.ccc.2020.08.004
0749-0704/21/Crown Copyright © 2020 Published by Elsevier Inc. All rights reserved.

review, the authors separate oncologic emergencies into treatment-related versus disease-related causes, focusing on the key aspects of pathophysiology, diagnosis, and management.

Disease-Related Emergencies

Hyperleukocytosis and leukostasis

Hyperleukocytosis is defined by a total white blood cell (WBC) count greater than 100 $\times$ 10^9/L, whereas leukostasis refers to end-organ hypoperfusion associated with the extreme WBC elevation.[2] Up to 30% of acute leukemia patients will present with hyperleukocytosis, with high mortalities if left untreated.[3,4] Leukostasis is more common in patients with acute myeloid leukemia (AML) than in patients with acute lymphoid leukemia (ALL) because of the relatively large size of the myeloid blasts. Approximately 1 in 4 patients with AML and hyperleukocytosis will develop clinical leukostasis,[5] whereas leukostasis does not typically occur in ALL until the WBC exceeds 400 $\times$ 10^9/L.[6]

Pathophysiology. Hyperleukocytosis occurs as leukemic blasts quickly multiply and lose affinity for the bone marrow.[7] It can result in leukostasis, which causes tissue hypoxemia, but the precise mechanism is not well understood. Pathology demonstrates leukemic cells occluding the microvasculature with or without hemorrhage, infarction, or edema. Risk factors for hyperleukocytosis are young age, T-cell ALL, monocytic or monoblastic subtypes of AML, acute promyelocytic leukemia, and specific chromosomal rearrangements.[8]

Clinical presentation and diagnosis. Leukostasis should be suspected in the presence of tissue hypoxia and a WBC greater than 100 $\times$ 10^9/L. However, it can occur at lower cell counts, particularly in the subgroup of monocytic or monoblastic AML.[9] Most patients present with respiratory compromise and/or neurologic symptoms,[5] but leukostasis may have a variety of clinical manifestations (**Fig. 1**).

There are additional considerations for the intensivist to recognize. Spurious laboratory abnormalities can confound the clinical picture because of ongoing metabolism of the leukemic cells in vitro: arterial P_{O_2} may be falsely lowered causing inaccurate measure of oxygenation; pseudohyperkalemia may be seen as blood clots after being drawn and blast cells release potassium; and lactic acidosis, out of keeping of end-organ hypoperfusion, has been reported due to anaerobic glycolysis and lactate production by malignant cells.[10] Finally, disseminated intravascular coagulation (DIC) and spontaneous tumor lysis syndrome (TLS) may also be present.

Management. The treatment should be focused on (1) reduction of blood viscosity, (2) emergent cytoreduction therapy, and (3) prophylaxis and monitoring for TLS.

All patients with hyperleukocytosis should receive fluid resuscitation with isotonic solutions to reduce blood viscosity and maintain adequate urine output. Red blood cell transfusions should be avoided unless symptomatic anemia develops, as they increase the hematocrit and blood viscosity and may worsen leukostasis. Similarly, diuretics should not be given in the absence of clinically important volume overload.

In addition to induction chemotherapy, hydroxyurea or leukapheresis may be pursued to urgently lower the WBC at the time of presentation. Hydroxyurea is an antimetabolite that inhibits DNA synthesis. It is typically started at 50 to 75 mg/kg/d divided into 3 or 4 oral doses with a reduction of WBC up to 80% at 48 hours.[11] Hydroxyurea may act as a temporizing measure to bridge the patient to transfer to an institution with tertiary oncologic care, or when the underlying diagnosis is unclear.

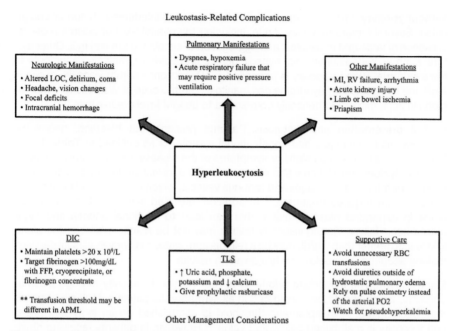

Fig. 1. Complications and management considerations of hyperleukocytosis. APML, acute promyelocytic leukemia; FFP, fresh frozen plasma; LOC, level of consciousness; MI, myocardial infarction; RBC, red blood cell; RV, right ventricular.

Despite rapidly lowering the WBC by 30% to 60% with a single session, leukapheresis has not been shown to improve mortality or reduce leukostasis-associated complications.[12] It may also be associated with worsening thrombocytopenia, bleeding, infection, and citrate toxicity.[13] Given the lack of evidence, the decision to pursue leukapheresis is center and patient dependent. However, it should not be offered in acute promyelocytic leukemia because of the significant coagulopathy.[14] Finally, some centers may initiate low-dose chemotherapy infusions if the WBC continues to increase, inducing organ dysfunction despite the use of hydroxyurea; this may be effective in minimizing end organ damage but could result in worsening tumor lysis parameters.

Patients should be closely observed for the development of DIC. It should be urgently treated with fresh frozen plasma, fibrinogen concentrate, or cryoprecipitate to maintain fibrinogen levels greater than 100 mg/dL.[15] Platelet counts should also be maintained greater than 20×10^9/L in nonbleeding patients and greater than 50×10^9/L in bleeding patients to avoid life-threatening hemorrhage until the hyperleukocytosis is treated.[16] These patients are also at risk of both spontaneous and treatment-induced TLS. Rasburicase should be started, and electrolytes must be followed closely.

Hyperviscosity syndrome

Hyperviscosity syndrome is a constellation of symptoms caused by increased blood viscosity. It is seen in 15% of Waldenstrom macroglobulinemia because of high levels of monoclonal immunoglobulin M (IgM) plasma protein.[17] Up to 6% of patients with multiple myeloma may also develop hyperviscosity syndrome, particularly IgA subtype.[18] If not recognized and rapidly treated, it can be fatal.

Pathophysiology. Hyperviscosity impairs blood flow and interferes with normal coagulation. Several factors may play a role, including the overall level of plasma proteins, presence of large IgM molecules, and aggregation of circulating IgA and IgG. Other factors, such as hypoalbuminemia, hyperlipidemia, and acidosis, may also contribute to the syndrome. Blood viscosity is normally 1.5 cP, and once serum viscosity exceeds 4 cP, the hyperviscosity syndrome can manifest.[19] In the case of Waldenstrom macroglobulinemia, this would generally correspond to an IgM level greater than 3 g/dL.[18]

Clinical presentation and diagnosis. Patients present with bleeding, neurologic changes, visual changes, and constitutional symptoms as outlined in **Table 1**.[20–22] The diagnosis is based on signs or symptoms of the disease and laboratory evidence of organ dysfunction. Patients should also undergo a formal funduscopic examination looking for retinal hemorrhages and tortuous vessels, which may signify clinical hyperviscosity that requires treatment.[23] In addition, elevated serum protein levels may result in expanded plasma volume that can lead to dilutional anemia and high-output heart failure. Serum viscosity testing may not be readily available; therefore, IgM levels greater than 3 g/dL may be a reliable surrogate.[22] However, clinical decision making should not be delayed while awaiting results.

Management. The immediate priority is to reduce blood viscosity through plasmapheresis, which should be considered in all symptomatic patients. Multiple sessions may be required. A symptomatic threshold is established on an individual basis, and viscosity is maintained below that value.[20] However, in patients receiving rituximab, there may be a transient spike in the monoclonal protein following treatment that can precipitate hyperviscosity syndrome. Therefore, in these patients, prophylactic plasmapheresis may be considered when pre–rituximab immunoglobulin levels are elevated (IgM $\geq$4 g/dL).[24] Blood transfusions should be avoided if possible until viscosity has been reduced. Initiating chemotherapy to address the underlying monoclonal protein production is also crucial.

Malignant pericardial effusion
Malignant pericardial effusions are a frequent complication of lung cancer, breast cancer, lymphoma, leukemia, sarcomas, and melanoma. They can become life-threatening if associated with cardiac tamponade. Malignant pericardial involvement may be found on autopsy in approximately 1 in 10 patients with cancer.[25]

Pathophysiology. Effusions may develop from metastases to the pericardium, side effects of chemotherapy, radiation toxicity, or infection. The volume may be enhanced by the blockage of lymphatic drainage in the mediastinum. As fluid accumulates, right

Table 1
Presenting signs, symptoms, and complications of hyperviscosity syndrome

Organ System	Signs and Symptoms
Neurologic	Altered level of consciousness, headache, tinnitus, ataxia, vertigo, delirium, seizures, coma, stroke
Ocular	Diplopia, blurry vision, central retinal vein occlusion, retinal detachment
Bleeding	Mucosal, nasal, cutaneous, gingival
Constitutional	Fatigue, malaise
Other	Acute kidney injury, dilutional anemia, high-output heart failure

Data from Refs.[20–22]

ventricular diastolic filling is impaired and intraventricular pressures begin to equalize, resulting in tamponade physiology. Given that malignant effusions can develop slowly over time, the effusion may be very large before patients become symptomatic.

Clinical presentation and diagnosis. Tachypnea, dyspnea on exertion, orthopnea, peripheral edema, chest discomfort or heaviness, palpitations, and nonspecific constitutional symptoms may be described. Findings supportive of a diagnosis of cardiac tamponade are outlined in **Box 1**.[26–28] Cardiac tamponade presents with the following signs in most patients: tachycardia, elevated jugular venous pressure, dyspnea, pulsus paradoxus, and enlargement of the cardiac silhouette on chest radiograph.[29] In severe cases, shock with multiorgan dysfunction is seen.

Pericardial effusion leading to hemodynamic compromise should be ruled out by transthoracic echocardiogram. Echocardiographic findings of right atrial and right ventricular diastolic collapse in the presence of an effusion are highly suggestive of cardiac tamponade.[30,31] Dilation of the inferior vena cava (IVC) is also seen. Ultimately, the diagnosis of cardiac tamponade is a clinical one and can be definitively diagnosed by improvement in hemodynamic status following pericardiocentesis.

Treatment. Drainage of pericardial fluid is the immediate priority. Even if hemodynamic compromise is not present, malignant pericardial effusions frequently progress over time, and pericardiocentesis may be considered to prevent future complications and establish a diagnosis. Percutaneous echo-guided drainage of malignant pericardial effusions has been shown to be safe and effective in a large case series and is the preferred method in the acute setting.[32] Guidelines recommend leaving the drain in situ until daily fluid output decreases to less than 30 mL.[33]

In the case of malignant effusions, the recurrence rate can be as high as 60%.[34] Options to prevent reaccumulation include instillation of sclerosing agents or chemotherapy into the pericardial space; systemic chemotherapy; radiation therapy; pericardiotomy; and pericardial window.[34] The patient's prognosis, treatment goals, and quality of life must be taken into account when deciding on a more definitive management approach.

Superior vena cava syndrome

Malignant superior vena cava (SVC) syndrome is caused by obstruction of the SVC, resulting in decreased blood return to the right atrium. It can occur in non-Hodgkin

---

Box 1
Findings supportive of a diagnosis of pericardial tamponade

Clinical signs and symptoms
- Hemodynamic instability: Hypotension, tachycardia
- Tachypnea, shortness of breath on exertion
- Muffled heart sounds
- Pulsus paradoxus
- Distended jugular venous pulse

Findings on investigation
- Chest radiograph: Cardiomegaly
- Electrocardiogram: Electrical alternans, low QRS voltage
- Transthoracic echocardiogram: Right atrial diastolic collapse, right ventricular diastolic collapse, dilated IVC
- Chest CT: Large size of the pericardial effusion; evidence of IVC dilation; bowing of intraventricular septum; compression of cardiac chambers

Data from Refs.[26–28]

lymphoma, non–small cell lung cancer, small cell lung cancer, thymoma, mediastinal germ cell tumors, and solid tumors that metastasize to the mediastinal lymph nodes. Of these, lung cancer is most common cause, and for many patients, SVC syndrome is the presenting feature. The prognosis in patients with SVC syndrome is generally poor.

Pathophysiology. The SVC is responsible for blood return from the head and upper body and can become obstructed by (1) external compression from a lung mass, mediastinal mass, or mediastinal lymphadenopathy; (2) invasion of an adjacent tumor into the SVC; or (3) thrombosis. As blood flow is progressively impaired, collaterals form to reestablish blood return via the azygous vein or IVC.[35] Blood vessels proximal to the area of occlusion become dilated, and symptoms related to impaired venous drainage develop.[35] SVC occlusion may develop rapidly in patients with cancer, resulting in inadequate collaterals to prevent a life-threatening increase in central venous pressure.

Clinical presentation and diagnosis. Signs and symptoms include facial swelling, arm swelling, dilated vessels across the upper chest, dyspnea, and cough. Patients may also develop pharyngeal or cerebral edema that can be life-threatening. Airway edema may present as stridor, hoarseness, dysphagia, or cough, whereas cerebral edema may lead to altered mental status, headaches, and visual changes. If cerebral edema is left untreated, fatal brainstem herniation can occur.

On chest radiograph, the presence of mediastinal widening or pleural effusion may be suggestive of an underlying mediastinal mass. Contrast-enhanced computed tomography (CT) venogram is the imaging modality of choice to determine the cause and degree of SVC obstruction as well as to identify any thrombus present.[36] MRI is also an option to define the precise location of the obstruction as well as the extent of collaterals.[36]

Management. The priority is identifying life-threatening symptoms, including signs of cerebral edema; evidence of severe laryngeal edema; and hemodynamic compromise. These patients must be urgently stabilized while a formal venogram and stenting are arranged. An overview of the approach to life-threatening SVC syndrome is outlined in **Fig. 2**.

Endovascular stenting has been shown to be safe and effective and may provide time to establish a tissue diagnosis and definitive treatment plan.[37] However, median symptom-free survival is only 6 months.[38] If thrombosis is present, the use of catheter-directed thrombolysis in combination with stenting may also be considered.[39] In the case of non-life-threatening symptoms, multidisciplinary input should be obtained before pursuing stenting.

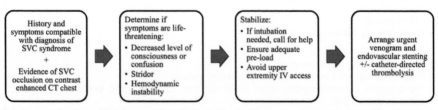

Fig. 2. Approach to life-threatening SVC syndrome. Suggested approach to the diagnosis, assessment, and stabilization of patients presenting with life-threatening symptoms is outlined. In the absence of life-threatening symptoms, a multidisciplinary discussion regarding treatment options should occur before an endovascular procedure.

Stabilizing patients with advanced SVC syndrome may present several challenges, and airway management may be particularly high risk. Important considerations include (1) potential cerebral edema and avoidance of hypotension to maintain cerebral perfusion pressure; (2) airway edema or compression making advancement of the endotracheal tube challenging or impossible; (3) need to maintain spontaneous respiration; and (4) location of intravenous (IV) access. With impaired venous drainage into the right atrium, preload may need to be augmented using lower-extremity IV access because infusion of fluids and medications from the upper limbs may be unreliable and worsen venous congestion.[40]

Before an intubation attempt, the location of a mediastinal mass should be reviewed on imaging to predict complications and optimal endotracheal tube depth. Administration of sedatives or paralytics may result in worsening hypotension, tracheal collapse from extrinsic compression with loss of spontaneous respiration, and an inability to intubate and ventilate if the airway edema or external compression is extensive.[41] Awake fiberoptic intubation with an armored tube and head of the bed elevated is the preferred approach,[40] but the airway plan should be a multidisciplinary discussion with the potential option for emergent cardiopulmonary bypass if the airway is lost in appropriate candidates.[42]

Syndrome of inappropriate antidiuretic hormone secretion

Hyponatremia has been reported to occur in almost 50% of hospitalized patients with cancer and is associated with poor outcomes, including increased morality.[43] Defined by a serum sodium less than 135 mEq/L, the primary cause for hyponatremia in this patient population is syndrome of inappropriate antidiuretic hormone secretion (SIADH). Although small cell lung cancer is the most common underlying cause, it can also be seen in a variety of other solid tumors as well as hematologic malignancies.

Pathophysiology. Antidiuretic hormone (ADH) is normally secreted from the posterior pituitary to enhance free water uptake in the renal collecting duct when there is an increase in serum osmolality or in response to decreased circulating blood volume. However, ectopic production of ADH by tumor cells results in inappropriately elevated ADH levels leading to excess water retention despite falling plasma osmolality. Other factors, such as medications (eg, vincristine, cyclophosphamide, opiates, antidepressants), intracranial pathology, such as brain metastases, nausea, pain, and stress, may also contribute to SIADH in patients with cancer.[44]

Clinical presentation and diagnosis. Hyponatremia may initially present with nonspecific symptoms, such as headache, nausea, vomiting, malaise, and confusion. However, when hyponatremia is severe or acute, it can result in cerebral edema with seizures, coma, and even death. Rapid evaluation of the patient's volume status, serum osmolality, urine sodium, and urine osmolality is critical. SIADH should be suspected in any patient with cancer presenting with hypoosmolar hyponatremia (serum osmolality <275 mOsm/kg) with normal volume status on examination, normal urine sodium (>30 mEq/L), and normal urine osmolality (>100 mOsm/kg).[44] Thyroid and adrenal dysfunction causing euvolemic hyponatremia should be ruled out along with diuretic use. Diagnostic features of additional causes of hypoosmolar hyponatremia are outlined in **Table 2**.[45,46]

Management. An approach to management is outlined in **Fig. 3**, based on European and American guidelines.[46,47] Most patients with SIADH should be assumed to have chronic hyponatremia (duration >48 hours). Care must be taken to avoid rapid

Table 2
Major causes of hyponatremia and associated laboratory features

Cause Based on Volume Status	Urine Sodium, mEq/L	Urine Osmolality, mEq/L
Hypovolemic		
Renal losses/diuretic use	>30	>100
Extrarenal losses	<20–30	>100
Euvolemic		
SIADH	>30	>100
Hypothyroidism	>30	>100
Adrenal insufficiency	>30	>100
Psychogenic polydipsia	<20	<100
Hypervolemic		
Congestive heart failure	<20–30	>100
Cirrhosis	<20–30	>100
Renal failure	>30	>100

Data from Milionis HJ, Liamis GL, Elisaf MS. The hyponatremic patient: a systematic approach to laboratory diagnosis. CMAJ. 2002;166(8):1056-1062 and Verbalis JG, Goldsmith SR, Greenberg A, et al. Diagnosis, evaluation, and treatment of hyponatremia: expert panel recommendations. Am J Med. 2013;126(10 Suppl 1):S1-42.

overcorrection and the devastating neurologic complication of osmotic demyelination syndrome. For patients with severe hyponatremia (Na $\leq$120 mEq/L), electrolytes should be monitored every 4 to 6 hours. Sodium levels should not increase by more than 8 mEq/L over the first 24 hours, or 18 mEq/L over the first 48 hours.[46] Patients

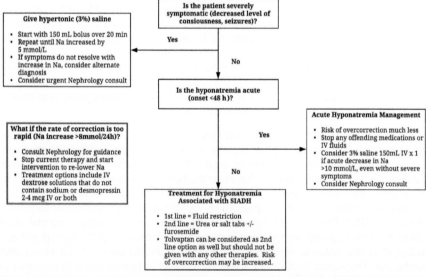

Fig. 3. Approach to management of hyponatremia secondary to SIADH.[46,47] (*Data from* Verbalis JG, Goldsmith SR, Greenberg A, et al. Diagnosis, evaluation, and treatment of hyponatremia: expert panel recommendations. *Am J Med.* 2013;126(10 Suppl 1):S1-42 and Spasovski G, Vanholder R, Allolio B, et al. Clinical practice guideline on diagnosis and treatment of hyponatraemia. *Intensive Care Med.* 2014;40(3):320-331.)

with coexisting liver disease, alcohol misuse, poor nutrition, or concurrent hypokalemia are more susceptible to osmotic demyelination syndrome, and excess caution must be taken.

Metastatic spinal cord compression
Up to 5% of malignancies may be complicated by spinal cord compression from metastatic disease, which may result in devastating neurologic deficits when not promptly recognized and treated.[48] Although lung, breast, and prostate cancers are most commonly implicated, it is also frequently seen in multiple myeloma, renal cell carcinoma, and non-Hodgkin lymphoma among others. Furthermore, metastatic spinal cord compression (MSCC) may be the initial feature of a previously undiagnosed malignancy in 20% of patients.[49]

Pathophysiology. MSCC occurs via 3 primary mechanisms: (1) hematogenous spread of cancer cells to the vertebra where the tumor may grow and impinge on the spinal canal. Furthermore, it may cause pathologic fracture and collapse of the vertebrae with resultant mass effect; (2) local spread from a tumor adjacent to the spine; or, in rare circumstances, (3) direct metastasis to the epidural space.[50] The thoracic spine is the most common site of MSCC, but many patients may have multilevel disease at the time of diagnosis.

Clinical presentation and diagnosis. MSCC often presents with pain as the initial symptom, but it can result in a range of neurologic sequelae, as outlined in **Table 3**.[48,51,52] A high index of suspicion must be maintained for any patient with known cancer presenting with new or worsening back pain. MRI is the imaging modality of choice. Given that multilevel disease may be present and the symptoms may not correlate with the level of the lesion, the entire spine should be imaged with and without contrast.[53] For patients in whom MRI is contraindicated, CT myelography can be performed.

Treatment. Early detection and treatment are key because neurologic prognosis largely depends on motor function at the time of diagnosis.[48] Urgent multidisciplinary

Table 3	
Clinical features of metastatic spinal cord compression	
Symptom	**Features**
Back pain	• Most common initial symptom (up to 95% of patients) • Can be localized or radicular • Often described as worse at night, with coughing/sneezing, with bending, or when lying flat • Location of pain poorly correlates with level of lesion
Motor weakness	• Typically occurs within 2 mo of pain onset • Initially limb weakness, clumsiness, heavy sensation • May progress to gait instability or paraplegia • Upper- or lower-motor neuron findings may be present
Sensory deficits	• Most patients have sensory symptoms at the time of diagnosis • Clear sensory level may or may not be present • Sensory level poorly predictive of lesion location
Bowel and bladder dysfunction	• Late finding associated with poor prognosis • Can present as urinary retention, constipation, urinary or fecal incontinence

Data from Refs.[48,51,52]

input is critical, and if the patient does not have a known cancer diagnosis, biopsy should be expedited. While awaiting definitive therapy, dexamethasone 10 to 16 mg IV should be administered and continued at 16 mg daily in divided doses.[53–55] In patients with suspected lymphoma, historically it was thought that the administration of corticosteroids could lead to a false negative biopsy result. However, this is controversial; therefore, emergent consultation with neurosurgery and a hematooncologist should be pursued in order to guide decision making surrounding diagnosis and treatment.[56]

Definitive management consists of surgical decompression followed by radiation therapy versus radiation therapy alone. Surgery is generally indicated in patients with spinal instability or severe compression on MRI with neurologic deficits; however, management decisions must be individualized, taking into account spinal stability, degree of neurologic compromise, radiosensitivity of the tumor, and the patient's overall health status and goals of care.[53,55] Important aspects of supportive care in patients with MSCC include multimodal analgesia for pain control, venous thromboembolism prophylaxis, bowel routine, and monitoring for urinary retention.

Treatment-Related Emergencies

Tumor lysis syndrome

TLS is a metabolic emergency arising from the rapid breakdown of tumor cells that is characterized by hyperuricemia, hyperkalemia, hyperphosphatemia, and hypocalcemia. Incidence estimates vary widely with reported rates up to 40% in some patients with hematologic malignancies.[57] Cancers that are characterized by a large disease burden and rapidly dividing cells represent the greatest risk of TLS. In-hospital mortalities have been estimated at approximately 20%.[58]

Pathophysiology. Rapid cell breakdown leads to the release of intracellular contents into the circulation. Large amounts of potassium and phosphate enter the extracellular compartment and cannot be effectively cleared in the urine. Purines are metabolized to uric acid via the xanthine oxidase pathway (**Fig. 4**).[59] As calcium phosphate crystals form, secondary hypocalcemia develops. Acute kidney injury (AKI) arises from uric acid deposition in the renal tubules; precipitation of calcium phosphate crystals;

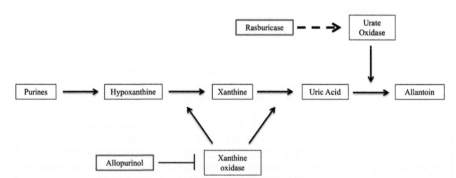

Fig. 4. Metabolism of purines to uric acid. Allopurinol and rasburicase, therapies to reduce uric acid levels, are shown in the red boxes. Allopurinol inhibits xanthine oxidase (*blocked line*), which reduces the metabolism of hypoxanthine and xanthine to uric acid. Rasburicase is recombinant urate oxidase (action depicted by *dotted arrow*), which promotes the metabolism of uric acid to allantoin. Allantoin is water soluble and can be safely excreted in urine.

and alteration in the renal vasculature. More than 50% of patients develop AKI and more than one-third may require dialysis.[60]

Although it can occur spontaneously, TLS is typically observed within 72 hours of treatment initiation.[61] In addition to cytotoxic chemotherapy, TLS can be precipitated by radiation therapy, biologic therapy, or steroids. Clinical trial data have also demonstrated significant rates of TLS for novel targeted therapies, including CAR T cells and kinase inhibitors.[62]

Malignancies that carry an increased risk of TLS are those with rapid cell turnover, high tumor burden, and sensitivity to chemotherapy. Patients with a high or intermediate risk of TLS based on expert consensus are outlined in **Table 4**.[63] Patient characteristics, such as preexisting renal disease, volume depletion, exposure to nephrotoxins, and baseline electrolyte abnormalities, may also make TLS more likely.

Clinical presentation and diagnosis. Symptoms include fatigue, anorexia, vomiting, diarrhea, and muscle cramps. However, patients may also present with tetany, seizures, heart failure, and life-threatening arrhythmias. It is important to distinguish between laboratory TLS and the clinical TLS syndrome. The diagnostic criteria based on the Cairo and Bishop classification are outlined in **Fig. 5**.[64]

Treatment. Major recommendations for the prevention and treatment of TLS from the British Society of Hematology Guidelines are outlined in **Box 2**.[65] Evaluating a patient's risk, and taking preventative measures, should be the first priority. All patients at risk of TLS should receive IV hydration to maintain urine output. Diuretics should be considered only if volume overload is present. Alkalinization of the urine as an adjunct therapy was historically advocated. However, evidence of efficacy is lacking, and it is no longer recommended for the treatment of TLS. Nonessential electrolyte replacement should also be avoided in at-risk patients; hold replacements for hypokalemia, hypocalcemia, or hypophosphatemia unless severe.

Allopurinol should be started before chemotherapy in all patients at intermediate risk of TLS and continued until tumor burden has decreased and laboratory parameters have normalized. The standard dosing is 300 mg/m^2/d in 3 divided oral doses with

Table 4
High and intermediate risk of tumor lysis syndrome by cancer type based on expert consensus[63]

Cancer Type	High-Risk Disease (>5% TLS Risk)	Intermediate-Risk Disease (1%–5% TLS Risk)
Leukemia	Acute leukemia with WBC ≥100 × 10^9/L ALL with WBC ≤100 × 10^9/L and lactate dehydrogenase (LDH) ≥2× upper limit of normal (ULN)	AML with WBC 25–100 × 10^9/L ALL with WBC ≤100 × 10^9/L and LDH ≤2× ULN CLL being treated with targeted therapies or biologics
Lymphoma	Diffuse large B-cell lymphoma (DLBCL), T-cell lymphomas, and transformed lymphomas with *elevated* LDH and bulky disease	DLBCL, T-cell lymphomas, and transformed lymphomas with *normal* LDH and bulky disease
Solid tumors	Neuroblastoma, germ-cell tumors, small cell lung cancer	

Abbreviation: DRESS, drug reaction with eosinophilia and systemic symptoms.

Data from Cairo MS, Coiffier B, Reiter A, Younes A, Panel TLSE. Recommendations for the evaluation of risk and prophylaxis of tumour lysis syndrome (TLS) in adults and children with malignant diseases: an expert TLS panel consensus. Br J Haematol. 2010;149(4):578-586.

Laboratory TLS

- Uric acid : $\geq$476 µmol/l or $\uparrow$ 25%
- Potassium: $\geq$6.0 mmol/l or $\uparrow$ 25%
- Phosphate: $\geq$1.45 mmol/l or $\uparrow$ 25%
- Calcium: $\leq$1.75 mmol/l or $\uparrow$ 25%

Clinical TLS

- Creatinine $\geq$ 1.5x ULN
- New onset seizure
- Cardiac arrhythmia or sudden death

Fig. 5. Diagnostic criteria for laboratory and clinical TLS. (*Data from* Cairo MS, Bishop M. Tumor lysis syndrome: new therapeutic strategies and classification. Br J Haematol. 2004;127(1):3-11.)

a 50% dose reduction in patients with renal dysfunction.[66] High-risk patients should be given rasburicase. Although rasburicase is safe and lowers uric acid levels more rapidly than allopurinol, the benefit in regard to clinical outcomes requires further study.[67] Importantly, rasburicase is contraindicated in patients with glucose-6-phosphate dehydrogenase deficiency.

Dialysis may be required for AKI or refractory metabolic abnormalities. Continuous renal replacement therapy (CRRT) with high dialysate flow rates may be required

---

Box 2
Major recommendations for the prevention and treatment of tumor lysis syndrome from the British Society of Hematology Guidelines[65]

Prevention of TLS
- All patients at risk of TLS should receive IV fluid hydration ($\sim$3 L/d)
- Urinary alkalinization is not recommended
- Intermediate-risk patients can be given allopurinol prophylaxis for up to 7 days
- High-risk patients should receive rasburicase prophylaxis
- Patients receiving rasburicase should not be prescribed allopurinol
- Urinary alkalinization is not recommended

Treatment of established TLS
- Rasburicase 0.2 mg/kg/d should be given with duration dependent on clinical response
- Dialysis indications include refractory electrolyte abnormalities or volume overload
- Target for urine output should be 100 mL/m^2/h with isotonic crystalloids
- Asymptomatic hypocalcemia should not be treated

Data from Jones GL, Will A, Jackson GH, Webb NJ, Rule S, British Committee for Standards in H. Guidelines for the management of tumour lysis syndrome in adults and children with haematological malignancies on behalf of the British Committee for Standards in Haematology. Br J Haematol. 2015;169(5):661-671.

because of the ongoing release of intracellular contents and in severe hyperphosphatemia, as phosphate clearance is time dependent. However, if life-threatening hyperkalemia has occurred, patients may initially need intermittent hemodialysis to rapidly clear potassium followed by CRRT.[68]

Adverse events associated with novel therapies

This section provides a brief overview of the adverse events associated with immune checkpoint inhibition and CAR T-cell therapy. For a full discussion of these novel therapies as they relate to critical care, please refer to C. Gutierrez and colleagues' article, "Toxicities Associated with Immunotherapy and Approach to Novel Cancer Therapies," in this issue.

Immune-related adverse events. Immune checkpoint inhibitors have transformed cancer treatment for a variety of malignancies. However, patients are at risk of immune-related adverse events (irAEs), and up to 1% may die from them.[69] Intensivists must be aware of the wide range of irAE clinical presentations because any organ system can be involved (**Table 5**).[70–72] irAEs may occur within weeks to months of treatment, and clinicians should consider that any rapid clinical changes could be immune mediated. A trial of ICU-level care in patients with organ failure is warranted, while the immune checkpoint inhibitor is held or permanently discontinued. A low threshold to administer empiric antibiotics and conduct an infectious workup is an important aspect of supportive care. The suggested workup and management of grade 3 or 4 (severe) irAEs with particular relevance to critical care are outlined in **Table 6**.[73]

Cytokine release syndrome. Cytokine release syndrome (CRS) is a life-threatening complication of CAR T-cell therapy that presents similarly to sepsis and is characterized by high levels of cytokines. CRS may initially appear to be a flulike illness; however, severe cases can result in a runaway immune response with vascular leak,

Table 5	
Organ involvement in immune-related adverse events associated with checkpoint inhibitor therapy	
Organ System	**Presentation**
Neuromuscular	Encephalitis, aseptic meningitis, peripheral or autonomic neuropathy, myasthenia gravis, Guillain-Barre syndrome, transverse myelitis
Endocrine	Hypophysitis, thyroiditis, hyperthyroidism or hypothyroidism, adrenal insufficiency, autoimmune diabetes
Dermatologic	Rash, bullous dermatoses, Stevens Johnson syndrome, toxic epidermal necrolysis, DRESS, uveitis, mucositis, vasculitis
Gastrointestinal	Colitis, hepatitis, pancreatitis, enteritis
Hematologic	Autoimmune hemolytic anemia, acquired thrombocytopenic purpura, hemolytic uremic syndrome, aplastic anemia, lymphopenia, acquired hemophilia, immune thrombocytopenia, venous thromboembolism
Ocular	Uveitis, iritis, episcleritis, blepharitis
Renal	Nephritis
Musculoskeletal	Inflammatory arthritis, polymyalgia-like syndrome
Respiratory	Pneumonitis
Cardiovascular	Myocarditis, pericarditis, arrhythmias, reduced ventricular function

Abbreviation: DRESS, drug reaction with eosinophilia and systemic symptoms.
Data from Refs.[70–72]

Table 6
Diagnostic management and workup of selected grade 3 or 4 immune-related adverse events according to the American Society of Clinical Oncology guidelines[73]

Immune-Related Reaction	Diagnostic Workup	Treatment
Colitis	Bloodwork in addition to routine studies: erythrocyte sedimentation rate, C-reactive protein, thyrotropin, cytomegalovirus testing Stool studies: Clostridium difficile, culture, ova, and parasite CT abdomen and pelvis Consider repeat lower endoscopy	Permanently discontinue immune checkpoint inhibitor Prednisone 1 to 2 mg/kg/d with escalation to IV if no improvement in 3–5 d Infliximab 5–10 mg/kg if no improvement with corticosteroids
Hepatitis	Viral serology, liver ultrasound with Doppler, imaging to rule out metastatic disease Can consider additional workup for elevated liver enzymes if clinically indicated	Permanently discontinue immune checkpoint inhibitor Methylprednisolone IV 1–2 mg/kg/d Consider mycophenolate mofetil or azathioprine if no improvement after 3 d Infliximab should be avoided (risk of liver failure) Consider Hepatology referral and transfer to tertiary care
Myocarditis	Eelectrocardiogram, troponin, brain natriuretic peptide, CXR, echocardiogram	Permanently discontinue immune checkpoint inhibitor Prednisone orally or methylprednisolone IV 1–2 mg/kg/d Consider pulse dose methylprednisolone (1 g IV daily) plus mycophenolate, infliximab, or antithymocyte globulin if no immediate response to steroids Consult Cardiology and consider admission to cardiac intensive care unit
Pneumonitis	CXR, chest CT, bronchoscopy with bronchoalveolar lavage ± transbronchial biopsy, sputum cultures, nasal swab, blood cultures	Permanently discontinue immune checkpoint inhibitor Empiric antibiotics Methylprednisolone IV 1–2 mg/kg/d Add infliximab 5 mg/kg, mycophenolate mofetil IV 1 g twice a day, intravenous immunoglobulin (IVIG) for 5 d, or cyclophosphamide if no improvement after 48 h
Encephalitis	Bloodwork in addition to routine studies: ESR, CRP, TSH MRI brain, lumbar puncture (send infectious workup ± paraneoplastic panel, autoimmune panel, oligoclonal bands and cytology), electroencephalogram	Hold immune checkpoint inhibitor Methylprednisolone IV 1–2 mg/kg/d For severe/progressive symptoms: methylprednisolone 1 g IV daily for 3-5 d + IVIG 2 g/kg over 5 d Consider empiric acyclovir until viral encephalitis ruled out Consult Neurology

vasodilatory shock, acute respiratory distress syndrome, multiorgan failure, and DIC.[74,75] CAR T-cell therapy may also cause immune-effector cell–associated neurotoxicity syndrome (ICANS), which presents as fever, apraxia, aphasia, dysgraphia, and lethargy, which can progress to decreased level of consciousness, and coma.

CRS and ICANS are reversible; ICU teams should be involved early, and threshold to admit should be low. Management is guided by CRS grading, which is measured on a scale of 1 to 4 based on the degree of fever, hypotension, hypoxemia, and organ damage. Tocilizumab, a monoclonal antibody against the interleukin-6 receptor, has been shown to be an effective treatment for severe CRS without an apparent impact on CAR T-cell function.[76] It is recommended for all patients with grade 3 or 4 CRS.[77] The first-line therapy in ICANS is corticosteroids, and when both CRS and ICANS are present, combination therapy with corticosteroids and tocilizumab should be given.[78]

SUMMARY

Early recognition and aggressive supportive care are crucial to improving outcomes across oncologic patients who develop critical illness. A multidisciplinary approach to patient care is also essential, including frequent collaboration with the oncology team.

DISCLOSURE

The authors have nothing to disclose.

REFERENCES

1. Soares M, Caruso P, Silva E, et al. Characteristics and outcomes of patients with cancer requiring admission to intensive care units: a prospective multicenter study. Crit Care Med 2010;38(1):9–15.
2. Ganzel C, Becker J, Mintz PD, et al. Hyperleukocytosis, leukostasis and leukapheresis: practice management. Blood Rev 2012;26(3):117–22.
3. Tien FM, Hou HA, Tsai CH, et al. Hyperleukocytosis is associated with distinct genetic alterations and is an independent poor-risk factor in de novo acute myeloid leukemia patients. Eur J Haematol 2018;101(1):86–94.
4. Shallis RM, Stahl M, Wei W, et al. Patterns of care and clinical outcomes of patients with newly diagnosed acute myeloid leukemia presenting with hyperleukocytosis who do not receive intensive chemotherapy. Leuk Lymphoma 2020;61(5): 1220–5.
5. Stahl M, Shallis RM, Wei W, et al. Management of hyperleukocytosis and impact of leukapheresis among patients with acute myeloid leukemia (AML) on short- and long-term clinical outcomes: a large, retrospective, multicenter, international study. Leukemia 2020. [Epub ahead of print].
6. Schwartz J, Padmanabhan A, Aqui N, et al. Guidelines on the use of therapeutic apheresis in clinical practice-evidence-based approach from the Writing Committee of the American Society for Apheresis: the Seventh Special issue. J Clin Apher 2016;31(3):149–62.
7. Gruszka AM, Valli D, Restelli C, et al. Adhesion deregulation in acute myeloid leukaemia. Cells 2019;8(1):66.
8. Giammarco S, Chiusolo P, Piccirillo N, et al. Hyperleukocytosis and leukostasis: management of a medical emergency. Expert Rev Hematol 2017;10(2):147–54.

9. Soares FA, Landell GA, Cardoso MC. Pulmonary leukostasis without hyperleuko-cytosis: a clinicopathologic study of 16 cases. Am J Hematol 1992;40(1):28–32.

10. Sillos EM, Shenep JL, Burghen GA, et al. Lactic acidosis: a metabolic complication of hematologic malignancies: case report and review of the literature. Cancer 2001;92(9):2237–46.

11. Mamez AC, Raffoux E, Chevret S, et al. Pre-treatment with oral hydroxyurea prior to intensive chemotherapy improves early survival of patients with high hyperleu-kocytosis in acute myeloid leukemia. Leuk Lymphoma 2016;57(10):2281–8.

12. Choi MH, Choe YH, Park Y, et al. The effect of therapeutic leukapheresis on early complications and outcomes in patients with acute leukemia and hyperleukocy-tosis: a propensity score-matched study. Transfusion 2018;58(1):208–16.

13. Korkmaz S. The management of hyperleukocytosis in 2017: do we still need leu-kapheresis? Transfus Apher Sci 2018;57(1):4–7.

14. Daver N, Kantarjian H, Marcucci G, et al. Clinical characteristics and outcomes in patients with acute promyelocytic leukaemia and hyperleucocytosis. Br J Haema-tol 2015;168(5):646–53.

15. Franchini M, Di Minno MN, Coppola A. Disseminated intravascular coagulation in hematologic malignancies. Semin Thromb Hemost 2010;36(4):388–403.

16. Barbui T, Falanga A. Disseminated intravascular coagulation in acute leukemia. Semin Thromb Hemost 2001;27(6):593–604.

17. Ghobrial IM, Witzig TE. Waldenstrom macroglobulinemia. Curr Treat Options On-col 2004;5(3):239–47.

18. Mehta J, Singhal S. Hyperviscosity syndrome in plasma cell dyscrasias. Semin Thromb Hemost 2003;29(5):467–71.

19. Crawford J, Cox EB, Cohen HJ. Evaluation of hyperviscosity in monoclonal gam-mopathies. Am J Med 1985;79(1):13–22.

20. Stone MJ, Bogen SA. Evidence-based focused review of management of hyper-viscosity syndrome. Blood 2012;119(10):2205–8.

21. Gertz MA. Acute hyperviscosity: syndromes and management. Blood 2018;132(13):1379–85.

22. Castillo JJ, Garcia-Sanz R, Hatjiharissi E, et al. Recommendations for the diag-nosis and initial evaluation of patients with Waldenstrom macroglobulinaemia: a task force from the 8th International Workshop on Waldenstrom Macroglobulinae-mia. Br J Haematol 2016;175(1):77–86.

23. Dumas G, Gabarre P, Bige N, et al. Hyperviscosity syndrome. Intensive Care Med 2018;44(7):1151–2.

24. Dimopoulos MA, Kastritis E, Owen RG, et al. Treatment recommendations for pa-tients with Waldenstrom macroglobulinemia (WM) and related disorders: IWWM-7 consensus. Blood 2014;124(9):1404–11.

25. Klatt EC, Heitz DR. Cardiac metastases. Cancer 1990;65(6):1456–9.

26. Spodick DH. Acute cardiac tamponade. N Engl J Med 2003;349(7):684–90.

27. Adler Y, Charron P, Imazio M, et al. 2015 ESC guidelines for the diagnosis and management of pericardial diseases: the task force for the diagnosis and man-agement of pericardial diseases of the European Society of Cardiology (ESC) endorsed by: the European Association for Cardio-Thoracic Surgery (EACTS). Eur Heart J 2015;36(42):2921–64.

28. Restrepo CS, Lemos DF, Lemos JA, et al. Imaging findings in cardiac tamponade with emphasis on CT. Radiographics 2007;27(6):1595–610.

29. Roy CL, Minor MA, Brookhart MA, et al. Does this patient with a pericardial effu-sion have cardiac tamponade? JAMA 2007;297(16):1810–8.

30. Klein AL, Abbara S, Agler DA, et al. American Society of Echocardiography clinical recommendations for multimodality cardiovascular imaging of patients with pericardial disease: endorsed by the Society for Cardiovascular Magnetic Resonance and Society of Cardiovascular Computed Tomography. J Am Soc Echocardiogr 2013;26(9):965–1012.e5.

31. Singh S, Wann LS, Schuchard GH, et al. Right ventricular and right atrial collapse in patients with cardiac tamponade–a combined echocardiographic and hemodynamic study. Circulation 1984;70(6):966–71.

32. Lekhakul A, Assawakawintip C, Fenstad ER, et al. Safety and outcome of percutaneous drainage of pericardial effusions in patients with cancer. Am J Cardiol 2018;122(6):1091–4.

33. Adler Y, Charron P, Imazio M, et al. 2015 ESC guidelines for the diagnosis and management of pericardial diseases. Rev Esp Cardiol (Engl Ed) 2015;68(12):1126.

34. Schusler R, Meyerson SL. Pericardial disease associated with malignancy. Curr Cardiol Rep 2018;20(10):92.

35. Wilson LD, Detterbeck FC, Yahalom J. Clinical practice. Superior vena cava syndrome with malignant causes. N Engl J Med 2007;356(18):1862–9.

36. Friedman T, Quencer KB, Kishore SA, et al. Malignant venous obstruction: superior vena cava syndrome and beyond. Semin Intervent Radiol 2017;34(4):398–408.

37. Urruticoechea A, Mesia R, Dominguez J, et al. Treatment of malignant superior vena cava syndrome by endovascular stent insertion. Experience on 52 patients with lung cancer. Lung Cancer 2004;43(2):209–14.

38. Lanciego C, Pangua C, Chacon JI, et al. Endovascular stenting as the first step in the overall management of malignant superior vena cava syndrome. AJR Am J Roentgenol 2009;193(2):549–58.

39. Rachapalli V, Boucher LM. Superior vena cava syndrome: role of the interventionalist. Can Assoc Radiol J 2014;65(2):168–76.

40. Chaudhary K, Gupta A, Wadhawan S, et al. Anesthetic management of superior vena cava syndrome due to anterior mediastinal mass. J Anaesthesiol Clin Pharmacol 2012;28(2):242–6.

41. Gardner JC, Royster RL. Airway collapse with an anterior mediastinal mass despite spontaneous ventilation in an adult. Anesth Analg 2011;113(2):239–42.

42. Goh MH, Liu XY, Goh YS. Anterior mediastinal masses: an anaesthetic challenge. Anaesthesia 1999;54(7):670–4.

43. Doshi SM, Shah P, Lei X, et al. Hyponatremia in hospitalized cancer patients and its impact on clinical outcomes. Am J Kidney Dis 2012;59(2):222–8.

44. Ellison DH, Berl T. Clinical practice. The syndrome of inappropriate antidiuresis. N Engl J Med 2007;356(20):2064–72.

45. Milionis HJ, Liamis GL, Elisaf MS. The hyponatremic patient: a systematic approach to laboratory diagnosis. CMAJ 2002;166(8):1056–62.

46. Verbalis JG, Goldsmith SR, Greenberg A, et al. Diagnosis, evaluation, and treatment of hyponatremia: expert panel recommendations. Am J Med 2013;126(10 Suppl 1):S1–42.

47. Spasovski G, Vanholder R, Allolio B, et al. Clinical practice guideline on diagnosis and treatment of hyponatraemia. Intensive Care Med 2014;40(3):320–31.

48. Bach F, Larsen BH, Rohde K, et al. Metastatic spinal cord compression. Occurrence, symptoms, clinical presentations and prognosis in 398 patients with spinal cord compression. Acta Neurochir (Wien) 1990;107(1–2):37–43.

49. Schiff D, O'Neill BP, Suman VJ. Spinal epidural metastasis as the initial manifestation of malignancy: clinical features and diagnostic approach. Neurology 1997; 49(2):452–6.

50. Gabriel K, Schiff D. Metastatic spinal cord compression by solid tumors. Semin Neurol 2004;24(4):375–83.

51. Helweg-Larsen S, Sorensen PS. Symptoms and signs in metastatic spinal cord compression: a study of progression from first symptom until diagnosis in 153 patients. Eur J Cancer 1994;30A(3):396–8.

52. Levack P, Graham J, Collie D, et al. Don't wait for a sensory level–listen to the symptoms: a prospective audit of the delays in diagnosis of malignant cord compression. Clin Oncol (R Coll Radiol) 2002;14(6):472–80.

53. Lawton AJ, Lee KA, Cheville AL, et al. Assessment and management of patients with metastatic spinal cord compression: a multidisciplinary review. J Clin Oncol 2019;37(1):61–71.

54. In: 2019 surveillance of metastatic spinal cord compression in adults: risk assessment, diagnosis and management (NICE guideline CG75). London: National Institute for Health and Care Excellence; 2019.

55. Al-Qurainy R, Collis E. Metastatic spinal cord compression: diagnosis and management. BMJ 2016;353:i2539.

56. Binnahil M, Au K, Lu JQ, et al. The influence of corticosteroids on diagnostic accuracy of biopsy for primary central nervous system lymphoma. Can J Neurol Sci 2016;43(5):721–5.

57. Howard SC, Jones DP, Pui CH. The tumor lysis syndrome. N Engl J Med 2011; 364(19):1844–54.

58. Durani U, Shah ND, Go RS. In-hospital outcomes of tumor lysis syndrome: a population-based study using the National Inpatient Sample. Oncologist 2017; 22(12):1506–9.

59. Maiuolo J, Oppedisano F, Gratteri S, et al. Regulation of uric acid metabolism and excretion. Int J Cardiol 2016;213:8–14.

60. Darmon M, Vincent F, Camous L, et al. Tumour lysis syndrome and acute kidney injury in high-risk haematology patients in the rasburicase era. A prospective multicentre study from the Groupe de Recherche en Reanimation Respiratoire et Onco-Hematologique. Br J Haematol 2013;162(4):489–97.

61. Davidson MB, Thakkar S, Hix JK, et al. Pathophysiology, clinical consequences, and treatment of tumor lysis syndrome. Am J Med 2004;116(8):546–54.

62. Howard SC, Trifilio S, Gregory TK, et al. Tumor lysis syndrome in the era of novel and targeted agents in patients with hematologic malignancies: a systematic review. Ann Hematol 2016;95(4):563–73.

63. Cairo MS, Coiffier B, Reiter A, et al. Recommendations for the evaluation of risk and prophylaxis of tumour lysis syndrome (TLS) in adults and children with malignant diseases: an expert TLS panel consensus. Br J Haematol 2010;149(4): 578–86.

64. Cairo MS, Bishop M. Tumour lysis syndrome: new therapeutic strategies and classification. Br J Haematol 2004;127(1):3–11.

65. Jones GL, Will A, Jackson GH, et al. Guidelines for the management of tumour lysis syndrome in adults and children with haematological malignancies on behalf of the British Committee for Standards in Haematology. Br J Haematol 2015; 169(5):661–71.

66. Criscuolo M, Fianchi L, Dragonetti G, et al. Tumor lysis syndrome: review of pathogenesis, risk factors and management of a medical emergency. Expert Rev Hematol 2016;9(2):197–208.

67. Lopez-Olivo MA, Pratt G, Palla SL, et al. Rasburicase in tumor lysis syndrome of the adult: a systematic review and meta-analysis. Am J Kidney Dis 2013;62(3): 481–92.
68. Wilson FP, Berns JS. Tumor lysis syndrome: new challenges and recent advances. Adv Chronic Kidney Dis 2014;21(1):18–26.
69. Wang DY, Salem JE, Cohen JV, et al. Fatal toxic effects associated with immune checkpoint inhibitors: a systematic review and meta-analysis. JAMA Oncol 2018; 4(12):1721–8.
70. Postow MA. Managing immune checkpoint-blocking antibody side effects. American Society of Clinical Oncology Educational Book 2015;35:76–83.
71. Vardhana S, Cicero K, Velez MJ, et al. Strategies for recognizing and managing immune-mediated adverse events in the treatment of Hodgkin lymphoma with checkpoint inhibitors. Oncologist 2019;24(1):86–95.
72. Baraibar I, Melero I, Ponz-Sarvise M, et al. Safety and tolerability of immune checkpoint inhibitors (PD-1 and PD-L1) in cancer. Drug Saf 2019;42(2):281–94.
73. Brahmer JR, Lacchetti C, Schneider BJ, et al. Management of immune-related adverse events in patients treated with immune checkpoint inhibitor therapy: American Society of Clinical Oncology clinical practice guideline. J Clin Oncol 2018;36(17):1714–68.
74. Shimabukuro-Vornhagen A, Godel P, Subklewe M, et al. Cytokine release syndrome. J Immunother Cancer 2018;6(1):56.
75. Bonifant CL, Jackson HJ, Brentjens RJ, et al. Toxicity and management in CAR T-cell therapy. Mol Ther Oncolytics 2016;3:16011.
76. Brudno JN, Kochenderfer JN. Toxicities of chimeric antigen receptor T cells: recognition and management. Blood 2016;127(26):3321–30.
77. Le RQ, Li L, Yuan W, et al. FDA approval summary: tocilizumab for treatment of chimeric antigen receptor T cell-induced severe or life-threatening cytokine release syndrome. Oncologist 2018;23(8):943–7.
78. Garcia Borrega J, Godel P, Ruger MA, et al. In the eye of the storm: immune-mediated toxicities associated with CAR-T cell therapy. Hemasphere 2019;3(2): e191.

Palliative, Ethics, and End-of-Life Care Issues in the Cancer Patient

Jamie C. Riches, DO*, Louis P. Voigt, MD, FCCP, MBE

KEYWORDS

- Bioethics • Cancer • Critical illness • Palliative care • End of life

KEY POINTS

- Cancer encompasses a range of disease processes with varying trajectories that include end of life (EOL).
- Patients favor their oncologists over other clinicians to explore their values, goals, and preferences, but too often, these discussions are initiated by hospital or critical care physicians.
- EOL care for patients with cancer often follows a sentinel event, limiting patient decision-making capacity and shifting the burden of decision making to unprepared surrogates.
- Absent institutional resources that promote high-quality palliative care, the provision of EOL care in the intensive care unit is fraught with ethical challenges that can impact patients'/surrogates' experience.

INTRODUCTION

Cancer is a complex array of diseases, with varying incidence, prevalence, and mortality. An estimated 18.1 million new cancer cases occurred worldwide in 2018, with 1 in 8 men and 1 in 10 women likely to be diagnosed with cancer during their lifetimes.[1,2] Disparities in access to effective interventions for the prevention, detection, and treatment of cancer persist globally, and mortality rates are either increasing or at best stabilizing for many cancer types in countries in developmental transition.[2] Incidence and survival rates are unbalanced among regional racial and ethnic groups.[3] Cancer is a leading cause of premature mortality (ie, deaths at ages 30–69 years) in more than 100 countries worldwide and is the second most common cause of death globally, accounting for an estimated 9.6 million deaths in 2018.[2] In the first 2 decades of the 21st century, cancer has replaced cardiovascular diseases as the leading cause of death in several affluent countries.[4]

Memorial Sloan Kettering Cancer Center, 1275 York Avenue, New York, NY 10065, USA
* Corresponding author.
E-mail address: richesj@mskcc.org

Crit Care Clin 37 (2021) 105–115
https://doi.org/10.1016/j.ccc.2020.08.005

Patients with cancer are prone to acute illnesses related to cancer, cancer-directed therapies, and other comorbid conditions. Yet, cancer is rarely cited as the primary reason for admission to the hospital or the intensive care unit (ICU).[5] The outcomes of these cancer-related admissions are often determined by the patient's characteristics (eg, frailty), the reversibility of the critical illness, and the social determinants of health.[6] Contrary to chronic illnesses associated with organ failures, most patients with cancer experience a trajectory of steady progression and a clear terminal phase.[7]

At the crossroads of oncology and acute illnesses, new relationships between patients and hospital and critical care medicine specialists emerge in the crucible of end-of-life (EOL) care. Regardless of prior therapeutic alliances with their oncologists, these new interactions between patients and hospitalists or intensivists can generate a plurality of ethical challenges (**Table 1**). Prognostic uncertainty, patients' willingness to undergo chemotherapy near the end of life, and physicians' discomfort or reluctance can interfere with candid explorations of patient's preferences.[8] In instances of advanced or multiply relapsed cancer, oncologists and patients may engage in a Sisyphean pursuit of disease control and become oblivious to sentinel events auguring fatal outcomes.[9] Families' anguish about the future and their influence on treatment decisions, patients' inaccurate expectations of chemotherapy, and physicians' proclivity to confirmation bias can lead to therapeutic misconception and illusion.[9–11] This article expands on the scope of the ethical conundrums that arise in the provision of EOL care to adult patients with cancer.

BARRIERS TO END-OF-LIFE CARE

The last 3 decades have borne many milestones in oncology and critical care medicine. The addition of checkpoint inhibitors and chimeric antigen receptor T-cell therapy has improved the longevity and quality of life of patients with advanced-stage melanoma, relapsed leukemia, and refractory lymphoma.[12–16] A remarkable reduction in hospital and ICU mortality is attributed to several factors: broader adherence to enhanced management of acute respiratory distress syndrome (ARDS) with low tidal volume ventilation strategies, better sepsis management and early initiation of appropriate antibiotics, and general improvement in ICU care with less liberal use of

| Table 1 |
| Range of ethical issues surrounding end of life care for critically ill patients with cancer |

Triggers	Patient-Related	Surrogate-Related	Provider-Related	Institution-Related
Request for NBI	Therapeutic misconception	Therapeutic illusion	Miscommunication	Laxed protocol
Excessive EOL care	Lack of understanding	Burden of decision	Tyranny of autonomy	Poor ICU triage
Refusal of Analgesics	Redemptive suffering	Guilt	Moral distress	Menu approach to EOL
WOLST	Confusing or lack of AD	Disregard to AD	Unaware of fiduciary	Lack of resources[a]
Informed refusal	Lack of decisional capacity	Limits of SDM	Ambiguous responsibilities	Confusing policies

Abbreviations: AD, advance directive; NBI, nonbeneficial interventions; SDM, surrogate decision making; WOLST, withholding or withdrawing of life-sustaining therapies.
[a] Resources = supportive care, social work, chaplaincy, ethics review, and legal services.

intravenous fluids and restrictive transfusion practices.[17–24] Compared with decades prior, higher survival rates were noted for cardiopulmonary resuscitation (CPR) in patients with cancer in the early years of the 21st century.[25] Paradoxically, cancer has become the leading cause of mortality in several high-income countries, in part because of concurrent progress in the care of patients with cardiovascular diseases.

The increased prevalence of cancer, combined with the improved survival associated with cancer, sepsis, ARDS, and CPR in many countries, has wrought ambiguity among many patients and physicians and erected new barriers to EOL care discussions.[26] Nuances between serious illness, severe illness, critical illness, and terminal illness; misperceptions about palliative medicine and hospice care; and confusion about the meaning of actively dying, terminal care, end of life, and comfort measures represent important hurdles to the delivery of care that is aligned to the patient's preferences and interests.[27,28] Oncologists have mixed perceptions of hospice enrollment because of inherent limitations in delivering round-the-clock care and supportive treatments such as blood transfusions.[29] As opposed to patients with advanced solid tumors, those with hematological malignancies characteristically experience a fluctuating illness trajectory leading to difficulties with prognostication. Often, deterioration is unpredictable and rapid, and can lead to a swift change in goals of care from curative to palliative.[30]

Prognostic heterogeneity for different types of cancer, lack of time and training, uninformed submission to the tyranny of autonomy, physicians' attitudes toward death in the ICU, cognitive biases, hardship by medical oncologists grieving patients' loss, surgical buy-in, and missed opportunities by oncologists, hospitalists, and intensivists contribute to delayed appraisal of prognosis and preparation of advance directives.[31–35]

Inadequate explorations of EOL care preferences by patients, surrogates, physicians, and nurses are manifestations of the human emotions and helplessness (see **Table 1**). Patients' reluctance to discuss death stems perhaps from a Panglossian outlook on life-limiting illnesses or lack of accurate information about prognosis, while hurried physicians may feel obligated to reassure worried patients.[9,36] Discussions about EOL care options tend to occur during sentinel events, in the acute hospital care setting, with providers other than oncologists, and late in the course of cancer.[37] Patients express preferences for discussing EOL care with their oncologists and for their primary physicians/oncologists to initiate the discussion during sentinel events (ie, hospitalizations, progression of the cancer, or when cancer-directed therapies are exhausted)[38] (**Table 2**).

Members of the ICU or inpatient team may not fully grasp the complexity of a cancer prognosis and treatment options. Similarly, oncologists may not appreciate the severity of the acute life-threatening illness and the associated grim prognosis. These 2 teams must work together to reach consensus on achievable goals. Progressive organ failure, despite an extensive range of life-supporting interventions, demonstrable lack of improvement, low to no chance of reversibility, or progression of cancer should prompt discussions between patients/surrogates and oncologists/hospitalists or intensivists of patients' prognosis and goals of care, and of exploration of patients' preferences and EOL treatment options.[39]

Physician-surrogate discordance is common and has been attributed to misunderstandings by surrogates about physicians' assessments of patients' prognoses, and to surrogates' convictions of their superior knowledge of patients' unique strengths, magical thinking, and religious beliefs.[40,41] In the ICU, surrogates with more hopeful beliefs correlated to longer use of life-supporting interventions and longer ICU stay at the end of life.[42]

Table 2
Barriers to optimal timing of end-of-life discussion

Barrier	Involved Populous	Potential Solutions
Reluctance to discuss death/ emotional toll of anticipated death	Patient, family/surrogate, oncologist, hospitalist, intensivist	Societal and organizational destigmatization- eliminate the battle mentality; involve religious/cultural leaders
Magical thinking/ dispositional optimism	Patient, family/surrogate, oncologist	Interdisciplinary communication teams, protocols for information sharing/truth telling; involve religious/cultural leaders
Prognostic uncertainty	Patient, family/surrogate, oncologist, hospitalist, intensivist	Interdisciplinary communication teams, protocols for information sharing/truth telling
Therapeutic misconception	Patient, family/surrogate	Interdisciplinary communication teams, protocols for information sharing/truth telling; informed consent
Uncertainty regarding optimal timing for EOL conversations	Patient, family/surrogate, oncologist	Early palliative care/interdisciplinary communication teams

BENEFITS OF END-OF-LIFE CARE EXPLORATIONS

Multiple randomized trials have shown that simultaneous delivery of palliative and oncology care in the outpatient setting improves patient-reported outcomes, and in 1 study involving patients with metastatic non-small-cell lung cancer, early palliative care led to longer survival.[43,44] In light of accruing evidence regarding its benefits, timely hospice enrollment is now endorsed as an indicator of high-quality EOL care.[29] So is dying at home. Hospice care in patients whose cancers carry a poor prognosis is associated with a lower incidence of hospital admissions, ICU admissions, and invasive procedures during the last year of life.[45] In the United States, for the first time since the early 20th century, home has surpassed the hospital as the most common place of death.[46]

Recognizing the multifaceted aspects and complexity of cancer care, the American Society of Clinical Oncology (ASCO) proposes consideration of palliative care throughout the cancer care trajectory and recommends that every adult patient with advanced cancer should be treated by a multidisciplinary palliative care team - in addition to her/his oncologist - within 8 weeks of diagnosis.[47,48] Both ASCO and the American Association of Hospice and Palliative Medicine endorse a more integrated model of high-quality palliative care.[49]

For many adult patients with metastatic, relapsed, or refractory cancers, and for those who cannot receive cancer-directed therapies because of poor performance status or underlying comorbid conditions, major challenges persist and center on access to high-quality palliative and hospice care, stigmatization and negative stereotyping, shortage of specialized providers, and lack of time and training for oncologists and for hospital and critical care medicine specialists. The term palliative care is perceived by medical oncologists and other cancer-care providers as more distressing and reducing hope to patients and families.[50] By 2030, the number of patients eligible for palliative care is expected to grow by over 20%, with a concurrent absolute increase of 1% in the number of palliative care physicians, resulting in a ratio of only 1 physician for every 26,000 patients.[51,52]

Early integration of an interdisciplinary palliative care team may result in a reduction of unnecessary ICU admissions, shorter ICU and hospital length of stay, and high-quality EOL care with expert management of distressing symptoms before/during withdrawal of life-sustaining interventions, discontinuation of monitoring, and dignity-preserving care.[39]

ETHICS OF END-OF LIFE CARE IN ONCOLOGY PRACTICE

Bioethics is a relatively new field in health sciences that analyzes concepts and practices through the prism of medical, professional, legal, and societal standards. The evolution of bioethics is intimately linked to advances in medical technologies and in life-sustaining therapies. In medicine, ethical dilemmas occur when patients, surrogates, and physicians are confronted with the need to choose among 2 or more morally acceptable options or between 2 or more equally unacceptable courses of action, when 1 choice prevents the selection of the other.[53] At the crossroads of critical care medicine, hospice and palliative medicine, and oncology research and practice, lie major ethical issues related to the patients, surrogate-decision makers, physicians and other members of the health care team, as well as the institution and society at large.

Ethical issues associated with the provision of EOL care for seriously or critically ill patients with cancer are multifaceted. They range from equitable ICU triage decision and avoidance of excessive ICU care to withholding/withdrawing of life-sustaining interventions and relief of suffering. Implicit in medical decision making is the principle of nonmaleficence: Do no harm. The doctrine of double effect, stemming from medieval theological ideology, frames the moral choice of an action based on the proportionality between bad effects and unrelated and unintended but foreseen and tolerated good effects (relief of suffering must not be directly caused by death).[54]

Some patients encounter difficulty in accepting the diagnosis of cancer and related prognosis, and they do not share their wishes with their surrogates. In the United States, patients are reluctant to articulate their values and preferences, and only one-third of the adult population has any types of advance directive.[55] Patients' values and preferences are by far the primary directives of decision making and a manifestation of respect for autonomy. In the absence of clear advance directives for patients with cancer who lack decisional capacity, the burden of EOL care choices falls on families. Aside from patient's known wishes documented in advance directives, the standards for surrogate decision making are substituted judgment and best interests and they are relevant for critically-ill patients who frequently lack decisional capacity. Substituted judgment implies an intimate knowledge of patients' preferences based on their personal or moral beliefs, while best interests prioritize patients' welfare.[56]

Some patients are altruistic, and their primary preoccupations are about minimizing emotional or other burdens on family members.[57] Therefore, physicians caring for critically ill incapacitated patients should be nimble in their interactions with surrogates; they should grant surrogates some latitude and be more supportive of their decisions. A different model of substituted interests and best judgment offers the potential of shared decisions that can be shouldered by both surrogates and physicians.[58] Clinical equipoise exists as to the benefits of this new model compared with the hierarchical standards of surrogate decision making.

Shared decision making improves health outcomes for multiple patient populations. The role of families in medical decision making varies by demographic factors, such as race, ethnicity, religion, marital status, and age.[10] Prognostic uncertainty can create discomfort for cancer care providers at the EOL and can limit communication between clinicians and patients and families. Most surrogates, however, see prognostic uncertainty as unavoidable and acceptable and desire a discussion of uncertain prognoses.[59]

Disagreements may arise among surrogates, among physicians, between patients and surrogates, between patients and physicians, and between surrogates and physicians (**Fig. 1**). These conflicts can be exacerbated by the emotional toll of anticipated death and by diverging assessments of patients' prognoses. An iterative process of thoughtful conversations with patients and surrogates, preferably in the outpatient setting, can help resolve these often-predictable conundrums. Major events such as admissions to the hospital or ICU offer opportunity to explore patients' preferences. Through nonjudgmental communication strategies, hospitalists, oncologists, and ICU physicians and nurses can mitigate the negative emotional toll on surrogates when making EOL care decisions.[57]

The presence of therapeutic misconception, misestimation, and dispositional optimism add complexity to the ability to accept cancer diagnoses and prognoses and to formulate objective preferences for EOL care.[9,60–62] Early discussions of patients' goals and values are prospectively associated with less aggressive care and greater use of hospice at EOL.[27] Current guidelines recommend that discussions about EOL care planning begin early in the disease course for patients with incurable cancer, during periods of relative medical stability rather than acute deterioration, and with physicians who know the patients well.[63]

The ethical dilemmas in the EOL care of patients with cancer are not limited to physicians. The most frequently reported ethical quandaries by oncology nurses include uncertainties and barriers to truth telling in the context of prognostic information, conflicting obligations to patients and family members, and futility (ie, the provision of nonbeneficial treatment).[64] Recurring exposure to such dilemmas, coupled with the

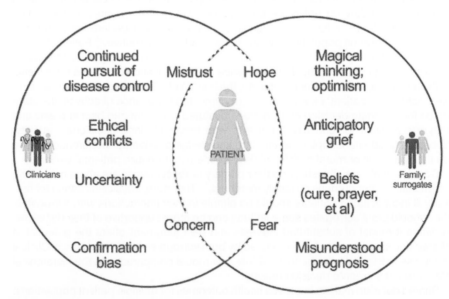

Fig. 1. Factors that complicate EOL discussions.

repeated exposure to death and dying, can, over, time give rise to maladaptive psycho-emotional states (eg, compassion fatigue, moral distress, or burnout) that negatively impact clinicians' well-being, professional quality of life, and job turnover.[65] A better ethical climate in the ICU can alleviate these predicaments.

Organizational ethics imposes on health care organizations the obligations for availing their staff with adequate resources for the safe and efficient delivery of care. ICU triage decisions can be influenced by the number of ICU beds[66] and can lead to agonizing decisions. When evaluating critically ill patients with cancer in need of ICU care, prognostic uncertainty and triage decisions can be additional sources of moral anguish for nurses, oncologists, hospitalists, and intensivists, since delay in ICU admission for patients deemed too-well to benefit carries an inappropriately high mortality rate.[67] Systematic processes of collaboration between oncologists, hospitalists, and intensivists on ICU triage decision can facilitate coherent communication with patients/families and cogent management of their expectations.[68] An institutional culture of frequent and transparent discussions between oncologists and members of the ICU team (intensivists, nurses, and pharmacists) is associated with improved mortality and efficient resource utilization.[69] Retention of ICU staff is more likely to occur in an ethical climate of professionalism, mutual respect, open interdisciplinary reflections, and EOL decisions that are not deferred or avoided.[70]

SUMMARY

Cancer is a broad diagnosis, encompassing a wide array of disease sites and processes, with varying therapeutic options and prognoses. Patients with advanced or relapsed/refractory cancers can develop acute and critical illnesses of multiple etiologies. Recent interests in studying the benefits of palliative care for patients with solid tumors enrolled in phase 1 clinical trials merit broad support.[71,72] These efforts should be expanded to patients with hematological malignancies. They are also likely to generate new controversies about the values and deontology of such practices.[73] The death trajectory for incurable cancer differs greatly from that of other advanced diseases, often with a steep decline over weeks to months prior to death.[7] Timing of EOL discussions is inconsistent, and best practice recommends early involvement of palliative care teams. Organizational cultures that promote strong interdisciplinary communication, awareness of internal barriers and biases, and early initiation of end-of-life discussions are essential to honoring patients' wishes for maintaining dignity in death.

REFERENCES

1. Bray F, Ferlay J, Soerjomataram I, et al. Global cancer statistics 2018: GLOBOCAN estimates of incidence and mortality worldwide for 36 cancers in 185 countries. CA Cancer J Clin 2018;68(6):394–424.
2. Wild CP, Weiderpass E, Stewart BW. World cancer report: cancer research for cancer prevention. Lyon (France): International Agency for Research on Cancer; 2020. Licence: CC BY-NC-ND 3.0 IGO. Available at: http://publications.iarc.fr/586. Accessed February 23, 2020.
3. DeSantis CE, Miller KD, Goding Sauer A, et al. Cancer statistics for African Americans, 2019. CA Cancer J Clin 2019;69(3):211–33.
4. Dagenais GR, Leong DP, Rangarajan S, et al. Variations in common diseases, hospital admissions, and deaths in middle-aged adults in 21 countries from five continents (PURE): a prospective cohort study. Lancet 2020;395(10226): 785–94.

5. Simpson HK, Clancy M, Goldfrad C, et al. Admissions to intensive care units from emergency departments: a descriptive study. Emerg Med J 2005;22(6):423–8.

6. McDaniel JT, Nuhu K, Ruiz J, et al. Social determinants of cancer incidence and mortality around the world: an ecological study. Glob Health Promot 2019; 26(1):41–9.

7. Murray SA, Kendall M, Boyd K, et al. Illness trajectories and palliative care. BMJ 2005;330(7498):1007–11.

8. Keating NL, Landrum MB, Rogers SO Jr, et al. Physician factors associated with discussions about end-of-life care. Cancer 2010;116(4):998–1006.

9. Weeks JC, Catalano PJ, Cronin A, et al. Patients' expectations about effects of chemotherapy for advanced cancer. N Engl J Med 2012;367(17):1616–25.

10. Hobbs GS, Landrum MB, Arora NK, et al. The role of families in decisions regarding cancer treatments. Cancer 2015;121(7):1079–87.

11. Casarett D. The science of choosing wisely–overcoming the therapeutic illusion. N Engl J Med 2016;374(13):1203–5.

12. Wolchok JD, Chiarion-Sileni V, Gonzalez R, et al. Overall survival with combined nivolumab and ipilimumab in advanced melanoma. N Engl J Med 2017;377(14): 1345–56.

13. Larkin J, Chiarion-Sileni V, Gonzalez R, et al. Five-year survival with combined nivolumab and ipilimumab in advanced melanoma. N Engl J Med 2019;381(16): 1535–46.

14. Siegel RL, Miller KD, Jemal A. Cancer statistics, 2020. CA Cancer J Clin 2020; 70(1):7–30.

15. Maude SL, Frey N, Shaw PA, et al. Chimeric antigen receptor T cells for sustained remissions in leukemia. N Engl J Med 2014;371(16):1507–17.

16. Schuster SJ, Bishop MR, Tam CS, et al. Tisagenlecleucel in adult relapsed or refractory diffuse large B-cell lymphoma. N Engl J Med 2019;380(1):45–56.

17. Kumar G, Kumar N, Taneja A, et al. Nationwide trends of severe sepsis in the 21st century (2000-2007). Chest 2011;140(5):1223–31.

18. Zambon M, Vincent JL. Mortality rates for patients with acute lung injury/ARDS have decreased over time. Chest 2008;133(5):1120–7.

19. Azoulay E, Lemiale V, Mokart D, et al. Acute respiratory distress syndrome in patients with malignancies. Intensive Care Med 2014;40(8):1106–14.

20. Erickson SE, Martin GS, Davis JL, et al. Recent trends in acute lung injury mortality: 1996-2005. Crit Care Med 2009;37(5):1574–9.

21. Rhodes A, Evans LE, Alhazzani W, et al. Surviving sepsis campaign: international guidelines for management of sepsis and septic shock: 2016. Intensive Care Med 2017;43(3):304–77.

22. Corl KA, Prodromou M, Merchant RC, et al. The restrictive IV fluid trial in severe sepsis and septic shock (RIFTS): a randomized pilot study. Crit Care Med 2019; 47(7):951–9.

23. Carson JL, Guyatt G, Heddle NM, et al. Clinical practice guidelines from the AABB: red blood cell transfusion thresholds and storage. JAMA 2016;316(19): 2025–35.

24. Cable CA, Razavi SA, Roback JD, et al. RBC transfusion strategies in the ICU: a concise review. Crit Care Med 2019;47(11):1637–44.

25. Champigneulle B, Merceron S, Lemiale V, et al. What is the outcome of cancer patients admitted to the ICU after cardiac arrest? Results from a multicenter study. Resuscitation 2015;92:38–44.

26. Allemani C, Matsuda T, Di Carlo V, et al. Global surveillance of trends in cancer survival 2000-14 (CONCORD-3): analysis of individual records for 37 513 025

patients diagnosed with one of 18 cancers from 322 population-based registries in 71 countries. Lancet 2018;391(10125):1023–75.

27. Parikh RB, Kirch RA, Smith TJ, et al. Early specialty palliative care–translating data in oncology into practice. N Engl J Med 2013;369(24):2347–51.

28. Hui D, Nooruddin Z, Didwaniya N, et al. Concepts and definitions for "actively dying," "end of life," "terminally ill," "terminal care," and "transition of care": a systematic review. J Pain Symptom Manage 2014;47(1):77–89.

29. Odejide OO, Cronin AM, Earle CC, et al. Why are patients with blood cancers more likely to die without hospice? Cancer 2017;123(17):3377–84.

30. Button E, Chan RJ, Chambers S, et al. A systematic review of prognostic factors at the end of life for people with a hematological malignancy. BMC cancer 2017; 17(1):213.

31. Granek L, Krzyzanowska MK, Tozer R, et al. Oncologists' strategies and barriers to effective communication about the end of life. J Oncol Pract 2013;9(4): e129–35.

32. Einstein DJ, Einstein KL, Mathew P. Dying for advice: code status discussions between resident physicians and patients with advanced cancer–A national survey. J Palliat Med 2015;18(6):535–41.

33. Visser M, Deliens L, Houttekier D. Physician-related barriers to communication and patient- and family-centred decision-making towards the end of life in intensive care: a systematic review. Crit Care 2014;18(6):604.

34. Schwarze ML, Bradley CT, Brasel KJ. Surgical "buy-in": the contractual relationship between surgeons and patients that influences decisions regarding life-supporting therapy. Crit Care Med 2010;38(3):843–8.

35. Curtis JR, Engelberg RA, Wenrich MD, et al. Missed opportunities during family conferences about end-of-life care in the intensive care unit. Am J Respir Crit Care Med 2005;171(8):844–9.

36. Mori M, Shimizu C, Ogawa A, et al. A national survey to systematically identify factors associated with oncologists' attitudes toward end-of-life discussions: what determines timing of end-of-life discussions? Oncologist 2015;20(11): 1304–11.

37. Mack JW, Cronin A, Taback N, et al. End-of-life care discussions among patients with advanced cancer: a cohort study. Ann Intern Med 2012;156(3):204–10.

38. Johnson S, Butow P, Kerridge I, et al. Advance care planning for cancer patients: a systematic review of perceptions and experiences of patients, families, and healthcare providers. Psychooncology 2016;25(4):362–86.

39. Kiehl MG, Beutel G, Boll B, et al. Consensus statement for cancer patients requiring intensive care support. Ann Hematol 2018;97(7):1271–82.

40. White DB, Ernecoff N, Buddadhumaruk P, et al. Prevalence of and factors related to discordance about prognosis between physicians and surrogate decision makers of critically ill patients. JAMA 2016;315(19):2086–94.

41. Azoulay E, Kentish-Barnes N, Nelson JE. Communication with family caregivers in the intensive care unit: answers and questions. JAMA 2016;315(19):2075–7.

42. White DB, Carson S, Anderson W, et al. A multicenter study of the causes and consequences of optimistic expectations about prognosis by surrogate decision-makers in ICUs. Crit Care Med 2019;47(9):1184–93.

43. Temel JS, Greer JA, El-Jawahri A, et al. Effects of early integrated palliative care in patients with lung and GI cancer: a randomized clinical trial. J Clin Oncol 2017; 35(8):834–41 (1527-7755 (Electronic)).

44. Temel JS, Greer JA, Muzikansky A, et al. Early palliative care for patients with metastatic non-small-cell lung cancer. N Engl J Med 2010;363(8):733–42 (1533-4406 (Electronic)).

45. Obermeyer Z, Makar M, Abujaber S, et al. Association between the Medicare hospice benefit and health care utilization and costs for patients with poor-prognosis cancer. JAMA 2014;312(18):1888–96 (1538-3598 (Electronic)).

46. Cross SH, Warraich HJ. Changes in the place of death in the United States. N Engl J Med 2019;381(24):2369–70 (1533-4406 (Electronic)).

47. Ferrell BR, Temel JS, Temin S, et al. Integration of palliative care into standard oncology care: ASCO clinical practice guideline update summary. J Clin Oncol 2017;13(2):119–21 (1935-469X (Electronic)).

48. Ferris FD, Bruera E, Cherny N, et al. Palliative cancer care a decade later: accomplishments, the need, next steps – from the American Society of Clinical Oncology. J Clin Oncol 2009;27(18):3052–8.

49. Bickel KE, McNiff K, Buss MK, et al. Defining high-quality palliative care in oncology practice: an American Society of Clinical Oncology/American Academy of Hospice and Palliative Medicine guidance statement. J Oncol Pract 2016; 12(9):e828–38.

50. Fadul N, Elsayem A, Palmer JL, et al. Supportive versus palliative care: what's in a name?: a survey of medical oncologists and midlevel providers at a comprehensive cancer center. Cancer 2009;115(9):2013–21 (0008-543X (Print)).

51. Kamal AH, Bull JH, Swetz KM, et al. Future of the palliative care workforce: preview to an impending crisis. Am J Med 2017;130(2):113–4.

52. Solutions. Pf. Chronic conditions: making the case for ongoing care. 2004. Available at: http://www.partnershipforsolutions.org/DMS/files/chronicbook2004.pdf.

53. Ong WY, Yee CM, Lee A. Ethical dilemmas in the care of cancer patients near the end of life. Singapore Med J 2012;53(1):11–6.

54. Brescia FJ. Philosophical oncology: calling on the principle of double effect. Natl Compr Canc Netw 2003;1(3):429–34 (1540-1405 (Print)).

55. Yadav KN, Gabler NB, Cooney E, et al. Approximately one in three US adults completes any type of advance directive for end-of-life care. Health Aff (Millwood) 2017;36(7):1244–51.

56. Pope TM. Legal fundamentals of surrogate decision making. Chest 2012;141(4): 1074–81.

57. Berger JT, DeRenzo EG, Schwartz J. Surrogate decision making: reconciling ethical theory and clinical practice. Ann Intern Med 2008;149(1):48–53.

58. Sulmasy DP, Snyder L. Substituted interests and best judgments: an integrated model of surrogate decision making. JAMA 2010;304(17):1946–7.

59. Evans LR, Boyd EA, Malvar G, et al. Surrogate decision-makers' perspectives on discussing prognosis in the face of uncertainty. Am J Respir Crit Care Med 2009; 179(1):48–53.

60. Lidz CW, Appelbaum PS, Grisso T, et al. Therapeutic misconception and the appreciation of risks in clinical trials. Soc Sci Med 2004;58(9):1689–97.

61. Pentz RD, White M, Harvey RD, et al. Therapeutic misconception, misestimation, and optimism in participants enrolled in phase 1 trials. Cancer 2012;118(18): 4571–8.

62. Jansen LA, Mahadevan D, Appelbaum PS, et al. Dispositional optimism and therapeutic expectations in early-phase oncology trials. Cancer 2016;122(8): 1238–46.

63. Mack JW, Cronin A, Keating NL, et al. Associations between end-of-life discussion characteristics and care received near death: a prospective cohort study. J Clin Oncol 2012;30(35):4387–95.
64. McLennon SM, Uhrich M, Lasiter S, et al. Oncology nurses' narratives about ethical dilemmas and prognosis-related communication in advanced cancer patients. Cancer Nurs 2013;36(2):114–21.
65. Austin CL, Saylor R, Finley PJ. Moral distress in physicians and nurses: impact on professional quality of life and turnover. Psychol Trauma 2017;9(4):399–406 (1942-969X (Electronic)).
66. Garrouste-Orgeas M, Montuclard L, Timsit JF, et al. Predictors of intensive care unit refusal in French intensive care units: a multiple-center study. Crit Care Med 2005;33(4):750–5.
67. Thiery G, Azoulay E, Darmon M, et al. Outcome of cancer patients considered for intensive care unit admission: a hospital-wide prospective study. J Clin Oncol 2005;23(19):4406–13.
68. Malak S, Sotto JJ, Ceccaldi J, et al. Ethical and clinical aspects of intensive care unit admission in patients with hematological malignancies: guidelines of the ethics commission of the French society of hematology. Adv Hematol 2014; 2014:704318.
69. Soares M, Bozza FA, Azevedo LC, et al. Effects of organizational characteristics on outcomes and resource use in patients with cancer admitted to intensive care units. J Clin Oncol 2016;34(27):3315–24.
70. Van den Bulcke B, Metaxa V, Reyners AK, et al. Ethical climate and intention to leave among critical care clinicians: an observational study in 68 intensive care units across Europe and the United States. Intensive Care Med 2020;46(1): 46–56.
71. Cassel JB, Del Fabbro E, Arkenau T, et al. Phase I cancer trials and palliative care: antagonism, irrelevance, or synergy? J Pain Symptom Manage 2016; 52(3):437–45.
72. Ferrell BR, Chung V, Koczywas M, et al. Palliative care and phase 1 trials: intervention to improve quality of life and provide education. Clin J Oncol Nurs 2017;21(4):473–9.
73. Adashek JJ, LoRusso PM, Hong DS, et al. Phase I trials as valid therapeutic options for patients with cancer. Nat Rev Clin Oncol 2019;16(12):773–8.

Section 2: Geriatric Critical Care

Preface

Caring for the Elderly in the Intensive Care Unit

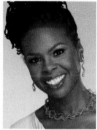

Wendy R. Greene, MD, FACS, FCCM   Maxwell A. Hockstein, MD

Editors

In this issue of Geriatric *Critical Care Clinics*, we focus on older adults admitted to the intensive care unit (ICU) and the importance of assessing their baseline states of health, understanding their unique physiology, and synthesizing appropriate care plans.

Adults greater than 65 years of age are an increasingly seen demographic in the ICU. Geriatric patients have unique physiology and certain predispositions to pathologic conditions. Common diagnoses such as malignancies, frailty, malnutrition, trauma, and dementia are some of the realities of this patient population which complicate critical illness amidst polypharmacy and social concerns. Moreover, rehabilitation of the critically ill geriatric patient population is complicated by an unlikely return to premorbid status once admitted to the ICU. Older adults in the ICU, regardless of the indication for admission or care trajectory, should have a goals-of-care conversation. Shared decision making is critical to align medical expertise and interventions with the patient's values.

The goal of the critical care team when caring for the older patient should be to first, respect the patient's (and/or family's) wishes, and second, to return the patient as close to their premorbid state as possible. Most importantly, the team needs to communicate with the patient and family the limitations and consequences of interventions often performed in the critical care arena. To accomplish this, the intensivist must understand the physiology of the older patient to provide adequate resuscitation when needed.

In the articles that follow, authors carefully review the impact of malignancies, frailty, malnutrition, traumatic injuries, dementia, and the rehabilitation considerations on geriatric patients admitted to the ICU.

Crit Care Clin 37 (2021) xvii–xviii
https://doi.org/10.1016/j.ccc.2020.10.002
0749-0704/21/© 2020 Published by Elsevier Inc.

criticalcare.theclinics.com

We hope that addressing these topics will help clinicians understand the unique challenges and opportunities in caring for the elderly patient in the ICU.

Wendy R. Greene, MD, FACS, FCCM
Department of Surgery
Emory University College of Medicine
1365 Clifton Road NE Building A, 4th Floor
Atlanta, GA 30322, USA

Maxwell A. Hockstein, MD
Department of Critical Care
MedStar Washington Hospital Center
110 Irving Street Northwest
Washington, DC 20010, USA

E-mail addresses:
wendy.ricketts.greene@emory.edu (W.R. Greene)
max.hockstein@gmail.com (M.A. Hockstein)

Rehabilitation Concerns in the Geriatric Critically Ill and Injured - Part 1

Corey X. Tapper, MD, MS[a],*, Kimberly Curseen, MD[b,c]

KEYWORDS

- Geriatric palliative care • Frailty • Delirium • Dementia • Pain • Constipation
- Rehabilitation • Prognostication

KEY POINTS

- Frailty is an independent risk factor for progressive physical dependence and mortality.
- Delirium is associated with poor long-term outcomes, including increased institutionalization, cognitive impairment, falls, and pneumonia.
- Hospitalized patients with dementia have increased short-term morbidity and mortality and do not return to previous baseline functional status after acute decompensation resolves.
- Prognostication tools and performance scales such as the Palliative Performance Scale should be used to help determine rehabilitation expectations.
- Goals of care should be determined before entering into a rehabilitation service.

INTRODUCTION

Geriatric patients who are critically ill have unique challenges that must be considered when attempting to prognosticate survival and determine expectations for rehabilitation and meaningful recovery. Furthermore, elderly patients with frailty present distinct rehabilitation and clinical challenges when suffering from critical illness. There are multiple symptoms and syndromes that negatively affect morbidity and mortality of elderly patients who require intensive care unit (ICU) management, including frailty, delirium, dementia, pain and constipation. Although long-term prognosis for elderly patients in the ICU may be poor, there are scenarios in which prognostic awareness is challenging. It is also important to consider options for physical rehabilitation after discharge based on the patient's functional status, care needs, and goals of care.

---

[a] Division of General Internal Medicine, Section of Palliative Medicine, Johns Hopkins University School of Medicine, 1830 East Monument Street, Suite 8021, Baltimore, MD 21287, USA;
[b] Department of Medicine, Emory University School of Medicine, Atlanta, GA, USA;
[c] Supportive and Palliative Care Outpatient Services, Emory Healthcare, 1821 Clifton Road, Northeast, Suite 1017, Atlanta, GA 30329, USA
* Corresponding author.
E-mail address: ctapper1@jhmi.edu

Crit Care Clin 37 (2021) 117–134
https://doi.org/10.1016/j.ccc.2020.08.012 **criticalcare.theclinics.com**
0749-0704/21/© 2020 The Authors. Published by Elsevier Inc. This is an open access article under
the CC BY-NC-ND license (http://creativecommons.org/licenses/by-nc-nd/4.0/).

DISCUSSION
Physiology of Aging

There are several natural changes that occur with aging that should be considered when medically managing elderly patients and creating long-term treatment plans after critical illness. An understanding of these age-related changes can help guide discussions with patients and families concerning long-term goals, practical expectation of recovery, and long-term survival.

There are several physiologic theories of aging ranging from destabilization of DNA integrity to reduction in physical reserves and energy metabolism.[1] What these theories have in common are progressive, irreversible, physiologic changes that lead to decline in both organ and physical function. These changes result in patients having less physiologic reserve to recover from an acute illness. The changes that occur in organs are at the molecular and cellular level and are specific to organ type and function.[2,3] Declines in plasma proteins, as well as renal and liver function, affect clearance of medications in the elderly. This results in narrowing of therapeutic windows for drugs used to treat and palliate critical illness, which can present challenges to meaningful recovery and rehabilitation.[4]

Nervous system

Changes in the nervous system lead to decreased fine motor control with aging and present challenges for elderly patients who develop muscle weakness from an acute illness, as they may not be able to recover fine motor skills that are required for certain activities of daily living such as dressing (ie, buttoning and zipping) even with adequate rehabilitation. Special attention may be required, with the addition of assist devices introduced early to assist patients with adaptation. For these patients, early planning for ongoing assistance may need to be considered.[5]

Musculoskeletal/Skin

Lean muscle mass decreases with aging. The rate of muscle mass decline is about 15% per decade up to age 50 years and then accelerates to about 30% per decade after age 60 years. The rate of replacing muscle tissue declines with advancing age. There is an increase in fat deposits and lipofuscin, which leads to loss of strength, tone, and contractility over time, which can result in an overall loss of strength and endurance.[2,3] This makes elderly patients more susceptible to sarcopenia, which is a syndrome characterized by loss of skeletal muscle mass correlating with physical debility, decline in quality of life, and death.[6] Elderly patients who are critically ill are usually confined to bed for extensive periods of time and have poor nutritional status, both risk factors for sarcopenia. With the addition of normal muscle aging, this can adversely affect an elderly patient's ability to rehabilitate back to baseline after a critical illness. Development of sarcopenia increases 1-year mortality.[3,6] The aging skeletal system can develop increased joint stiffness and reduced flexibility, which can result in restricted movements and the development of chronic pain; this can limit an elder's functional recovery. The loss of skin elasticity and thickness increases the risk of pressure wounds.[3,5]

Cardiovascular

Age-related changes in the cardiovascular system, including increased myocardial stiffness, fat deposition, and reduction in response to cardiovascular agents, can lead to difficulties in compensation to cardiac stressors, and this can manifest as increased risk of arrhythmias and diastolic heart failure. Pacemaker cells decline at a rate of 10% per decade. Fibrosis, lipofuscin, and calcium deposition in the myocardium, secondary to aging, can manifest as prolonged QTc and PR intervals, contributing to arrhythmias under stress. Arteries become dilated and rigid, affecting responses to cardiovascular agents.[7–9]

Pulmonary
The changes in pulmonary tissue with aging result in decreased exercise tolerance and pulmonary reserve, which can present a challenge for elders recovering from an acute pulmonary insult. These patients may require longer, less intensive rehabilitation, which can optimize recovery of function and return to independence. By 80 years of age, the average person develops reductions in vital capacity, surface area of the lung, and forced vital capacity/forced expiratory capacity ratio by about 30%. Subsequently, elders develop increased residual volumes, decreased skeletal muscle mass and strength, reduction in lung elastic recoil, and decreased efforts in dependent and independent respiration, which can result in challenges to weaning and managing respiratory assist devices. There is a higher risk of both hypoxia and hypercapnia. Age-related changes of kyphosis can lead to narrowing of the intercostal spaces, which can contribute a restrictive physiology.[1,3,10]

Immune responses
Changes that occur in immunity with normal aging result in atrophy of the thymus, which contributes to decreases in T lymphocytes, natural killer cells, cytokines, and B-cell function. There is a decline in immune function with aging, which can blunt primary and secondary responses to new pathogens. As aging occurs, more time and stimulus are required to mount immune responses. This can make elderly patients more vulnerable to infections and their sequela.[1,9,11]

Cognitive decline
There are normal cognitive changes associated with aging that can include diminished spatial orientation, decline in perceptual speed, numeric ability, verbal memory, and slower problem solving. When patients are suffering from critical illness, these declines increase the risk for delirium and require consideration in developing rehabilitation plans. Patients may require more assistance during the recovery period with activities of independent living as they attempt to cognitively recover. Cognitive recovery can be prolonged. If an elder has an acute neurologic injury, the ceiling of recovery may be lower than that of a younger patient secondary to a decline in cognitive reserves.[3,12,13]

Sensory/Endocrine function
The natural decline of vision, hearing, and taste functions can have profound effects on recovering from an acute illness. Patients with sensory impairment are at higher risk for delirium when suffering from acute illness or injury. Also, sensory disturbances can present challenges to participation in rehabilitation leading to functional recovery.[3,14] There are also age-related changes in the endocrine system that can lead to alterations in stress responses and declines in functional capacity.[2,3,15] These changes likely contribute to the development of sarcopenia and frailty. See **Table 1** for further details regarding hormonal changes in aging.

When faced with physiologic stressors, the elderly may have more difficulty maintaining homeostasis secondary to homeostenosis, a narrowing of reserve capacity. Older patients with excellent premorbid status may struggle to recover and rehabilitate back to baseline or have increased mortality secondary to the decline in reserve capacity.[2] This difficulty stresses the importance of starting early, acute care interventions focused on preserving function, decreasing physiologic and emotional stress when managing frail elders in the acute care setting extending into rehabilitation.[16]

Table 1	
Effects of aging on the endocrine system	
Hormone Reductions	**Hormone Increases**
• Melatonin	• Atrial natriuretic peptide
• Growth hormone	• Parathyroid hormone
• Testosterone	• Norepinephrine
• Estrogen	• Erythropoietin
• Leptin	
• Cortisol	
• Aldosterone	
• Prolactin	
• DHEA	

Frailty

Frailty is a syndrome that is characterized by dysregulation and reduction of physiologic, physical, and cognitive reserve, which culminates in decline across several physiologic systems. Alterations in cellular processes affect the body's energy regulation and production, resulting in decreased reserve and resistance to stress causing a patient to be at risk for adverse outcomes.[17,18] The frailty phenotype identified by Fried and Walston is composed of weakness, slowness, exhaustion, low activity, and weight loss.[19] A consensus statement in 2013 characterized frailty as *"diminished strength, endurance, and reduced physiologic function that increases an individual's vulnerability for developing increased dependency and death."*[18]

Primary frailty is characterized by sarcopenia as its major manifestation and is independent of a comorbidity. Secondary frailty occurs when a patient has serious illness such as heart failure or chronic obstructive pulmonary disease and subsequently develops the frailty phenotype.[18,20,21]

There are several validated tools to identify frailty in the geriatric population. Frailty in older adults is associated with poor health outcomes, disability, worsening mobility, falls, emergency room visits, and hospitalizations. Frailty is an independent risk factor for progressive physical dependency and mortality. The prevalence of frailty has been noted to be about 7% to 10% in community-dwelling elders.[18,22,23]

Screening for frailty helps to identify patients at risk for poor outcomes in the surgical, hospital, skilled nursing, home, and ICU settings. Patients who have been identified as frail with end-stage renal disease have been associated with increased rates of falls, hospitalizations, and mortality.[23] Frailty screening tools have been used in the evaluation for renal transplant. Frailty predicts all-cause and postoperative mortality and chemotherapy intolerance in patients with cancer. In cardiac surgery, frailty screening tools have been used in preoperative risk assessments, medical decision-making, and palliative care consultation. Patients admitted to the ICU who have been identified as frail have worse health outcomes. In a systematic review, frail patients admitted to the ICU were less likely to be discharged to home and have increased mortality compared with nonfrail patients.[18,21] Refer to **Table 2** for details on validated frailty screening instruments.[18]

For patients who are critically ill and frail, it is appropriate to facilitate early discussions concerning goals of care with patients and their family. These discussions should identify surrogate decision makers, code status, and patient/family perception of an acceptable quality of life. Palliative Care and Geriatric consultations should be considered to assist with advanced care planning, prognostication, family meetings, and support. Prognostic information should be given in a compassionate and clear

Table 2
Validated frailty scales

Frailty Tool	Scoring	Tool Characteristics
Frailty Index (FI)	Scoring: 0–0.7 0.2–0.45: Frail 0.45–0.7: Severely frail	Based on a comprehensive geriatric assessment scale
Frailty Phenotype (FP)	FP ≥3 signifies frailty *Scoring*: 5 phenotypic criteria—weakness, slowness, low level of physical activity, self-reported exhaustion, unintentional weight loss	Objective and self-reported criteria, excludes cognition
Clinical Frailty Scale (CFS)	Scoring: 1–9 1–4: Nonfrail 5–6: Mild-to-moderately frail 7–8: Severely frail 9: Terminally ill	Subjective assessment of functional status

manner, focusing not only on immediate physical recovery from the acute illness but also long-term outcomes including expectations of physical and cognitive recovery.[20,21] The concept of frailty may be difficult for patients and families to understand and accept as reasons for poor clinical outcomes. This can especially be true if a patient is doing poorly secondary to primary frailty or if they developed the syndrome secondary to an acute illness but had excellent premorbid status.[24,25] Early identification of a surrogate and engaging them in collaborative decision-making during the patients treatment course will be key to achieve appropriate outcomes and establish trust when trying to explain this difficult concept.[18,20,26]

Delirium

Delirium is a neuropsychiatric syndrome that occurs in acutely ill individuals whose core features are inattention, acute onset, and fluctuating course that cannot be explained by a preexisting neurocognitive disorder.[27,28] Delirium is a clinical diagnosis based on comprehensive history and evaluation of cognitive function. In the elderly and critical care population, it is considered an emergency.[29] **Table 3** shows details regarding the diagnostic criteria of delirium according to the Diagnostic and Statistical Manual of Mental Disorders, Fifth Edition (DSM-V).[27]

Delirium is a widely underdiagnosed syndrome. It is among the most common complications in hospitalized patients aged 65 years and older.[30] Delirium affects 2.6 million elderly patients in the United States each year.[28,31] In the intensive care setting, the incidence of delirium is estimated to reach 20% to 50% of the general ICU patient population and up to 80% of those on mechanical ventilation.[28,32,33] Because of its insidious features, the hypoactive form of delirium is likely routinely unidentified in more than two-thirds of hospitalized patients.[34]

Although it can be caused by one insult, delirium is often multifactorial, especially in elderly patients. Elderly patients are more vulnerable to factors that predispose for delirium. The risk of delirium is increased if multiple factors are present.[28] Patients with underlying dementia are at increased risk for developing delirium with odds ratios (OR) ranging from 6.3 (95% confidence interval [CI]: 2.9–13.8) to 11.5 (95% CI: 6.1–20.1).[35,36] **Box 1** shows risk factors for ICU delirium.[31]

Table 3
Diagnostic criteria of delirium based on Diagnostic and Statistical Manual of Mental Disorders, Fifth Edition

Criteria	Explanation
Disturbance in attention	Decreased ability to direct, focus, shift, or sustain attention; easily distracted; impaired orientation to self or environment
Acute onset	Develops over a short period of time (hours to days); waxing/waning fluctuation in course
At least one other domain affected	Disorganized thinking; altered level of consciousness; altered memory and learning; alteration in language; perceptual distortions (eg,: hallucinations, delusions)

Supporting Features: altered sleep-wake cycle; emotional disturbances (eg, anxiety, agitation, apathy)

Data from Diagnostic and statistical manual of mental disorders: DSM-5. In. 5th ed. Washington, D.C.: American Psychiatric Association; 2013.

Given the incidence of delirium in hospitalized patients, especially those who are elderly and admitted to the ICU, it is important to proactively screen patients for this syndrome. Two of the most commonly used instruments for delirium screening in the ICU are the Confusion Assessment Method for the ICU (CAM-ICU)[37] and the Intensive Care Delirium Screening Checklist (ICDSC).[38] These instruments were specifically designed for patients with limited communication abilities. In 2012, a systematic review and meta-analysis showed the CAM-ICU had a pooled sensitivity of 80% and pooled specificity of 95.9%, whereas the ICDSC had a pooled sensitivity of 74% and pooled specificity of 81.9%.[39] These data suggest that although both instruments can be used as screening tools for delirium in the ICU setting, the CAM-ICU is the superior diagnostic instrument. However, not all studies show consistency in the diagnosis of delirium via these 2 tools. In 2017, a validation study compared these 2 instruments against the DSM-IV criteria for delirium. The CAM-ICU had moderate concurrent validity and sensitivity of 50% but high specificity of 95%. The ICDSC also had

Box 1
Risk factors for intensive care unit delirium

Comorbidity or severity of illness

Older age (≥75 years)

Sedative or hypnotic use

Increased serum urea

Metabolic acidosis

Infection

Neurosurgery

Trauma admission

Urgent admission

Coma

Data from Inouye SK, Westendorp RG, Saczynski JS. Delirium in elderly people. Lancet. 2014;383(9920):911-922.

moderate concurrent validity and sensitivity of 63% but high specificity of 95%. Between the 2 tools, the concurrent validity was moderate. The ICDSC yielded higher sensitivity and specificity of 78% and 83%, respectively.[32]

Delirium screening should be performed at multiple points throughout hospitalization, given its waxing/waning course and potentially subtle features. Consistently using the same instrument to assess for this syndrome allows for comparison over time. Furthermore, these tools should be used in conjunction with patient history, as well as collateral history from family and friends.

Delirium causes significant harm to hospitalized patients, especially those requiring ICU care. In a 2010 meta-analysis, delirium was found to have an increased risk of death compared with controls over a two-year follow-up period.[30] Other studies have also found delirium to be associated with increased mortality anywhere from 6 months[34] to 5 years.[28,29] Patients with delirium who are admitted to a postacute facility have a five-fold increased risk of six-month mortality.[40]

Delirium often occurs in patients who have other serious preexisting conditions. Delirium is associated with poor long-term outcomes in both cognitive and functional domains. Patients are at increased risk of institutionalization.[30,41] Patients with delirium have increased risk of dementia over a four-year follow-up period.[30] Patients with delirium have longer hospital length of stay, including post-ICU length of stay. These patients spend, on average, 10 more days in the hospital than those without delirium.[41] Delirious patients also have fewer ventilator-free days and increased cognitive impairment at hospital discharge.[34] In hospitalized delirious patients discharged to a postacute facility, there were higher rates of rehospitalization, falls, and pneumonia. There were lower rates of eventual discharge to the community.[40] Delirium is associated with chronic functional impairment up to 18 months after the episode.[28,30] These complications pose significant limitations to the potential rehabilitation of elderly patients.

Delirium severity and duration are independently associated with increased morbidity and mortality among older medical inpatients.[42,43] **Box 2** shows predictors of poor outcomes in the setting of delirium based on a 2015 systematic review.[44]

It is well established that patients treated in the ICU, for any reason, have significant incidences of posttraumatic stress disorder (PTSD) ranging from 14% to 44%. There are now case reports of hallucinations and delusions during episodes of delirium being linked by patients to PTSD.[45] In fact, a small study has suggested that one-third of all patients who suffer from delirium eventually develop PTSD.[46] Patients have higher risk of depression after an episode of delirium, although there is no apparent increased risk of anxiety.[47] Further research is warranted in these domains, especially regarding the onset of PTSD in ICU patients with delirium.

Box 2
Predictors of poor outcomes in delirium

Duration of delirium episode

Hypoactive subtype

Delirium severity

Preexisting neuropsychiatric morbidity with depression or dementia

Data from Jackson TA, Wilson D, Richardson S, Lord JM. Predicting outcome in older hospital patients with delirium: a systematic literature review. Int J Geriatr Psychiatry. 2016;31(4):392-399.

Efforts should be taken to aid in delirium prevention in hospitalized patients, given the known negative impacts of delirium on morbidity and mortality. The Hospital Elder Life Program (HELP) is an intervention strategy for delirium prevention. These interventions include several behavioral and environmental modifications such as reality orientation, minimization of psychoactive medications, use of a non-pharmacologic sleep protocol, early mobilization, and attention to feeding and nutrition.[48] A recent meta-analysis assessing delirium prevention models based on HELP showed significant reductions in delirium incidence with an OR of 0.47 (95% CI: 0.38–0.58).[49]

Dementia

Dementia includes a constellation of cognitive and behavioral impairments in multiple domains: memory; executive function (reasoning, planning, judgment); visuospatial ability; language; and personality/behavior. A diagnosis of dementia is made when sustained impairments are witnessed in at least 2 of these domains.[50] Given the progressive decline in patients with dementia, prognostication is often challenging. Further, the chronicity of this disease makes it difficult to conceptualize as a terminal condition. However, experts encourage that dementia be viewed similarly to cancer or other chronic organ failure. Patients with dementia experience functional decline, frailty, and cachexia with a median survival of 5 years from diagnosis.[51]

A 2013 systematic review attempted to identify accurate prognostic indicators of mortality in patients with advanced dementia.[52] Unfortunately, reliable predictors were not found in the literature. However, the most common prognostic variables encountered related to nutrition and nourishment including decreased appetite, anorexia, eating less than 25% of meals, and cachexia. The National Hospice and Palliative Care Organization recommends the use of the Functional Assessment Staging scale for use in prognostication for hospice eligibility in patients with dementia.[53,54] At stage 7, patients are believed to have a prognosis of 6 months or less if they also have a listed medical complication. At this stage, patients depend on all activities of daily living, are incontinent of bowel and bladder, and speech vocabulary is limited to no more than 6 words. Medical complications include aspiration pneumonia, upper urinary tract infection, stage III or IV pressure wound, greater than 10% weight loss over the span of 6 months or albumin less than 2.5 g/dL.[51,55]

Patients with dementia often have recurrent acute decompensations such as urosepsis, aspiration pneumonia, dehydration, falls, and delirium.[51] Hospitalization is a warning sign for short-term morbidity and mortality.[56,57] In fact, when patients with dementia recover from acute illness, the progression of their underlying dementia continues without returning to their previous baseline functionality. Identifying the type of dementia present is important. For example, patients with Alzheimer dementia have significantly decreased mobility at advanced stages; patients with Lewy body dementia exhibit parkinsonism.[58] These considerations have significant implications on the physical rehabilitation potential of critically ill elderly patients with dementia. Therefore, there has been renewed interest in patient and family education regarding the clinical course of dementia. Greater efforts are being made with patients regarding advance care planning and identifying a surrogate decision maker or health care agent to help make care choices based on the patient's values when acute and critical illness occurs. This caregiver education and preparation is a foundation of managing dementia.[51] These discussions are most valuable when performed in the early stages of dementia so that patients can participate and speak to their preferences. Patients with dementia who have surrogate decision makers who have awareness of prognostic information and clinical course are likely to receive less aggressive care at the end of life.[59]

Pain

Elderly populations tend to experience pain at higher rates than younger people, affecting up to two-thirds of patients. Further, pain prevalence increases in critical illness and at the end of life.[60–62] Despite this, there are often misconceptions and lack of knowledge among clinicians on how to best manage pain in this patient population.[63]

The most important step in the management of pain is an initial, thorough pain assessment. In elderly patients, it is essential to also assess for cognitive and sensory impairment. Pain is a common cause of suffering for patients with advanced dementia and even when identified, it is often undertreated.[51,64] One of the most widely used pain assessment tools in nonverbal dementia patients is the Pain Assessment in Advanced Dementia Scale.[65,66] This scale uses various observational metrics such as breathing, negative vocalization, facial expression, body language, and consolability in order to rate pain.

Uncontrolled pain may contribute to the development of frailty. It can also cause increased falls and functional impairment, potentially leading to increased trauma and ICU admissions, affecting future rehabilitation potential.[60] Although opioids can be safe and effective at low doses for moderate and severe pain, they should only be used as first-line therapy in cancer-related pain. When used, steps to mitigate side effects should be taken. In other pain syndromes, adjuvant medications are preferred first. For example, in elderly patients, up to 3 g of acetaminophen can be used daily. If there is concomitant liver injury, up to 2 g can be used daily.[67] Further, topical analgesics may be used for musculoskeletal pain. In patients with advanced dementia, it is recommended to provide analgesics on a scheduled basis, as these patients are unable to ask for as-needed medications.[51,68] Inadequate pain control may impair rehabilitation. Therefore, it is important to start pain interventions early in the treatment course.

When adjuvant analgesics are inadequate in managing pain in elderly patients, the use of opioids is warranted. When opioids are ineffectively and inadvisably used, delirium may result in elderly patients. A similar situation is also true: uncontrolled pain can also cause and exacerbate delirium.[60] Cognitively intact patients with uncontrolled pain are 9 times more likely to develop delirium.[69]

Constipation

The prevalence of constipation is higher in the elderly, affecting about 20% of the population, which increases to 50% in the nursing home patient population.[70] The pathophysiology of constipation in this population includes age-related cellular dysfunction that affects plasticity, compliance, macroscopic structural changes, altered control of the pelvic floor, and altered colonic motility due to age-related neuronal loss.[71] It is especially important to manage constipation in the elderly ICU population. Constipation is a risk factor for delirium and can contribute to nausea and decreased oral intake.[72] A recent observational study found that up to 75% of ICU patients suffer from constipation. In fact, as ICU length of stay increases and number of mechanical ventilation days increase, constipation becomes more common and severe. In the ICU setting, constipation is best managed with the use of osmotic laxatives such as polyethylene glycol or stimulant laxatives such as sennosides or bisacodyl. In the setting of fecal impaction, manual disimpaction, water enemas, and mineral oil enemas may be used.[70] Docusate, a stool softening agent, should not be used. It has not been shown to be effective for the management of constipation and often contributes to polypharmacy in the elderly population.[73]

Prognostication Scales

Prognosticating how a geriatric patient will recover after critical illness can be difficult. In a study evaluating advanced age (>85 years) geriatric patients, unplanned surgical ICU admissions had higher mortality than general medical admissions. In patients who survived to ICU discharge, they had the potential to return to population-based norms by 1 year after discharge from the ICU. Patients reached premorbid physical status 25% of the time. The physical gains plateaued after 9 months. Baseline functional status of patients can be a determining factor in the ability to survive and/or to reach pre-acute illness baseline function.[14] In a study evaluating ICU discharges for patients older than 75 years, short-term mortality correlated to the severity of the acute illness and long-term mortality to the preadmission cognitive status, functional status, and number of comorbidities. In the study, one-third of patients had moderate-to-severe disability requiring significant family support on discharge. Even in patients with high premorbid function, 40% were dependent at hospital discharge, with some improvement by 3 months, with plateauing, again, at 9 months.[74] In another study the survival rate of baseline healthy elderly medical patients 12 months postdischarge from the ICU was 49% with functional status and quality of life returning close to base-line in most of the survivors. However, they did experience a two-fold increase in the prevalence of geriatric syndromes.[75]

When determining expectations for rehabilitation in these patients, prognostication tools can be helpful. These tools can also serve as triggers for involving palliative care services and facilitating goal of care discussions with patients and families when prognosis is poor or goals cannot be met.[14] The Palliative Performance Scale (PPS) was developed by Anderson and Downing in 1996. It is a modification of the Karnofsky Performance Scale (KPS) used to assess a patient's functional performance and to determine progression toward end of life.[76] The KPS and PPS can be used interchangeably.[77] In a study evaluating trauma patients with a mean age of 70 years, if the preinjury PPS was low ($\leq$70), this correlated with hospital mortality and poor outcomes for survivors at 6 months. Low PPS predicted poor functional outcomes at 6 months, whereas age and the Injury Severity Score did not. Patients with lower scores who had functional improvement often continued to have persistent pain and anxiety/depression. Patients with low PPS scores plateaued in improvement compared with patients with higher scores.[78,79] In another retrospective study of elderly trauma patients admitted to a surgical ICU, a PPS of 80 or less was an independent risk factor for mortality, discharge to skilled care, and poor functional outcomes.[26]

Postintensive Care Unit Care and Rehabilitation

Healthy elderly patients with good baseline functional status have a possibility, with rehabilitation and management and prevention of geriatric syndromes, to functionally recover after acute illness. Patients start to develop muscle atrophy and skin pressure areas on the first day of hospitalization bedrest. By the eighth day, patients can start to develop bone degradation.[80] When a patient is showing clinical improvement, introducing physical and occupational therapy early in the acute care setting can improve patient outcomes. Also, taking measures to identify and avoid delirium and maximizing nutrition improve outcomes. After discharge from the ICU, frail elderly patients should transition to specialized care units for the elderly, if available. The Acute Care for Elders units have trained nurses and therapists in geriatric care and principles; these units improve outcomes for frail hospitalized elders. These units result in increased adherence to evidence-based geriatric care, improved patient function at time of hospital discharge, and reductions in length of stay and costs compared with usual care.[81]

For patients who do not exhibit functional recovery, or if it is determined that goals of treatment are not going to provide the patient with an acceptable quality of life, a palliative care consultation should be requested. This may also be an appropriate time to introduce hospice as an option to provide the patient with comfort and preserve dignity. The concept of hospice as an acceptable option should be introduced early if there is a concern that the patient's prognosis will be poor. Even if the goal is to pursue aggressive interventions, allowing patients and their family to become familiar with hospice, as a reasonable option can help with transition if it were to be needed. Geriatric patients who survive the ICU have high symptom burdens and care needs after discharge. Fatigue and pain are primary symptoms that can trigger outpatient palliative care consultations for symptom management and ongoing goals of care discussions.[20]

Patients are able to be discharged to a rehabilitation facility or home with rehabilitation services. There are 4 major types of interventions to improve health outcomes of frail elders: exercise, nutritional intervention, multicomponent interventions, and individually tailored geriatric care models.[80,82] Exercise interventions should focus on balance, flexibility, resistance, and endurance. The exercise program should focus first on flexibility and balance training, followed by resistance and endurance training with a gradual increase of exercise intensity. Resistance training can start to rebuild the lean muscle mass that was lost during illness (sarcopenia). In one study, frail women with advanced age and those living in long-term care facilities tend to benefit the most from these interventions.[82] These interventions can start before leaving the acute care setting. Multicomponent interventions include nutrition, attention to emotional/physiologic distress, and management of distressing symptoms (ie, pain, constipation, delirium, nausea, reducing polypharmacy).

Disposition

If a patient is able to tolerate 3 hours of nonconsecutive physical therapy, then transition to an acute rehabilitation facility, which provides intensive rehabilitation with medical supervision, should be considered. The average length of stay is 12 to 16 days. If a patient cannot tolerate 3 hours of nonconsecutive rehabilitation daily, then transfer to a skilled nursing facility (SNF) for subacute rehabilitation services should be considered. Subacute rehabilitation in SNFs is performed over a longer period of time and allows for lower intensity and a slower pace. The average length of stay is 21 to 28 days. Both are covered by Medicare and Medicare Advantage programs if a patient meets the qualifications based on hospital physical therapy recommendation, documentation, and clinical history.[16] For patients requiring extended hospitalization, long-term acute care (LTAC) hospitals specialize in treating patients requiring extended hospitalization who may have more than one serious condition and who have hope of return to home and/or meaningful recovery. LTAC hospitals are appropriate for patients who may require long-term ventilator weaning, extensive wound care, and antibiotic care that cannot be provided on an outpatient basis, in addition to rehabilitation.[83] Patients may also elect to be discharged to home with home health to provide rehabilitation. In a cohort study of Medicare data, patients discharged to home with home health were associated with higher 30-day readmission rates than were discharges to SNF. However, there were no significant differences between functional outcomes or 30-day mortality rates between these dispositions.[84] Refer to **Table 4** for details on outpatient rehabilitation options.[16,83,84]

Table 4
Outpatient rehabilitation options

Outpatient Rehabilitation	Average Length of Stay	Requirements	Notes
Home health	41.5 d	Patient must be homebound Require skilled care on a part-time or intermittent basis to improve, maintain, prevent, or further slow your health condition Rehab services in home 1–3 d per wk based on need and availability	Medicare authorizes 60 d
Skilled nursing facility	21–28 d	Services cannot be provided at lower level One or more skilled therapies are needed Rehab can be tolerated 1 h/d, if needed	Medicare certification SNF within 30 d of leaving the hospital and receive care for the same condition treated for during your hospital stay
Acute rehabilitation facility	12–16 d	Patient must be able to tolerate 3 nonconsecutive hours of therapy daily over 5-d period or 15 h over 7 d	Requires 24-h physician availability with specialized rehabilitation training. Requires 24-h availability of nurses with specialized rehabilitation training

For patients who are not showing clinical improvement and experiencing recurrent hospitalizations, progressive decline, and/or persistent symptom burden, palliative care consultation should be considered to clarify goals of care and manage symptoms. Outpatient palliative care consultation may be available through the facility or provided by independent agencies.[20] For patients with a prognosis with 6 months or less, referral to hospice is appropriate. The eligibility under the Medicare hospice benefit is based on the prognosis of the individual and not on the diagnosis.[85]

SUMMARY

Natural, physiologic changes occur with aging that make rehabilitation and return to baseline functional status more challenging and potentially prolonged in the setting of critical illness. These physiologic changes occur in multiple organ systems: nervous system, skin, musculoskeletal, cardiovascular, pulmonary, and immune system. Frailty culminates in decline across several systems causing risk for adverse outcomes including increased falls, emergency department visits, and hospitalizations. Delirium is a geriatric emergency and is widely underdiagnosed. Most of the mechanically ventilated ICU patients experience delirium. Dementia is characterized by progressive cognitive and behavioral deficits. The prevalence of pain is increased in critical illness and at the end of life. Constipation occurs in most of the critical care patients. These symptoms and syndromes have negative impacts on morbidity and mortality. Prognostication is challenging with most critically ill elderly patients. Multiple options exist for physical rehabilitation based on the patient's clinical recovery, including long-term acute care, acute rehabilitation, subacute rehabilitation, and home therapy.

CLINICS CARE POINTS

- Frailty is an independent risk factor for progressive physical dependence and mortality.
- Screening for delirium should occur at multiple points during hospitalization, given its waxing/waning course and potentially subtle features. Prevention strategies should be enacted.
- Patients with delirium have increased mortality up to 5 years after the episode.
- Delirium is associated with poor long-term outcomes, including increased institutionalization, cognitive impairment, falls, and pneumonia.
- Hospitalized patients with dementia have increased short-term morbidity and mortality. These patients do not return to previous baseline functional status after the acute decompensation resolves.
- Uncontrolled pain can contribute to frailty and delirium.
- Constipation is associated with increased days on mechanical ventilation and increased ICU length of stay. Treat constipation with scheduled osmotic and stimulant laxatives.
- Prognostication tools and performance scales such as the PPS should be used to help determine rehabilitation expectations.
- If functional recovery is not achieved or if continued disease-directed therapy will not provide adequate quality of life for the patient, hospice enrollment should be considered.

DISCLOSURE

The authors have nothing to disclose.

REFERENCES

1. Moskalev A, Aliper A, Smit-McBride Z, et al. Genetics and epigenetics of aging and longevity. Cell Cycle 2014;13(7):1063–77.
2. Shega JW, Dale W, Andrew M, et al. Persistent pain and frailty: a case for homeostenosis. J Am Geriatr Soc 2012;60(1):113–7.
3. Brooks SE, Peetz AB. Evidence-based care of geriatric trauma patients. Surg Clin North Am 2017;97(5):1157–74.
4. Waring R, Harris R, Mitchell S. Drug metabolism in the elderly: a multifactorial problem? Maturitas 2017;100:27–32.
5. Sleimen-Malkoun R, Temprado J-J, Hong SL. Aging induced loss of complexity and dedifferentiation: consequences for coordination dynamics within and between brain, muscular and behavioral levels. Front Aging Neurosci 2014;6:140.
6. Kou H-W, Yeh C-H, Tsai H-I, et al. Sarcopenia is an effective predictor of difficult-to-wean and mortality among critically ill surgical patients. PLoS One 2019;14(8): e0220699.

7. Avery MD, Martin RS, Chang MC. Effect of aging on cardiac function plus monitoring and support. In: Luchette FA, Yelon JA, editors. Geriatric trauma and critical care. New York: Springer; 2017. p. 9–16.

8. Martin RS, Farrah JP, Chang MC. Effect of aging on cardiac function plus monitoring and support. Surg Clin North Am 2015;95(1):23–35.

9. De Cecco M, Criscione SW, Peterson AL, et al. Transposable elements become active and mobile in the genomes of aging mammalian somatic tissues. Aging (Albany NY) 2013;5(12):867.

10. Ramly E, Kaafarani HM, Velmahos GC. The effect of aging on pulmonary function: implications for monitoring and support of the surgical and trauma patient. Surg Clin 2015;95(1):53–69.

11. Burns EA, Goodwin JS. Effects of aging on immune function. In: Rosenthal RA, Zenilman ME, Katlic MR, editors. Principles and practice of geriatric surgery. New York: Springer; 2001. p. 46–64.

12. Mosti CB, Rog LA, Fink JW. Differentiating mild cognitive impairment and cognitive changes of normal aging. In: Ravdin LD, Katzan HL, editors. Handbook on the neuropsychology of aging and dementia. New York: Springer; 2019. p. 445–63.

13. Abdulle AE, de Koning ME, van der Horn HJ, et al. Early predictors for long-term functional outcome after mild traumatic brain injury in frail elderly patients. J Head Trauma Rehabil 2018;33(6):E59–67.

14. Reece G, Poojara L. The elderly in intensive care. In: Nagaratnum N, Nagaratnum K, Cheuk G, editors. Advanced age geriatric care. New York: Springer; 2019. p. 101–9.

15. van den Beld AW, Kaufman J-M, Zillikens MC, et al. The physiology of endocrine systems with ageing. Lancet Diabetes Endocrinol 2018;6(8):647–58.

16. Achterberg WP, Cameron ID, Bauer JM, et al. Geriatric rehabilitation—state of the art and future priorities. J Am Med Dir Assoc 2019;20(4):396–8.

17. Clegg A, Young J, Iliffe S, et al. Frailty in elderly people. Lancet 2013;381(9868): 752–62.

18. Muscedere J, Waters B, Varambally A, et al. The impact of frailty on intensive care unit outcomes: a systematic review and meta-analysis. Intensive Care Med 2017; 43(8):1105–22.

19. Fried LP, Tangen CM, Walston J, et al. Frailty in older adults: evidence for a phenotype. J Gerontol A Biol Sci Med Sci 2001;56(3):M146–57.

20. Pollack LR, Goldstein NE, Gonzalez WC, et al. The frailty phenotype and palliative care needs of older survivors of critical illness. J Am Geriatr Soc 2017;65(6): 1168–75.

21. Montgomery CL, Rolfson DB, Bagshaw SM. Frailty and the association between long-term recovery after intensive care unit admission. Crit Care Clin 2018;34(4): 527–47.

22. O'Caoimh R, Costello M, Small C, et al. Comparison of frailty screening instruments in the emergency department. Int J Environ Res Public Health 2019; 16(19):3626.

23. Walston J, Buta B, Xue Q-L. Frailty screening and interventions: considerations for clinical practice. Clin Geriatr Med 2018;34(1):25–38.

24. Kendall M, Carduff E, Lloyd A, et al. Different experiences and goals in different advanced diseases: comparing serial interviews with patients with cancer, organ failure, or frailty and their family and professional carers. J Pain Symptom Manage 2015;50(2):216–24.

25. Lindhardt T, Hallberg IR, Poulsen I. Nurses' experience of collaboration with relatives of frail elderly patients in acute hospital wards: a qualitative study. Int J Nurs Stud 2008;45(5):668–81.
26. McGreevy CM, Bryczkowski S, Pentakota SR, et al. Unmet palliative care needs in elderly trauma patients: can the Palliative Performance Scale help close the gap? Am J Surg 2017;213(4):778–84.
27. American Psychiatric Association. Diagnostic and statistical manual of mental disorders : DSM-5. 5th edition. Washington, DC: American Psychiatric Association; 2013.
28. Hshieh TT, Inouye SK, Oh ES. Delirium in the elderly. Psychiatr Clin North Am 2018;41(1):1–17.
29. Tosun Tasar P, Sahın S, Akcam NO, et al. Delirium is associated with increased mortality in the geriatric population. Int J Psychiatry Clin Pract 2018;22(3):200–5.
30. Witlox J, Eurelings LS, de Jonghe JF, et al. Delirium in elderly patients and the risk of postdischarge mortality, institutionalization, and dementia: a meta-analysis. JAMA 2010;304(4):443–51.
31. Inouye SK, Westendorp RG, Saczynski JS. Delirium in elderly people. Lancet 2014;383(9920):911–22.
32. Boettger S, Nuñez DG, Meyer R, et al. Delirium in the intensive care setting: a reevaluation of the validity of the CAM-ICU and ICDSC versus the DSM-IV-TR in determining a diagnosis of delirium as part of the daily clinical routine. Palliat Support Care 2017;15(6):675–83.
33. Pun BT, Ely EW. The importance of diagnosing and managing ICU delirium. Chest 2007;132(2):624–36.
34. Ely EW, Shintani A, Truman B, et al. Delirium as a predictor of mortality in mechanically ventilated patients in the intensive care unit. JAMA 2004;291(14):1753–62.
35. National Clinical Guideline Centre. Delirium: Diagnosis, Prevention and Management. London: National Institute for Health and Clinical Excellence; 2010.
36. van Roessel S, Keijsers CJPW, Romijn MDM. Dementia as a predictor of morbidity and mortality in patients with delirium. Maturitas 2019;125:63–9.
37. Ely EW, Inouye SK, Bernard GR, et al. Delirium in mechanically ventilated patients: validity and reliability of the confusion assessment method for the intensive care unit (CAM-ICU). JAMA 2001;286(21):2703–10.
38. Devlin JW, Fong JJ, Schumaker G, et al. Use of a validated delirium assessment tool improves the ability of physicians to identify delirium in medical intensive care unit patients. Crit Care Med 2007;35(12):2721–4 [quiz: 2725].
39. Gusmao-Flores D, Salluh JI, Chalhub R, et al. The confusion assessment method for the intensive care unit (CAM-ICU) and intensive care delirium screening checklist (ICDSC) for the diagnosis of delirium: a systematic review and meta-analysis of clinical studies. Crit Care 2012;16(4):R115.
40. Marcantonio ER, Kiely DK, Simon SE, et al. Outcomes of older people admitted to postacute facilities with delirium. J Am Geriatr Soc 2005;53(6):963–9.
41. Siddiqi N, House AO, Holmes JD. Occurrence and outcome of delirium in medical in-patients: a systematic literature review. Age Ageing 2006;35(4):350–64.
42. McCusker J, Cole M, Abrahamowicz M, et al. Delirium predicts 12-month mortality. Arch Intern Med 2002;162(4):457–63.
43. Lindroth H, Khan BA, Carpenter JS, et al. Delirium severity trajectories and outcomes in ICU patients: defining a dynamic symptom phenotype. Ann Am Thorac Soc 2020;17(9):1094–103.

44. Jackson TA, Wilson D, Richardson S, et al. Predicting outcome in older hospital patients with delirium: a systematic literature review. Int J Geriatr Psychiatry 2016;31(4):392–9.

45. DiMartini A, Dew MA, Kormos R, et al. Posttraumatic stress disorder caused by hallucinations and delusions experienced in delirium. Psychosomatics 2007; 48(5):436–9.

46. Grover S, Sahoo S, Chakrabarti S, et al. Post-traumatic stress disorder (PTSD) related symptoms following an experience of delirium. J Psychosom Res 2019; 123:109725.

47. Langan C, Sarode DP, Russ TC, et al. Psychiatric symptomatology after delirium: a systematic review. Psychogeriatrics 2017;17(5):327–35.

48. Inouye SK. Delirium-A framework to improve acute care for older persons. J Am Geriatr Soc 2018;66(3):446–51.

49. Hshieh TT, Yue J, Oh E, et al. Effectiveness of multicomponent nonpharmacological delirium interventions: a meta-analysis. JAMA Intern Med 2015;175(4): 512–20.

50. McKhann GM, Knopman DS, Chertkow H, et al. The diagnosis of dementia due to Alzheimer's disease: recommendations from the National Institute on Aging-Alzheimer's Association workgroups on diagnostic guidelines for Alzheimer's disease. Alzheimers Dement 2011;7(3):263–9.

51. Stewart JT, Schultz SK. Palliative care for dementia. Psychiatr Clin North Am 2018;41(1):141–51.

52. Brown MA, Sampson EL, Jones L, et al. Prognostic indicators of 6-month mortality in elderly people with advanced dementia: a systematic review. Palliat Med 2013; 27(5):389–400.

53. Medical guidelines for determining prognosis in selected non-cancer diseases. The National Hospice Organization. Hosp J 1996;11(2):47–63.

54. Organization NH, Palliative C. The medicare hospice benefit, regulations, quality reporting, and public policy. 2016. Available at: https://www.nhpco.org/wp-content/uploads/2019/08/Hospice_Policy_Compendium.pdf. Accessed June 9, 2020.

55. Sclan SG, Reisberg B. Functional assessment staging (FAST) in Alzheimer's disease: reliability, validity, and ordinality. Int Psychogeriatr 1992;4(Suppl 1):55–69.

56. Sampson EL, Candy B, Davis S, et al. Living and dying with advanced dementia: a prospective cohort study of symptoms, service use and care at the end of life. Palliat Med 2018;32(3):668–81.

57. Agar M, Phillips J. Palliative medicine and care of the elderly. In: Cherny N, Fallon M, Kaasa S, et al, editors. Oxford textbook of palliative medicine. 5th edition. Oxford (UK): Oxford University Press; 2015. p. 1044–55.

58. Widera E, Covinsky KE. What is the clinical course of advanced dementia?. In: Goldstein N, Morrison RS, editors. Evidence-based practice of palliative medicine. Philadelphia: Elsevier Saunders; 2013. p. 290–4.

59. Mitchell SL, Teno JM, Kiely DK, et al. The clinical course of advanced dementia. N Engl J Med 2009;361(16):1529–38.

60. Malec M, Shega JW. Pain management in the elderly. Med Clin North Am 2015; 99(2):337–50.

61. Shega JW, Tiedt AD, Grant K, et al. Pain measurement in the National Social life, health, and aging Project: presence, intensity, and location. J Gerontol B Psychol Sci Soc Sci 2014;69(Suppl 2):S191–7.

62. Smith AK, Cenzer IS, Knight SJ, et al. The epidemiology of pain during the last 2 years of life. Ann Intern Med 2010;153(9):563–9.

63. Pargeon KL, Hailey BJ. Barriers to effective cancer pain management: a review of the literature. J Pain Symptom Manage 1999;18(5):358–68.
64. Scherder E, Oosterman J, Swaab D, et al. Recent developments in pain in dementia. BMJ 2005;330(7489):461–4.
65. Leong IY, Chong MS, Gibson SJ. The use of a self-reported pain measure, a nurse-reported pain measure and the PAINAD in nursing home residents with moderate and severe dementia: a validation study. Age Ageing 2006;35(3): 252–6.
66. Warden V, Hurley AC, Volicer L. Development and psychometric evaluation of the pain assessment in advanced dementia (PAINAD) scale. J Am Med Dir Assoc 2003;4(1):9–15.
67. Persons AGSPoPPiO. The management of persistent pain in older persons. J Am Geriatr Soc 2002;50(6 Suppl):S205–24.
68. Haasum Y, Fastbom J, Fratiglioni L, et al. Pain treatment in elderly persons with and without dementia: a population-based study of institutionalized and home-dwelling elderly. Drugs Aging 2011;28(4):283–93.
69. Morrison RS, Magaziner J, Gilbert M, et al. Relationship between pain and opioid analgesics on the development of delirium following hip fracture. J Gerontol A Biol Sci Med Sci 2003;58(1):76–81.
70. Mounsey A, Raleigh M, Wilson A. Management of constipation in older adults. Am Fam Physician 2015;92(6):500–4.
71. Vazquez Roque M, Bouras EP. Epidemiology and management of chronic constipation in elderly patients. Clin Interv Aging 2015;10:919–30.
72. Weckmann M, Morrison RS. What is delirium?. In: Goldstein N, Morrison RS, editors. Evidence-based practice of palliative medicine. Philadelphia: Elsevier Saunders; 2013. p. 198–204.
73. Ahmedzai SH, Boland J. Constipation in people prescribed opioids. BMJ Clin Evid 2010;2010:2407.
74. Villa P, Pintado MC, Luján J, et al. Functional status and quality of life in elderly intensive care unit survivors. J Am Geriatr Soc 2016;64(3):536–42.
75. Sacanella E, Perez-Castejon JM, Nicolas JM, et al. Functional status and quality of life 12 months after discharge from a medical ICU in healthy elderly patients: a prospective observational study. Crit Care 2011;15(2):R105.
76. Anderson F, Downing GM, Hill J, et al. Palliative performance scale (PPS): a new tool. J Palliat Care 1996;12(1):5–11.
77. de Kock I, Mirhosseini M, Lau F, et al. Conversion of Karnofsky performance status (KPS) and eastern cooperative oncology group performance status (ECOG) to palliative performance scale (PPS), and the interchangeability of PPS and KPS in prognostic tools. J Palliat Care 2013;29(3):163–9.
78. Hwang F, Pentakota SR, McGreevy CM, et al. Preinjury Palliative Performance Scale predicts functional outcomes at 6 months in older trauma patients. J Trauma Acute Care Surg 2019;87(3):541–51.
79. Javali RH, Krishnamoorthy AP, Srinivasarangan M, et al. Comparison of injury severity score, new injury severity score, revised trauma score and trauma and injury severity score for mortality prediction in elderly trauma patients. Indian J Crit Care Med 2019;23(2):73.
80. Giambattista L, Howard R, Porto RR, et al. NICHE recommended care of the critically ill older adult. Crit Care Nurs Q 2015;38(3):223–30.
81. Flood KL, Booth K, Vickers J, et al. Acute care for elders (ACE) team model of care: a clinical overview. Geriatrics 2018;3(3):50.

82. Cesari M, Vellas B, Hsu F-C, et al. A physical activity intervention to treat the frailty syndrome in older persons—results from the LIFE-P study. J Gerontol A Biol Sci Med Sci 2015;70(2):216–22.

83. Makam AN, Tran T, Miller ME, et al. The clinical course after long-term acute care hospital admission among older Medicare beneficiaries. J Am Geriatr Soc 2019; 67(11):2282–8.

84. Werner RM, Coe NB, Qi M, et al. Patient outcomes after hospital discharge to home with home health care vs to a skilled nursing facility. JAMA Intern Med 2019;179(5):617–23.

85. Oberoi-Jassal R, Pope J, Jassal N. Hospice care. In: Abd-Elsayed A, editor. Pain. New York: Springer; 2019. p. 937–9.

The Effect of Aging Physiology on Critical Care

Dijoia B. Darden, MD[a], Frederick A. Moore, MD, MCCM[a],
Scott C. Brakenridge, MD, MSCS[a], Eduardo B. Navarro, BHS[a], Stephen D. Anton, PhD[b],
Christiaan Leeuwenburgh, PhD[b], Lyle L. Moldawer, PhD[a], Alicia M. Mohr, MD, FCCM[a],
Philip A. Efron, MD, FCCM[a], Robert T. Mankowski, PhD[b],*

KEYWORDS

- Aging • Geriatrics • Critical care • Physiology • Sepsis • Trauma
- Chronic critical illness

KEY POINTS

- Older adults demonstrate lower physiologic reserves of major organs such as brain, cardiopulmonary, renal, musculoskeletal, and intestinal systems and impaired immunity.
- Because of lower physiologic reserves, older adults are more susceptible to critical illness and are at high risk of poor short-term and long-term outcomes with failure to recover.
- Intensivists should take into account compromised physiology in the critical care management.
- In-hospital and ambulatory interventions are needed to improve the function of the majorly affected organs due to critical illness in older adults to improve in-hospital outcomes and importantly prevent chronic critical illness.

INTRODUCTION

The number of older adults, defined as individuals older than or equal to 65 years, are rapidly increasing in the United States and are projected to reach 84 million by the year 2050.[1] Although there is a difference between chronologic and physiologic aging,[2] older adult populations tend to have a weaker physiologic phenotype compared with a younger population.[3] In addition, older adults account for nearly 50% of intensive care unit (ICU) admissions and 60% of all ICU days.[4,5]

Funding: Supported, in part, by National Institutes Health grants: American Heart Association 18CDA34080001 (R.T. Mankowski) and National Institutes of General Medical Sciences R01 GM-040586 and R01 GM-104481 (L.L. Moldawer), NIGMS R01 GM-113945 (P.A. Efron), NIGMS P50 GM-111152 (F.A. Moore, S.C. Brakenridge, L.L. Moldawer, P.A. Efron, A.M. Mohr), and in a postgraduate training grant T32 GM-008721 in burns, trauma, and perioperative injury (D.B. Darden).
[a] Department of Surgery, University of Florida College of Medicine, 1600 SW Archer Road, Gainesville, FL 32610, USA; [b] Department of Aging and Geriatric Research, University of Florida, 2004 Mowry Road, Gainesville, FL 32611, USA
* Corresponding author.
E-mail address: r.mankowski@ufl.edu

Crit Care Clin 37 (2021) 135–150
https://doi.org/10.1016/j.ccc.2020.08.006
0749-0704/21/© 2020 Elsevier Inc. All rights reserved.

One of the main biological processes of systemic deterioration that contributes to development of organ dysfunctions in aging are immunosenescence (age-associated gradual deterioration of protective immunity) and inflammaging (chronic subclinical systemic inflammation). Both of these detrimental processes lower the efficacy of the immune system, leading to higher vulnerability to infections and susceptibility to inflammatory conditions[6,7] and thus higher susceptibilities for critical illness and dismal outcomes.[8] Other cellular processes such as elevated oxidative stress and apoptosis, as well as declines in autophagy are hallmarks of the aging deterioration process that contribute to susceptibility to infections and worse outcomes in critical illness.[9–12]

Reactive oxygen species are produced in the normal aging process at the cellular level in all systems as mediators of cell differentiation and growth and are scavenged by antioxidant enzymes in order to maintain homeostasis.[13,14] The aging process is associated with a less efficient free radical scavenging process and overproduction of free radicals elevating oxidative stress, cell damage, and death—necrosis.[15,16] Aging is also associated with a higher level of apoptosis, programmed death, and decline in autophagy, a cellular process where dysfunctional and cytotoxic parts of the cell are digested and removed by lysosomes.[17,18] These detrimental processes contribute to the development of comorbidities in older adults such as cardiovascular disease, neurodegenerative diseases, physical disability, and cancers.

The main purpose of this review is to briefly summarize the age-specific changes in the main physiologic systems (**Fig. 1**) that occur in critically ill older adults that can have implications in clinical management. Special considerations for clinical management of older patients in the ICU need to be considered[3,5] due to different physiologic and biological profile especially when considering the management of sepsis and

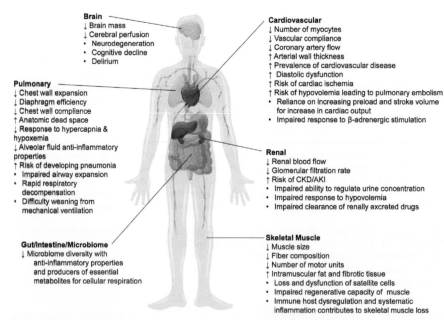

Brain
↓ Brain mass
↓ Cerebral perfusion
• Neurodegeneration
• Cognitive decline
• Delirium

Pulmonary
↓ Chest wall expansion
↓ Diaphragm efficiency
↓ Chest wall compliance
↑ Anatomic dead space
↓ Response to hypercapnia & hypoxemia
↓ Alveolar fluid anti-inflammatory properties
↑ Risk of developing pneumonia
• Impaired airway expansion
• Rapid respiratory decompensation
• Difficulty weaning from mechanical ventilation

Cardiovascular
↓ Number of myocytes
↓ Vascular compliance
↓ Coronary artery flow
↑ Arterial wall thickness
↑ Prevalence of cardiovascular disease
↑ Diastolic dysfunction
↑ Risk of cardiac ischemia
↑ Risk of hypovolemia leading to pulmonary embolism
• Reliance on increasing preload and stroke volume for increase in cardiac output
• Impaired response to β-adrenergic stimulation

Renal
↓ Renal blood flow
↓ Glomerular filtration rate
↑ Risk of CKD/AKI
• Impaired ability to regulate urine concentration
• Impaired response to hypovolemia
• Impaired clearance of renally excreted drugs

Gut/Intestine/Microbiome
↓ Microbiome diversity with anti-inflammatory properties and producers of essential metabolites for cellular respiration

Skeletal Muscle
↓ Muscle size
↓ Fiber composition
↓ Number of motor units
↑ Intramuscular fat and fibrotic tissue
• Loss and dysfunction of satellite cells
• Impaired regenerative capacity of muscle
• Immune host dysregulation and systematic inflammation contributes to skeletal muscle loss

Fig. 1. Summary of the effect of aging on various physiologic systems.

trauma, which may result in a relatively new phenotype, prevalent in older critical illness survivors, classified as chronic critical illness (CCI).[19]

Brain

Aging is associated with neurodegeneration, neuroinflammation, and decreased perfusion of the cerebrovascular circulation that contributes to cognitive decline, dementia, and Alzheimer disease.[20] Interpersonal degrees of alterations in the brain are highly variable, but the largest changes are observed in the frontal and temporal cortex. The frontal cortex is responsible for attention and memory and also speech production.[21] The temporal cortex is involved in auditory and visual recognition such as language recognition.[22] Older adults with preexisting cognitive impairment are more susceptible to an amplified burden of critical illness leading to delirium in the ICU.[23] Delirium is an acute state of confusion that affects most of the older patients and develops within hours or days after the ICU admission and leads to alterations in consciousness and cognition.[24] A medical team should distinguish between delirium and dementia or other psychiatric disorders and implement reduction of factors that triggered delirium and apply medication treatment for those at risk of harming themselves.[25]

Cardiovascular

Advanced age is associated with a change in cardiac structure such as a loss in the number of myocytes, increased arterial wall thickness, increase in collagen deposition, and reduced vascular compliance.[26,27] These changes contribute to the higher prevalence of cardiovascular disease in older adults such as hypertension, atrial fibrillation, heart failure, myocardial infarction, stroke, and peripheral arterial disease.[28,29] However, the addition of the stress of critical illness accentuates the cardiac dysfunction in the elderly requiring special consideration in hemodynamic support in the ICU.[30]

Coronary artery flow is also diminished in the elderly population, which is secondary to increased prevalence of coronary artery disease, increased arterial wall thickness, and increased pulse pressure.[31,32] During critical illness, these changes lead to increased risk for cardiac ischemia in the elderly.[33] Finally, increased age is also an independent risk factor for the development of arrhythmias as a result of the conduction system dysfunction caused by an increase in collagen, inflammation, and fat deposition as well as decreased myocyte number.[34–37] New onset atrial fibrillation secondary to acute critical illness is more common in the elderly and is associated with increased mortality in the ICU.[38]

During aging, cellular loss and increases in myocardial collagen deposits lead to a decreased response to β-adrenergic stimulation,[39,40] and this translates to a decreased heart rate response to stressors.[41] Therefore, the aging heart relies on increasing preload and stroke volume for increase in cardiac output, which makes this population sensitive to hypovolemic states.[26,42] In addition, these changes lead to a diastolic dysfunction, secondary to impaired early left ventricular filling and decreased ventricular compliance.[43] Therefore, the critical care practitioner must pay special attention to volume resuscitation in the older adult population.[26] A small amount of hypovolemia can compromise cardiac function, whereas a small amount of hypervolemia can precipitate pulmonary edema.[26] Bedside transthoracic echocardiography has become a very important noninvasive tool and is now routinely used for assessing the cardiac function and hemodynamic evaluation that is used in clinical management decisions in older ICU patients.[44,45]

Pulmonary

Age-related changes in chest wall rigidity and lung parenchyma contribute to decreased respiratory reserve in older adults as well as many ICU-related respiratory complications in elderly patients. Chest wall compliance can decrease up to 30% by the age of 75 years and respiratory muscle strength can decline nearly 50% in older patients, both ultimately resulting in decreased chest wall expansion.[4,46] The diaphragm also flattens and becomes less efficient.[47–49] Full airway expansion cannot occur unless the geriatric patient is in the standing position, which is difficult to achieve in the ICU setting, resulting in a propensity for atelectasis.[48,50] Geriatric patients who depend on mechanical ventilation have to work harder because of the diaphragm muscle weakness and decreased chest wall compliance, which can result in difficulties weaning from a ventilator.[51]

Aging is also associated with a decreased host response to hypoxemia and hypercapnia.[52] Therefore, with decreased respiratory reserve, older patients are likely to seem normal during respiratory decline and can decompensate very quickly.[4] Decreased alveolar fluid antiinflammatory proteins and decreased ability for airway clearance result in a higher risk of developing pneumonia.[53–55] Pneumonia is associated with more complications, frequently requires ICU admission and mechanical ventilation, and can lead to death in older adults.[56–58] Although the treatment is the same regardless of age, consideration of the abovementioned physiology can aid the intensivist in adjuvant treatment and even prevention of pneumonia in their older patients.

Renal

Normal aging is associated with nearly a 45% decrease in glomerular filtration rate secondary to a 50% decrease in renal blood flow and loss of functional parenchyma.[59,60] Also, with aging there is an impaired ability to regulate sodium and hydrogen ions and thus, a decreased ability to manage acid-base status.[61] There is also impaired ability to maximally dilute or concentrate urine that is exacerbated under stress conditions.[62] This renal dysfunction is partially responsible for the inability of older adults to respond to hypovolemia.[61] In addition, older adults' kidneys have a decreased filtering ability, and this requires careful consideration for drug levels that are renally excreted and those that can cause nephrotoxicity such as vancomycin, amphotericin B, nonsteroidal antiinflammatory drugs, or aminoglycosides.[63,64]

Age greater than 65 years is an independent risk factor for acute kidney injury (AKI). The cause of AKI in critically ill aged patients is usually multifactorial with ischemia, hypovolemia, drug- or contrast-induced nephrotoxicity, and/or acute urinary obstruction often co-existing.[64–66] Preexisting cardiovascular and chronic kidney disease, as well as iatrogenic injury from contrast exposure and various drugs, are among the common causes of AKI in critically ill patients.[67] Also, renal recovery rates are significantly lower in older patients.[66] A recent study suggests that early initiation of renal replacement therapy was associated with increased renal recovery, attenuated kidney-specific and non-kidney organ injury, and decreased risk of all-cause mortality.[68] However, prevention of AKI remains the most important factor in management.[65] Intensivists should maintain appropriate blood pressure and volume status and limit drug and imaging contrast toxicity to reduce increased morbidity and mortality associated with AKI in older patients.[69] In addition, intensivists should keep in mind that because older patients have lower muscle mass[70,71] and creatinine is formed almost exclusively in the muscles,[72] creatinine is a less reliable biomarker of baseline renal function and the development of AKI in this population.[73]

Gut/Intestine

The intestinal microbiome consists of trillions of organisms and its metabolites and plays an important role in maintaining the immune system homoeostasis.[74] Importantly, microbiome alterations occur with normal aging as well as contribute to maintaining chronic low-grade inflammation (inflammaging) and immunosenescence. Thus, the microbiome is thought to be involved in the risk for and the development of chronic diseases, as well those conditions associated with these chronic diseases and aging (eg, sepsis).[75,76]

Sepsis is thought to lead to a complete "collapse" of the intestinal microbiome, with an accompanying emergence of a "pathobiome," both of which contribute significantly to the pathology of sepsis.[77] In particular, during aging and in response to critical illness, the gut microbiome loses its microbial diversity. This includes the disappearance of microbes that represent an important part of the microbiota of healthy individuals with antiinflammatory properties, as well as those producing short-chain fatty acids from digested fibers, essential metabolites for cellular energy production.[74,78]

The aging-related gut microbiome dysbiosis and pathobiome in critical illness have been linked to peripheral organ dysfunctions such as brain, liver, kidney, cardiovascular system, pancreas, and skeletal muscle.[76] Therefore, improving the gut microbiome may be a target to prevent aging-related comorbidities, lower the susceptibility of these individuals to infections, and improve their outcomes to critical illness.[76] For example, gut microbiota can be modulated by supplementing specific beneficial microbial communities deficient in disease states with prebiotics and probiotics as well as fecal microbiota transplantation (FMT).[79,80] FMT is thought to supply underrepresented microorganisms with probiotics or increasing the diversity of the microbiome and decreasing the pathobiome. Recolonizing particular microbes and the whole microbiota of the older adult host holds promise as approaches to prevent and treat age-related pathologic conditions.[78]

Skeletal Muscle

Gradual loss of muscle mass, strength, and function with aging is natural, but the clinically significant loss of muscle mass and function could be considered as a disease.[81] Sarcopenia is described as a progressive skeletal muscle disorder characterized by decrease in muscle size, fiber composition, number of motor units, and increase of intramuscular fat fibrotic tissue and is associated with increased likelihood of adverse outcomes including falls, fractures, physical disability, and mortality.[82] Age-related contributing factors to the development of sarcopenia are denervated motor units resulting from disuse atrophy, malnutrition, hormonal changes, and increase of inflammation and oxidative stress.[82]

Acute and chronic immune host dysregulation and systemic inflammation contribute to rapid loss of skeletal muscle and lead to the ICU-acquired weakness (ICU-AW). The main risk factors contributing to the development of ICU-AW include the severity of critical illness, immobilization, hyperglycemia, and the use of some medications, including steroids and neuromuscular agents.[83] The pathophysiology of sepsis-induced myopathy involves mitochondrial dysfunction leading to a bioenergetic failure, oxidative stress, and inflammatory cell infiltration protein catabolism, mainly related to an activation of the ubiquitin-proteasome pathway, muscle fibrosis, and satellite cell loss and dysfunction.[84–86] Satellite cells are progenitor cells that differentiate to myoblasts and fuse to myofibers as part of muscle regeneration.[87]

Loss and dysfunction of satellite cells in response to critical illness impairs the regenerative capacity of muscle and ameliorates weaning from the ICU.[87,88]

Given the acute and chronic muscle wasting and impaired regeneration, clinical management should include early postdischarge rehabilitation and nutritional strategies to stimulate anabolic processes and muscle regeneration. Consideration should be given to a high protein diet paired with resistance exercise training, as this therapy combination has been shown to reverse sarcopenia.[89,90]

Implications for Clinical Management of Older Trauma Patients

Geriatric trauma accounts for one-third of all trauma health care costs in the United States.[91] Elderly trauma patients present with worse injuries, have longer hospital stays, and have 3 times higher mortality rate than young trauma patients.[92] One study demonstrated that geriatric trauma patients that present with severe injuries (Injury Severity Score>15) and low systolic blood pressure had an odds of 2.16 for mortality compared with young patients with the same injury severity.[93] In a different multicenter cohort study, advanced age was found to be strongly associated with poor outcomes such as severe organ failure, secondary infectious complications, intensive care utilization, ventilator days, and poor discharge disposition or loss of independent living status (long-term acute care facility, skilled nursing facility, hospice etc.).[94] In addition, elderly trauma patients older than 74 years have a 1.67 odds of mortality compared with trauma patients aged 65 to 74 years.[93]

Falls are the most common mechanism of injury in geriatric trauma patients.[95] In fact, same level falls are responsible for more severe injury (30-fold) and for an increased cause of death (10-fold) in older adult patients compared with younger cohorts.[96,97] Motor vehicle accidents are the second most common mechanism of injury and the leading cause for mortality in geriatric trauma patients.[98,99]

The association of advancing age with increasing frailty has been described as a main contributor to increased risk of short- and long-term poor outcomes after trauma.[100–102] Frailty syndrome is defined as a "decreased reserve and resistance to stressors, resulting from cumulative declines across multiple physiologic systems, and causing vulnerability to adverse outcomes" and can be found in more than one-third of geriatric trauma patients.[100,102–104] Diminished reserves and decreased ability to compensate, as described earlier, leads to significant morbidity and mortality even with minor injuries after trauma.[97,105–107] Diminished respiratory reserve and diminished response to hypoxia and hypercapnia pose a challenge for management of the geriatric patient after chest trauma.[108] In addition, traditional physiologic parameters of systolic blood pressure (SBP) 90 or heart rate greater than 120 do not accurately reflect clinical decline for elderly trauma patients.[109,110] Therefore, CDC guidelines recommend transport to trauma center for patients older than or equal to 65 years with SBP 110.[111]

Implications for Clinical Management of Older Patients with Sepsis

Sepsis is the leading cause of death in US hospitals, with studies estimating more than 5 million deaths per year worldwide.[112,113] There has been an improvement in mortality over the last 3 decades.[114–117] The reduction in short-term mortality can be largely credited to the improvements in sepsis screening, evidence-based resuscitation strategies, and standardized critical care, starting with the "Surviving Sepsis Campaign" in 2004.[118] These improvements include increased compliance with evidence-based strategies including early fluid administration, broad-spectrum antibiotic therapy, and vasopressor support to restore end-organ perfusion.[119–122] However, older adults continue to have increased susceptibility and mortality to sepsis.[123] One single-center study revealed that critically ill patients older than or equal to 55 years with sepsis have greater organ dysfunction, 8-fold higher hospital mortality, and even higher 6-month mortality secondary to persistent immunosuppression and catabolism.[124]

This predisposition to sepsis in older patients can be partially explained by the aged immune system's inability to mount an effective immune response to pathogens, which is in part due to inflammaging and immunosenescence.[82,125–127] Studies in aged humans and mice reveal that the immune dysfunction associated with aging extends to both innate and adaptive immunity.[128–130] The aging bone marrow has been noted to produce fewer well-functioning innate cells (eg, granulocytes, macrophages, and dendritic cells) and more immature, less effective myeloid-derived suppressor cells (MDSCs).[131] MDSCs are immature myeloid cells that have the ability to suppress acute inflammatory responses, including lymphocyte proliferation, and resolve inflammation.[132–134] Sepsis induces emergency myelopoiesis that amplifies expansion of MDSCs.[133,135–137] Although younger patients are more capable of returning to a balanced state of innate and adaptive immunity after infection, older patients have difficulty returning to homeostasis.[124,128,138,139] The ongoing animal and human studies at the University of Florida Sepsis and Critical Illness Research Center suggest that the long-term, persistent MDSC expansion and infiltration resulting from geriatric post-sepsis *dyshomeostasis* plays a major role in the simultaneous low-grade inflammation (promoting catabolism and anabolic resistance) and immunosuppression (increasing the risk of secondary infections), which is a major contributor to increased morbidity and mortality.[3,124,128,140,141]

Chronic Critical Illness as a Result of Improved Intensive Care Unit Care Management

Improvements in critical care for all ages have led to a decline in inpatient mortality.[142,143] Improvements in 30-day mortality after critical illness for trauma and sepsis have led to a larger focus on long-term outcomes, including postdischarge mortality.[19] Among those that survive severe injury or sepsis, there are 2 clinical trajectories—CCI and rapid recovery.[144,145] CCI is defined as prolonged intensive care utilization and/or transfer to inpatient facility postdischarge ($\geq$14 days) and persistent organ dysfunction.[146] CCI seems to be driven by a persistence in immune dysfunction.[146–148] Many studies have shown a prolonged elevation of circulating inflammatory cytokines and persistent lymphopenia postsepsis.[133,140,148–150] However, older patients are noted to have a longer persistence of this pattern of immune dysfunction with higher levels of soluble programmed death ligand 1 and decreased absolute lymphocyte counts out to 28 days, whereas young patients returned to normal levels by day 14.[124]

It is estimated that CCI accounts for more than \$25 billion in health care expenses.[151] Patients older than 55 years are more likely to have an inpatient disposition (long-term acute care, skilled nursing facilities, inpatient facility, hospice), which is associated with higher 1-year mortality rates.[100,124,152] Importantly, CCI disproportionately affects elderly patients.[151,153,154] In fact, age greater than or equal to 55 year has been found to be predictive of CCI after severe trauma.[155]

SUMMARY

Although older age is a risk factor for susceptibility to developing critical illness and poor outcomes in the ICU, it is important to recognize that patient's outcome is still determined primarily by the severity of their critical illness. The authors have highlighted age-specific changes in physiologic systems majorly affected by critical illness (see **Fig. 1**), especially because it pertains to sepsis and trauma, which can lead to chronic critical illness. Clinical management decisions should take into account that older adults have lower physiologic reserves and impaired immunity and are at high risk of nonrecovery from critical illness. Besides customized, life-saving acute clinical management, there is a need for in-hospital and ambulatory interventions to improve the function of the majorly affected systems due to critical illness in older adults, and thus improve in-hospital outcomes, and importantly prevent chronic critical illness.

AUTHOR CONTRIBUTIONS

D.B. Darden, E.B. Navarro, P.A. Efron, and R.T. Mankowski contributed extensively to the drafting of the article, revision of its content, and approval of the article in its final form. F.A. Moore, .S.C. Brakenridge, S.D. Anton, C. Leeuwenburgh, L.L. Moldawer, and A.M. Mohr provided revisions and critical feedback.

ACKNOWLEDGMENTS

Not applicable.

DISCLOSURE

The authors declare that the research was conducted in the absence of any commercial or financial relationships that could be construed as a potential conflict of interest.

REFERENCES

1. Kingston A, Comas-Herrera A, Jagger C, et al. Forecasting the care needs of the older population in England over the next 20 years: estimates from the Population Ageing and Care Simulation (PACSim) modelling study. Lancet Public Health 2018;3(9):e447–55.
2. Lowsky DJ, Olshansky SJ, Bhattacharya J, et al. Heterogeneity in healthy aging. J Gerontol A Biol Sci Med Sci 2014;69(6):640–9.
3. Mankowski RT, Anton SD, Ghita GL, et al. Older sepsis survivors suffer persistent disability burden and poor long-term survival. J Am Geriatr Soc 2020. [Epub ahead of print].
4. Menaker J, Scalea TM. Geriatric care in the surgical intensive care unit. Crit Care Med 2010;38(9 Suppl):S452–9.
5. Prescott HC, Angus DC. Enhancing recovery from sepsis: a review. JAMA 2018; 319(1):62–75.
6. Schulz AR, Malzer JN, Domingo C, et al. Low thymic activity and dendritic cell numbers are associated with the immune response to primary viral infection in elderly humans. J Immunol 2015;195(10):4699–711.
7. Metcalf TU, Cubas RA, Ghneim K, et al. Global analyses revealed age-related alterations in innate immune responses after stimulation of pathogen recognition receptors. Aging Cell 2015;14(3):421–32.
8. Gruver AL, Hudson LL, Sempowski GD. Immunosenescence of ageing. J Pathol 2007;211(2):144–56.
9. Al-Zamil WM, Yassin SA. Recent developments in age-related macular degeneration: a review. Clin Interv Aging 2017;12:1313–30.
10. Horiguchi H, Loftus TJ, Hawkins RB, et al. Innate immunity in the persistent inflammation, immunosuppression, and catabolism syndrome and its implications for therapy. Front Immunol 2018;9:595.
11. Martin TR, Nakamura M, Matute-Bello G. The role of apoptosis in acute lung injury. Crit Care Med 2003;31(4 Suppl):S184–8.

12. Tardif N, Polia F, Tjader I, et al. Autophagy flux in critical illness, a translational approach. Sci Rep 2019;9(1):10762.
13. Calabrese EJ, Mattson MP. How does hormesis impact biology, toxicology, and medicine? NPJ Aging Mech Dis 2017;3:13.
14. Zhang H, Davies KJA, Forman HJ. Oxidative stress response and Nrf2 signaling in aging. Free Radic Biol Med 2015;88(Pt B):314–36.
15. Khan SS, Singer BD, Vaughan DE. Molecular and physiological manifestations and measurement of aging in humans. Aging Cell 2017;16(4):624–33.
16. Hoeijmakers JH. DNA damage, aging, and cancer. N Engl J Med 2009;361(15): 1475–85.
17. Dutta D, Xu J, Dirain ML, et al. Calorie restriction combined with resveratrol induces autophagy and protects 26-month-old rat hearts from doxorubicin-induced toxicity. Free Radic Biol Med 2014;74:252–62.
18. Marzetti E, Calvani R, Cesari M, et al. Mitochondrial dysfunction and sarcopenia of aging: from signaling pathways to clinical trials. Int J Biochem Cell Biol 2013; 45(10):2288–301.
19. Gardner AK, Ghita GL, Wang Z, et al. The development of chronic critical illness determines physical function, quality of life, and long-term survival among early survivors of sepsis in surgical ICUs. Crit Care Med 2019;47(4):566–73.
20. Harada CN, Natelson Love MC, Triebel KL. Normal cognitive aging. Clin Geriatr Med 2013;29(4):737–52.
21. Gabrieli JD, Poldrack RA, Desmond JE. The role of left prefrontal cortex in language and memory. Proc Natl Acad Sci U S A 1998;95(3):906–13.
22. Bartzokis G, Beckson M, Lu PH, et al. Age-related changes in frontal and temporal lobe volumes in men: a magnetic resonance imaging study. Arch Gen Psychiatry 2001;58(5):461–5.
23. Peterson JF, Pun BT, Dittus RS, et al. Delirium and its motoric subtypes: a study of 614 critically ill patients. J Am Geriatr Soc 2006;54(3):479–84.
24. Hayhurst CJ, Pandharipande PP, Hughes CG. Intensive care unit delirium: a review of diagnosis, prevention, and treatment. Anesthesiology 2016;125(6): 1229–41.
25. Bienvenu OJ, Neufeld KJ, Needham DM. Treatment of four psychiatric emergencies in the intensive care unit. Crit Care Med 2012;40(9):2662–70.
26. Oxenham H, Sharpe N. Cardiovascular aging and heart failure. Eur J Heart Fail 2003;5(4):427–34.
27. Picca A, Mankowski RT, Burman JL, et al. Mitochondrial quality control mechanisms as molecular targets in cardiac ageing. Nat Rev Cardiol 2018;15(9): 543–54.
28. Damluji AA, Forman DE, van Diepen S, et al. Older adults in the cardiac intensive care unit: factoring geriatric syndromes in the management, prognosis, and process of care: a scientific statement from the American Heart Association. Circulation 2020;141(2):e6–32.
29. Writing Group M, Mozaffarian D, Benjamin EJ, et al. Executive summary: heart disease and stroke statistics–2016 update: a report from the American Heart Association. Circulation 2016;133(4):447–54.
30. Morley JE, Reese SS. Clinical implications of the aging heart. Am J Med 1989; 86(1):77–86.
31. Benetos A, Waeber B, Izzo J, et al. Influence of age, risk factors, and cardiovascular and renal disease on arterial stiffness: clinical applications. Am J Hypertens 2002;15(12):1101–8.

32. Joyner MJ. Effect of exercise on arterial compliance. Circulation 2000;102(11): 1214–5.

33. Shinmura K. Cardiac senescence, heart failure, and frailty: a triangle in elderly people. Keio J Med 2016;65(2):25–32.

34. Hu YF, Chen YJ, Lin YJ, et al. Inflammation and the pathogenesis of atrial fibrillation. Nat Rev Cardiol 2015;12(4):230–43.

35. Kim SC, Stice JP, Chen L, et al. Extracellular heat shock protein 60, cardiac myocytes, and apoptosis. Circ Res 2009;105(12):1186–95.

36. Aviles RJ, Martin DO, Apperson-Hansen C, et al. Inflammation as a risk factor for atrial fibrillation. Circulation 2003;108(24):3006–10.

37. Bellumkonda L, Tyrrell D, Hummel SL, et al. Pathophysiology of heart failure and frailty: a common inflammatory origin? Aging Cell 2017;16(3):444–50.

38. Chen AY, Sokol SS, Kress JP, et al. New-onset atrial fibrillation is an independent predictor of mortality in medical intensive care unit patients. Ann Pharmacother 2015;49(5):523–7.

39. Stratton JR, Cerqueira MD, Schwartz RS, et al. Differences in cardiovascular responses to isoproterenol in relation to age and exercise training in healthy men. Circulation 1992;86(2):504–12.

40. Jones SA, Boyett MR, Lancaster MK. Declining into failure: the age-dependent loss of the L-type calcium channel within the sinoatrial node. Circulation 2007; 115(10):1183–90.

41. Boillot A, Massol J, Maupoil V, et al. Alterations of myocardial and vascular adrenergic receptor-mediated responses in Escherichia coli-induced septic shock in the rat. Crit Care Med 1996;24(8):1373–80.

42. Strait JB, Lakatta EG. Aging-associated cardiovascular changes and their relationship to heart failure. Heart Fail Clin 2012;8(1):143–64.

43. Swinne CJ, Shapiro EP, Lima SD, et al. Age-associated changes in left ventricular diastolic performance during isometric exercise in normal subjects. Am J Cardiol 1992;69(8):823–6.

44. Patel AR, Patel AR, Singh S, et al. Cardiac ultrasound in the intensive care unit: a review. Cureus 2019;11(5):e4612.

45. McLean AS. Echocardiography in shock management. Crit Care 2016;20:275.

46. Estenne M, Yernault JC, De Troyer A. Rib cage and diaphragm-abdomen compliance in humans: effects of age and posture. J Appl Physiol (1985) 1985;59(6):1842–8.

47. Vaz Fragoso CA, Gill TM. Respiratory impairment and the aging lung: a novel paradigm for assessing pulmonary function. J Gerontol A Biol Sci Med Sci 2012;67(3):264–75.

48. Watsford ML, Murphy AJ, Pine MJ. The effects of ageing on respiratory muscle function and performance in older adults. J Sci Med Sport 2007;10(1):36–44.

49. Polkey MI, Hamnegard CH, Hughes PD, et al. Influence of acute lung volume change on contractile properties of human diaphragm. J Appl Physiol (1985) 1998;85(4):1322–8.

50. Kelly NG, McCarter RJ, Barnwell GM. Respiratory muscle stiffness is age- and muscle-specific. Aging (Milano) 1993;5(3):229–38.

51. Aghasafari P, Heise RL, Reynolds A, et al. Aging effects on alveolar sacs under mechanical ventilation. J Gerontol A Biol Sci Med Sci 2019;74(2):139–46.

52. Kronenberg RS, Drage CW. Attenuation of the ventilatory and heart rate responses to hypoxia and hypercapnia with aging in normal men. J Clin Invest 1973;52(8):1812–9.

53. Moliva JI, Rajaram MV, Sidiki S, et al. Molecular composition of the alveolar lining fluid in the aging lung. Age (Dordr) 2014;36(3):9633.
54. Ho JC, Chan KN, Hu WH, et al. The effect of aging on nasal mucociliary clearance, beat frequency, and ultrastructure of respiratory cilia. Am J Respir Crit Care Med 2001;163(4):983–8.
55. Svartengren M, Falk R, Philipson K. Long-term clearance from small airways decreases with age. Eur Respir J 2005;26(4):609–15.
56. Kaplan V, Angus DC, Griffin MF, et al. Hospitalized community-acquired pneumonia in the elderly: age- and sex-related patterns of care and outcome in the United States. Am J Respir Crit Care Med 2002;165(6):766–72.
57. Tong S, Amand C, Kieffer A, et al. Trends in healthcare utilization and costs associated with pneumonia in the United States during 2008-2014. BMC Health Serv Res 2018;18(1):715.
58. Fry AM, Shay DK, Holman RC, et al. Trends in hospitalizations for pneumonia among persons aged 65 years or older in the United States, 1988-2002. JAMA 2005;294(21):2712–9.
59. Denic A, Lieske JC, Chakkera HA, et al. The substantial loss of nephrons in healthy human kidneys with aging. J Am Soc Nephrol 2017;28(1):313–20.
60. Fuiano G, Sund S, Mazza G, et al. Renal hemodynamic response to maximal vasodilating stimulus in healthy older subjects. Kidney Int 2001;59(3):1052–8.
61. Musso CG. Geriatric nephrology and the 'nephrogeriatric giants. Int Urol Nephrol 2002;34(2):255–6.
62. Sands JM. Urine concentrating and diluting ability during aging. J Gerontol A Biol Sci Med Sci 2012;67(12):1352–7.
63. Denic A, Mathew J, Lerman LO, et al. Single-nephron glomerular filtration rate in healthy adults. N Engl J Med 2017;376(24):2349–57.
64. Musso CG, Liakopoulos V, Ioannidis I, et al. Acute renal failure in the elderly: particular characteristics. Int Urol Nephrol 2006;38(3–4):787–93.
65. Baldea AJ. Effect of aging on renal function plus monitoring and support. Surg Clin North Am 2015;95(1):71–83.
66. Schmitt R, Coca S, Kanbay M, et al. Recovery of kidney function after acute kidney injury in the elderly: a systematic review and meta-analysis. Am J Kidney Dis 2008;52(2):262–71.
67. Cheung CM, Ponnusamy A, Anderton JG. Management of acute renal failure in the elderly patient: a clinician's guide. Drugs Aging 2008;25(6):455–76.
68. Wang C, Lv LS, Huang H, et al. Initiation time of renal replacement therapy on patients with acute kidney injury: a systematic review and meta-analysis of 8179 participants. Nephrology (Carlton) 2017;22(1):7–18.
69. Chronopoulos A, Rosner MH, Cruz DN, et al. Acute kidney injury in elderly intensive care patients: a review. Intensive Care Med 2010;36(9):1454–64.
70. Lynch GS. Update on emerging drugs for sarcopenia - age-related muscle wasting. Expert Opin Emerg Drugs 2008;13(4):655–73.
71. Moretti C, Frajese GV, Guccione L, et al. Androgens and body composition in the aging male. J Endocrinol Invest 2005;28(3 Suppl):56–64.
72. Heymsfield SB, Arteaga C, McManus C, et al. Measurement of muscle mass in humans: validity of the 24-hour urinary creatinine method. Am J Clin Nutr 1983;37(3):478–94.
73. Coca SG. Acute kidney injury in elderly persons. Am J Kidney Dis 2010;56(1):122–31.
74. Honda K, Littman DR. The microbiota in adaptive immune homeostasis and disease. Nature 2016;535(7610):75–84.

75. Grosicki GJ, Fielding RA, Lustgarten MS. Gut microbiota contribute to age-related changes in skeletal muscle size, composition, and function: biological basis for a gut-muscle Axis. Calcif Tissue Int 2018;102(4):433–42.

76. Haak BW, Wiersinga WJ. The role of the gut microbiota in sepsis. Lancet Gastroenterol Hepatol 2017;2(2):135–43.

77. Alverdy JC, Krezalek MA. Collapse of the microbiome, emergence of the pathobiome, and the immunopathology of sepsis. Crit Care Med 2017;45(2):337–47.

78. Haak BW, Prescott HC, Wiersinga WJ. Therapeutic potential of the gut microbiota in the prevention and treatment of sepsis. Front Immunol 2018;9:2042.

79. Nakov R, Segal JP, Settanni CR, et al. Microbiome: what intensivists should know. Minerva Anestesiol 2020;86(7):777–85.

80. Cook DJ, Johnstone J, Marshall JC, et al. Probiotics: prevention of severe pneumonia and endotracheal colonization trial-PROSPECT: a pilot trial. Trials 2016; 17:377.

81. Curtis E, Litwic A, Cooper C, et al. Determinants of muscle and bone aging. J Cell Physiol 2015;230(11):2618–25.

82. Brummel NE, Balas MC, Morandi A, et al. Understanding and reducing disability in older adults following critical illness. Crit Care Med 2015;43(6):1265–75.

83. Jolley SE, Bunnell AE, Hough CL. ICU-acquired weakness. Chest 2016;150(5): 1129–40.

84. Puthucheary ZA, Rawal J, McPhail M, et al. Acute skeletal muscle wasting in critical illness. JAMA 2013;310(15):1591–600.

85. Hasselgren PO, Alamdari N, Aversa Z, et al. Corticosteroids and muscle wasting: role of transcription factors, nuclear cofactors, and hyperacetylation. Curr Opin Clin Nutr Metab Care 2010;13(4):423–8.

86. Klaude M, Fredriksson K, Tjader I, et al. Proteasome proteolytic activity in skeletal muscle is increased in patients with sepsis. Clin Sci (Lond) 2007;112(9): 499–506.

87. Rocheteau P, Chatre L, Briand D, et al. Sepsis induces long-term metabolic and mitochondrial muscle stem cell dysfunction amenable by mesenchymal stem cell therapy. Nat Commun 2015;6:10145.

88. Dos Santos C, Hussain SN, Mathur S, et al. Mechanisms of chronic muscle wasting and dysfunction after an intensive care unit stay. A pilot study. Am J Respir Crit Care Med 2016;194(7):821–30.

89. Liao CD, Tsauo JY, Wu YT, et al. Effects of protein supplementation combined with resistance exercise on body composition and physical function in older adults: a systematic review and meta-analysis. Am J Clin Nutr 2017;106(4): 1078–91.

90. Phillips SM, Dickerson RN, Moore FA, et al. Protein turnover and metabolism in the elderly intensive care unit patient. Nutr Clin Pract 2017;32(1_suppl): 112S–20S.

91. Weir S, Salkever DS, Rivara FP, et al. One-year treatment costs of trauma care in the USA. Expert Rev Pharmacoecon Outcomes Res 2010;10(2):187–97.

92. Keller JM, Sciadini MF, Sinclair E, et al. Geriatric trauma: demographics, injuries, and mortality. J Orthop Trauma 2012;26(9):e161–5.

93. Hashmi A, Ibrahim-Zada I, Rhee P, et al. Predictors of mortality in geriatric trauma patients: a systematic review and meta-analysis. J Trauma Acute Care Surg 2014;76(3):894–901.

94. Vanzant EL, Hilton RE, Lopez CM, et al. Advanced age is associated with worsened outcomes and a unique genomic response in severely injured patients with hemorrhagic shock. Crit Care 2015;19:77.

95. Labib N, Nouh T, Winocour S, et al. Severely injured geriatric population: morbidity, mortality, and risk factors. J Trauma 2011;71(6):1908–14.
96. Bergeron E, Clement J, Lavoie A, et al. A simple fall in the elderly: not so simple. J Trauma 2006;60(2):268–73.
97. Sterling DA, O'Connor JA, Bonadies J. Geriatric falls: injury severity is high and disproportionate to mechanism. J Trauma 2001;50(1):116–9.
98. Bonne S, Schuerer DJ. Trauma in the older adult: epidemiology and evolving geriatric trauma principles. Clin Geriatr Med 2013;29(1):137–50.
99. Lee WY, Cameron PA, Bailey MJ. Road traffic injuries in the elderly. Emerg Med J 2006;23(1):42–6.
100. Joseph B, Orouji Jokar T, Hassan A, et al. Redefining the association between old age and poor outcomes after trauma: the impact of frailty syndrome. J Trauma Acute Care Surg 2017;82(3):575–81.
101. Joseph B, Pandit V, Zangbar B, et al. Validating trauma-specific frailty index for geriatric trauma patients: a prospective analysis. J Am Coll Surg 2014;219(1): 10–7.e11.
102. Fried LP, Tangen CM, Walston J, et al. Frailty in older adults: evidence for a phenotype. J Gerontol A Biol Sci Med Sci 2001;56(3):M146–56.
103. Walston J, Hadley EC, Ferrucci L, et al. Research agenda for frailty in older adults: toward a better understanding of physiology and etiology: summary from the American Geriatrics Society/National Institute on Aging Research conference on frailty in older adults. J Am Geriatr Soc 2006;54(6):991–1001.
104. Hamerman D. Toward an understanding of frailty. Ann Intern Med 1999;130(11): 945–50.
105. Bardes JM, Benjamin E, Schellenberg M, et al. Old age with a traumatic mechanism of injury should be a trauma team activation criterion. J Emerg Med 2019; 57(2):151–5.
106. Caterino JM, Valasek T, Werman HA. Identification of an age cutoff for increased mortality in patients with elderly trauma. Am J Emerg Med 2010;28(2):151–8.
107. Demetriades D, Sava J, Alo K, et al. Old age as a criterion for trauma team activation. J Trauma 2001;51(4):754–6 [discussion: 756–7].
108. Sharma G, Goodwin J. Effect of aging on respiratory system physiology and immunology. Clin Interv Aging 2006;1(3):253–60.
109. Heffernan DS, Thakkar RK, Monaghan SF, et al. Normal presenting vital signs are unreliable in geriatric blunt trauma victims. J Trauma 2010;69(4):813–20.
110. Martin JT, Alkhoury F, O'Connor JA, et al. Normal' vital signs belie occult hypoperfusion in geriatric trauma patients. Am Surg 2010;76(1):65–9.
111. Sasser SM, Hunt RC, Faul M, et al. Guidelines for field triage of injured patients: recommendations of the National expert panel on field triage, 2011. MMWR Recomm Rep 2012;61(RR-1):1–20.
112. Center for Disease Control and Prevention. Sepsis, data & reports. 2016. Available at: https://www.cdc.gov/sepsis/datareports/index.html. Accessed April 10, 2020.
113. Fleischmann C, Scherag A, Adhikari NK, et al. Assessment of global incidence and mortality of hospital-treated sepsis. Current estimates and limitations. Am J Respir Crit Care Med 2016;193(3):259–72.
114. Fleischmann C, Thomas-Rueddel DO, Hartmann M, et al. Hospital incidence and mortality rates of sepsis. Dtsch Arztebl Int 2016;113(10):159–66.
115. Kumar G, Kumar N, Taneja A, et al. Nationwide trends of severe sepsis in the 21st century (2000-2007). Chest 2011;140(5):1223–31.

116. Martin GS, Mannino DM, Eaton S, et al. The epidemiology of sepsis in the United States from 1979 through 2000. N Engl J Med 2003;348(16):1546–54.

117. Stevenson EK, Rubenstein AR, Radin GT, et al. Two decades of mortality trends among patients with severe sepsis: a comparative meta-analysis*. Crit Care Med 2014;42(3):625–31.

118. Dellinger RP, Carlet JM, Masur H, et al. Surviving Sepsis Campaign guidelines for management of severe sepsis and septic shock. Intensive Care Med 2004; 30(4):536–55.

119. Castellanos-Ortega A, Suberviola B, Garcia-Astudillo LA, et al. Impact of the Surviving Sepsis Campaign protocols on hospital length of stay and mortality in septic shock patients: results of a three-year follow-up quasi-experimental study. Crit Care Med 2010;38(4):1036–43.

120. Gao F, Melody T, Daniels DF, et al. The impact of compliance with 6-hour and 24-hour sepsis bundles on hospital mortality in patients with severe sepsis: a prospective observational study. Crit Care 2005;9(6):R764–70.

121. Levy MM, Rhodes A, Phillips GS, et al. Surviving Sepsis Campaign: association between performance metrics and outcomes in a 7.5-year study. Crit Care Med 2015;43(1):3–12.

122. Rhodes A, Phillips G, Beale R, et al. The surviving sepsis campaign bundles and outcome: results from the international multicentre prevalence study on sepsis (the IMPreSS study). Intensive Care Med 2015;41(9):1620–8.

123. Angus DC, Linde-Zwirble WT, Lidicker J, et al. Epidemiology of severe sepsis in the United States: analysis of incidence, outcome, and associated costs of care. Crit Care Med 2001;29(7):1303–10.

124. Brakenridge SC, Efron PA, Stortz JA, et al. The impact of age on the innate immune response and outcomes after severe sepsis/septic shock in trauma and surgical intensive care unit patients. J Trauma Acute Care Surg 2018;85(2): 247–55.

125. Pinheiro da Silva F, Machado MCC. Septic shock and the aging process: a molecular comparison. Front Immunol 2017;8:1389.

126. Baldwin MR. Measuring and predicting long-term outcomes in older survivors of critical illness. Minerva Anestesiol 2015;81(6):650–61.

127. Solana R, Pawelec G, Tarazona R. Aging and innate immunity. Immunity 2006; 24(5):491–4.

128. Nacionales DC, Gentile LF, Vanzant E, et al. Aged mice are unable to mount an effective myeloid response to sepsis. J Immunol 2014;192(2):612–22.

129. Cao JN, Gollapudi S, Sharman EH, et al. Age-related alterations of gene expression patterns in human CD8+ T cells. Aging Cell 2010;9(1):19–31.

130. Tarazona R, DelaRosa O, Alonso C, et al. Increased expression of NK cell markers on T lymphocytes in aging and chronic activation of the immune system reflects the accumulation of effector/senescent T cells. Mech Ageing Dev 2000; 121(1–3):77–88.

131. Schefold JC, Bierbrauer J, Weber-Carstens S. Intensive care unit-acquired weakness (ICUAW) and muscle wasting in critically ill patients with severe sepsis and septic shock. J Cachexia Sarcopenia Muscle 2010;1(2): 147–57.

132. Stortz JA, Mira JC, Raymond SL, et al. Benchmarking clinical outcomes and the immunocatabolic phenotype of chronic critical illness after sepsis in surgical intensive care unit patients. J Trauma Acute Care Surg 2018;84(2): 342–9.

133. Mathias B, Delmas AL, Ozrazgat-Baslanti T, et al. Human myeloid-derived suppressor cells are associated with chronic immune suppression after severe sepsis/septic shock. Ann Surg 2017;265(4):827–34.

134. Cuenca AG, Moldawer LL. Myeloid-derived suppressor cells in sepsis: friend or foe? Intensive Care Med 2012;38(6):928–30.

135. Darcy CJ, Minigo G, Piera KA, et al. Neutrophils with myeloid derived suppressor function deplete arginine and constrain T cell function in septic shock patients. Crit Care 2014;18(4):R163.

136. Delano MJ, Scumpia PO, Weinstein JS, et al. MyD88-dependent expansion of an immature GR-1(+)CD11b(+) population induces T cell suppression and Th2 polarization in sepsis. J Exp Med 2007;204(6):1463–74.

137. Janols H, Bergenfelz C, Allaoui R, et al. A high frequency of MDSCs in sepsis patients, with the granulocytic subtype dominating in gram-positive cases. J Leukoc Biol 2014;96(5):685–93.

138. Nacionales DC, Szpila B, Ungaro R, et al. A detailed characterization of the dysfunctional immunity and Abnormal myelopoiesis induced by severe shock and trauma in the aged. J Immunol 2015;195(5):2396–407.

139. Bueno V, Sant'Anna OA, Lord JM. Ageing and myeloid-derived suppressor cells: possible involvement in immunosenescence and age-related disease. Age (Dordr) 2014;36(6):9729.

140. Hollen MK, Stortz JA, Darden D, et al. Myeloid-derived suppressor cell function and epigenetic expression evolves over time after surgical sepsis. Crit Care 2019;23(1):355.

141. Mira JC, Brakenridge SC, Moldawer LL, et al. Persistent inflammation, immunosuppression and catabolism syndrome. Crit Care Clin 2017;33(2):245–58.

142. Dellinger RP, Levy MM, Rhodes A, et al. Surviving sepsis campaign: international guidelines for management of severe sepsis and septic shock: 2012. Crit Care Med 2013;41(2):580–637.

143. Iwashyna TJ, Cooke CR, Wunsch H, et al. Population burden of long-term survivorship after severe sepsis in older Americans. J Am Geriatr Soc 2012;60(6):1070–7.

144. Lamas D. Chronic critical illness. N Engl J Med 2014;370(2):175–7.

145. Cox CE. Persistent systemic inflammation in chronic critical illness. Respir Care 2012;57(6):859–64 [discussion: 864-6].

146. Hawkins RB, Raymond SL, Stortz JA, et al. Chronic critical illness and the persistent inflammation, immunosuppression, and catabolism syndrome. Front Immunol 2018;9:1511.

147. Efron PA, Mohr AM, Bihorac A, et al. Persistent inflammation, immunosuppression, and catabolism and the development of chronic critical illness after surgery. Surgery 2018;164(2):178–84.

148. Mira JC, Gentile LF, Mathias BJ, et al. Sepsis pathophysiology, chronic critical illness, and persistent inflammation-immunosuppression and catabolism syndrome. Crit Care Med 2017;45(2):253–62.

149. Minejima E, Bensman J, She RC, et al. A dysregulated balance of proinflammatory and anti-inflammatory host cytokine response early during therapy predicts persistence and mortality in Staphylococcus aureus Bacteremia. Crit Care Med 2016;44(4):671–9.

150. Drewry AM, Samra N, Skrupky LP, et al. Persistent lymphopenia after diagnosis of sepsis predicts mortality. Shock 2014;42(5):383–91.

151. Kahn JM, Le T, Angus DC, et al. The epidemiology of chronic critical illness in the United States*. Crit Care Med 2015;43(2):282–7.

152. Davidson GH, Hamlat CA, Rivara FP, et al. Long-term survival of adult trauma patients. JAMA 2011;305(10):1001–7.
153. Nelson JE, Cox CE, Hope AA, et al. Chronic critical illness. Am J Respir Crit Care Med 2010;182(4):446–54.
154. Carson SS, Bach PB. The epidemiology and costs of chronic critical illness. Crit Care Clin 2002;18(3):461–76.
155. Mira JC, Cuschieri J, Ozrazgat-Baslanti T, et al. The epidemiology of chronic critical illness after severe traumatic injury at two level-one trauma centers. Crit Care Med 2017;45(12):1989–96.

The Frailty Syndrome
A Critical Issue in Geriatric Oncology

Christina A. Minami, MD, MS[a,b], Zara Cooper, MD, MSc[c,*]

KEYWORDS

- Frailty • Oncology • Surgery • Radiation • Chemotherapy • Systemic therapy
- Geriatric assessment • Outcomes

KEY POINTS

- Frailty is defined as an age-related condition characterized by decreased physiologic reserves, loss of adaptive capacity, and an increased vulnerability to stressors.
- The presence of frailty is associated with worse survival and, in some cases, higher postoperative complication rates in patients undergoing surgery for an oncologic indication.
- The relationship between frailty and noncompletion of radiation and/or radiation toxicity is ill defined.
- Components of the geriatric assessment may be predictive of chemotherapy toxicity.
- Geriatric-specific assessments in older adults with cancer is recommended, as they identify potential areas for interventions.

INTRODUCTION

Given the relationship between cancer and aging, it is not surprising that as a growing proportion of the US population ages, the incidence of cancer increases.[1] In recent years, more than 50% of new cancers diagnosed have occurred in people aged 65 years and older.[2] The aging baby boomer generation represents a shifting demographic who requires a nuanced approach for the care of older adults with cancer. Older adults are often burdened by varying degrees of physical and mental comorbidities, disabilities, and a state of frailty. Physicians require a better understanding of the associations between patients' baseline state of health and potential treatment complications.

Frailty's role in clinical decision-making is evolving. Frailty is defined as an age-related condition characterized by decreased physiologic reserves, loss of adaptive

[a] Division of Breast Surgery, Department of Surgery, Brigham and Women's Hospital, Boston, MA, USA; [b] Breast Oncology Program, Dana-Farber Cancer Institute, 450 Brookline Avenue, Yawkey 1274, Boston, MA 02215, USA; [c] Division of Trauma, Burn, and Critical Care, Department of Surgery, Brigham and Women's Hospital, 1620 Tremont Street, Suite 2-016, Boston, MA 02120, USA
* Corresponding author.
E-mail address: zcooper@bwh.harvard.edu

Crit Care Clin 37 (2021) 151–174
https://doi.org/10.1016/j.ccc.2020.08.007
0749-0704/21/© 2020 Elsevier Inc. All rights reserved.

criticalcare.theclinics.com

capacity, and an increased vulnerability to stressors. Frailty can often coexist with disability and chronic disease but may exist independent of these.[3-7] The gold standard for frailty evaluation is the comprehensive geriatric assessment (CGA), which is a multidimensional, interdisciplinary evaluation that uses validated tools to assess domains crucial to determining physiologic age. The aforementioned domains include comorbidity, functional status, nutritional status, polypharmacy, social support, cognition, and psychological status.[8] Although many oncologists routinely assess comorbidities and functional status, evaluation of the remaining domains are often neglected.

Interest in both defining and measuring frailty has increased in recent years. Additional effort has been set forth to quantify the association of frailty with morbidity and mortality after oncologic treatment. Frailty incidence has been estimated to be 10% to 20% in patients aged 65 years or older and up to 20% to 40% in those aged 85 years or older.[9,10] Frailty has been shown to be associated with adverse outcomes in oncology patients: both disease-related (ie, progression and death) as well as treatment-related (ie, postoperative complications and chemotherapy toxicity).[3,11-17] In this section, the authors review cancer-specific geriatric assessments, the existing data on the significance of frailty in oncology patients, and current initiatives to integrate geriatric assessment data into cancer care.

CANCER-SPECIFIC GERIATRIC ASSESSMENTS

Oncologists have developed several rigorous, cancer-specific geriatric assessments (CGSAs) to aid evaluation and counseling of older adults with cancer. The authors review a current list of assessments available to oncologists.

Cancer-Specific Geriatric Assessment

The CSGA is a multidimensional assessment that uses both patient-completed and health care provider–administered questionnaires to evaluate geriatric domains. Developed in a cohort of patients aged 65 years and older with lymphoma, breast, colon, and lung cancer by Hurria and colleagues,[18] the CSGA was designed to be a brief, mainly self-administered, and comprehensive assessment. The specific components of the CSGA can be found in **Table 1**. There are 112 items in the CSGA, and the mean time-to-completion in the original feasibility study was 27 minutes.[18] The CSGA is able to identify deficits in patients with a normal Karnofsky performance status, a commonly used measure in oncology to quantify functional impairment, and is also predictive of treatment-related toxicities in older adults with cancer.[19]

Carolina Frailty Index

The Carolina frailty index (CFI) was developed based on the principles of deficit accumulation described by Rockwood and Mitnitski.[20] Thirty-six items are included in the assessment, most of which are patient-reported single-item questions. Health care practitioner assessment items include the Timed Up and Go test and Blessed Orientation-Memory-Concentration test. The CFI was validated in a cohort of patients with cancer from the Carolina Senior: University of North Carolina Registry for Older Patients, which contains geriatric assessment data from patients aged 65 years of age and older diagnosed with cancer between 2009 and 2014. Guerard and colleagues[21] demonstrated that frailty as measured by a CFI greater than or equal to 0.4 had a greater than 2-fold increase in risk of overall mortality compared with robust patients (CFI<0.2).

Table 1
Cancer-specific geriatric assessments

Instrument/Method	Domains/Items Assessed
Cancer-Specific Geriatric Assessment[18]	Functional status (ADL/IADL) Karnofsky physician-rated and self-rated performance rating scale Timed Up and Go test Falls Comorbidity (Physical Health Section) Cognition (Blessed Orientation-Memory-Concentration test) Psychological (Hospital Anxiety and Depression Scale) Social functioning (MOS Social Activity Limitations Measure) Social support (MOS Social Support survey) Seeman and Berkman Social Ties Nutrition (body mass index and percent unintentional weight loss in the last 6 mo)
Carolina Frailty Index[21]	IADLs Self-reported health Physical function (Timed Up and Go test and falls) Comorbidities Vision Hearing Nutrition Mental health Social activity Medications Cognition (Blessed Orientation-Memory-Concentration test)
Chemotherapy Risk Assessment Scale for High-Age Patients (CRASH)[22]	Chemotherapy Risk: Examples of toxicity of various chemotherapy regimens: • 0: cisplatin/pemetrexed, dacarbazine, docetaxel weekly, paclitaxel weekly • 1: topotecan weekly, gemcitabine/irinotecan, capecitabine, 2.5 g, carboplatin/pemetrexed • 2: cisplatin/etoposide, doxorubicin q3 weeks, irinotecan q3 weeks, docetaxel q3 weeks Hematologic Risk Factors: • Diastolic blood pressure • IADL • LDH Nonhematologic Risk Factors: • ECOG PS • Mini-Mental Health Status • Mini-Nutritional Assessment
Cancer and Aging Research Group (CARG)[23]	Age Cancer type Planned chemotherapy dose Planned number of chemotherapy drugs

(continued on next page)

Table 1 (continued)	
Instrument/Method	**Domains/Items Assessed**
	Hemoglobin level
	Creatinine clearance
	Falls in the past 6 months
	Need for assistance with daily medications
	Ability to walk one block
	Limitations in social activities
	Hearing ability

Abbreviations: ADL, activities of daily living; ECOG PS, Eastern Cooperative Oncology Group performance status; IADL, instrumental activities of daily living; LDH, lactate dehydrogenase; MOS, medical outcomes study.

Chemotherapy Risk Assessment Scale for High-Age Patients

The Chemotherapy Risk Assessment Scale for High-Age Patients (CRASH) score is designed for patients aged 70 years and older and predicts grade 3 hematologic and grade 3 to 4 nonhematologic chemotherapy toxicity.[22] The specifics of chemotherapy toxicity grading encompass multiple measures in a variety of organ systems, and as such, CRASH integrates factors from different geriatric assessment tools (function, nutrition, and cognition). In general, Grade 1 toxicities are deemed mild, Grade 2 moderate, Grade 3 severe, Grade 4 life-threatening, and Grade 5 denoting treatment-related death. The CRASH assessment takes approximately 20 to 30 minutes to perform and can be found through the Senior Adult Oncology Program at Moffitt Cancer Center's Website.[8]

Cancer and Aging Research Group

The Cancer and Aging Research Group (CARG) score is an 11-item predictive model for chemotherapy toxicity in adults aged 65 years and older.[23,24] The model was demonstrated to have a better discrimination of chemotherapy toxicity risk in older adults with solid tumors than the Karnofsky performance status.[23,25] This tool estimates the risk of a grade 3 to 5 toxicity and takes less than 5 minutes to complete.[23,24]

FRAILTY AND OUTCOMES IN LOCOREGIONAL THERAPY
Surgical Outcomes

Although both the populations and the interventions studied have been heterogeneous, studies that examined the association between frailty and postoperative outcomes demonstrated that frailty is often associated with an increased risk of complications and mortality. **Table 2** reviews the oncologic studies to date examining the association between various frailty indicators and surgical outcomes. Many studies used the CGA, which requires medical, functional, psychosocial, geriatric syndrome, and nutritional assessments; however, it also allows physicians to choose from a multitude of validated tools to assess each domain. Studies using the American College of Surgeons National Surgical Quality Improvement Program (ACS NSQIP) database have used the modified frailty index (mFI). The mFI is a 11-factor measure that was based on the Canadian Study of Health and Aging Frailty Index and was developed to be used in conjunction with NSQIP. The mFI has since been simplified to a 5-factor version. Both versions have shown associations with increased postoperative morbidity and mortality.[26]

Table 2
Frailty and surgical practice pattern changes and outcomes in older patients with cancer

Cancer Type	Author, Year	Study Population	Study Outcome Measure	Frailty Assessment	Results
Breast	Clough-Gorr et al,[58] 2010	660 women, stage I–IIIa, age ≥65 y, who underwent surgery	Treatment tolerance, all-cause mortality	CSGA	GA domains are associated with poor treatment tolerance and predict mortality at 7 y of posttreatment follow-up, independent of age and stage of disease.
Breast	Clough-Gorr,[13] 2012	660 women with stage I–IIIa, age ≥65 y, who underwent surgery	Survival	CSGA	Women with ≥3 CSGA deficits had poorer 5- and 10-y overall survival (HR 1.87 and 1.74, respectively) and breast-cancer specific survival (HR 1.95 and 1.99).
Breast	Extermann et al,[59] 2004	15 women who underwent surgery for stage I–II breast cancer, age ≥70 y	Geriatric problems "amenable to intervention"	CGA	CGA directly influenced treatment decisions in 4/11 cases, and, overall, identified opportunities for preventative interventions
Breast	Stotter et al,[60] 2015	328 women, early stage estrogen-receptor (ER)-+ breast cancer in whom there were concerns regarding fitness to receive standard treatment	3-y overall survival	CGA	Comorbidity, MMSE, poor functional status, and ASA class was associated with 3-y mortality (30% of the cohort had died within 3 y)
Breast	Okonji et al,[61] 2017	326 women, stage I–III breast cancer, age ≥70 y	Receipt of therapy	CGA	Lower proportion of unfit patients underwent resection (100% of fit pts vs 91% of unfit) and received

(continued on next page)

Table 2
(continued)

Cancer Type	Author, Year	Study Population	Study Outcome Measure	Frailty Assessment	Results
					chemotherapy (51% of fit vs 20% of unfit)
Breast	Parks et al,[62] 2015	47 women stage I–II breast cancer, age ≥70 y	Receipt of therapy	CGA	Age ≥80 y, ≥4 comorbidities of daily medications (P = .002), and slower (≥19 s) TUG score were significantly associated with nonoperative treatment. No correlation found between QOL scores and treatment modality
Colorectal	Tan et al,[16] 2012	83 patients, age ≥75 y, undergoing colorectal resection	Major complications (Clavien-Dindo class II and higher)	Phenotypic (Fried)	Frailty was associated with postoperative major complications (OR 4.083; 95% CI 1.433–11.638)
Colorectal	Kristjansson et al,[12] 2010	178 patients, age ≥70 y, undergoing elective colorectal cancer operations	OS, postoperative complications (Clavien-Dindo class II and higher)	CGA	33% of fit patients, 36% of intermediate patients, 62% of frail patients (P = .002) experienced severe postoperative complications
Gastric	Lu et al,[17] 2017	165 patients, age ≥80 y, who underwent surgery for gastric cancer	Postoperative complications, survival	Preoperative frailty, inflammation-based prognostic scores	Preoperative frailty was independently associated with OS (OR 1.613; 95% CI 1.052–2.473; P = .028), RFS (OR 1.859; 95% CI 1.279–2.703; P = .001), and CSS (OR 1.859; 95% CI 1.279–2.703; P = .001).

				Phenotypic (Fried)	
Gynecologic	Courtney-Brooks, et al,[30] 2012	40 patients, age ≥65 y, undergoing gynecologic oncology procedures	Postoperative complications, nonhome discharge, 30-d readmission		Rate of 30-d surgical complications increased with frailty score and was 24% vs 67% for women who were not frail as compared with the frail ($P = .04$), no difference in nonhome discharge or 30-d readmission
GI	Buettner et al,[27] 2016	1326 patients, age ≥18 y, undergoing elective hepatobiliary, pancreatic, or colorectal surgery	1-y mortality	Sarcopenia, mFI	Independent risk factors for 1-y mortality: increasing age (65–75 y: HR 1.81, 95% CI 1.05–3.14; ≥75 y: HR 2.79, 95% CI 1.55–5.02), preoperative anemia hemoglobin <12.5 g/dL (HR 1.68, 95% CI 1.17–2.40), and preoperative sarcopenia (HR 1.98, 95% CI 1.36–2.88; all $P<.05$)
GI	Peng et al,[28] 2012	557 patients, undergoing pancreatic resection for adenocarcinoma	90-d, 1- and 3-y mortality	Sarcopenia	Sarcopenia was found to be associated with an increased risk of death at 3 y (HR = 1.63, 95% CI 1.28–2.07, $P<.001$)
Head and Neck	Abt et al,[63] 2016	1193 patients undergoing head and neck cancer operations	Clavien-Dindo grade IV complications, 30-d mortality	mFI	mFI associated with postoperative critical care support but was not associated with overall mortality
Pancreas	Mogal et al,[31] 2017	9986 patients who underwent pancreaticoduodenectomy	Postop morbidity, 30-d mortality	mFI	High mFI is an independent preoperative predictor of postoperative morbidity (OR 1.544; 95% CI 1.289–1.850; $P<.0001$) and 30-d mortality

(continued on next page)

Table 2
(continued)

Cancer Type	Author, Year	Study Population	Study Outcome Measure	Frailty Assessment	Results
Urologic	Lascano et al,[33] 2015	41,681 undergoing surgery for presumed urologic malignancy	Complications, 30-d mortality	Proposed 15-variable mFI, ASA class	(OR 1.536; 95% CI 1.049–2.248; P = .027) Patients with a high frailty index score had higher odds of a Clavien-Dindo IV event (OR 3.7, CI: 2.865–4.788, P<.0005) and of 30-d mortality (OR 5.95, CI: 3.72–9.51, P<.0005) compared with nonfrail patients. The proposed mFI combined with ASA was most predictive of major complications and 30-d mortality
Urologic	Chappidi et al,[64] 2016	2679 patients, undergoing cystectomy	Complications, 30-d mortality	mFI	Predictors of Clavien-Dindo grade 4 or 5 complications were age ≥80 y (OR 1.58 [1.11–2.27]), mFI score ≥2 (OR = 1.84 [1.28–2.64]), and mFI ≥3 (OR = 2.58 [1.47–4.55])

Abbreviations: ASA, American Society of Anesthesiologists; ECOG PS, Eastern Cooperative Oncology Group performance status; GA, geriatric assessment; HR, hazard ratio; mFI, modified frailty index; MMSE, mini-mental status examination; OR, odds ratio; OS, overall survival; TUG, timed up and go test.

The association between frailty and impaired survival has been demonstrated across multiple malignancies. In patients with breast cancer, Clough-Gorr and colleagues[13] showed that women with 3 or more cancer-specific geriatric assessment deficits had poorer 10-year overall survival (OS) (hazard ratio [HR] 1.74, 95% confidence interval [CI]: 1.35–2.15) and breast –cancerspecific survival (HR 1.99, 95% CI: 1.21–3.28). Lu and colleagues[17] similarly demonstrated in patients older than 80 years and undergoing gastric cancer resection that frailty, as defined by preoperative albumin (<3.4 g/dL), hematocrit (<35%), and creatinine level (>2 mg/dL), was associated with worse OS (HR 1.613, 95% CI 1.052–2.473, P = .028) and disease-specific survival (HR 1.859, 95% CI 1.279–2.703, P = .001). Buettner and colleagues[27] also found that sarcopenia (defined by psoas density, occasionally used as a marker of frailty) was independently associated with a higher risk of 1-year postoperative mortality (HR 1.98, 95% CI 1.36–2.99, P<.001).[28,29] Sarcopenia, however, was not uniformly associated with frailty as measured by the mFI in this study.

The relationship between frailty and postoperative complications is complex. Lu and colleagues,[17] in their study of older adults with gastric cancer, found that although frail patients were at a significantly increased risk for systemic complications (OR 6.063, 95% CI 1.758–20.911), they were not at risk for local complications (OR 1.650, 95% CI 0.649–4.196). Courtney-Brooks and colleagues[30] observed in a small series of 37 patients with gynecologic cancers that the rate of 30-day surgical complications (urinary tract infection, surgical site infection, and pneumonia) increased with phenotypic frailty score but also found that there was no difference in the rate of nonhome discharge or 30-day hospital readmission.

Studies using the mFI in the NSQIP database demonstrate that although increased mFI scores are associated with higher odds of postoperative complications, the magnitude of the association varies by the patient population, the mFI cut-off point that defines "frail," and the outcome measure. For instance, Mogal and colleagues[31] found that in patients undergoing pancreaticoduodenectomy, a high mFI (defined as a score of 0.27 or higher) predicted Clavien-Dindo class III–IV complications (odds ratio [OR] 1.544, 95% CI 1.289–1.850) on multivariate analyses. The Clavien-Dindo classification is a scale of postoperative complications graded from I–V (class I: any deviation from the normal postoperative course without intervention to class V: death).[32] In patients undergoing surgery of a presumed urologic malignancy, however, Lascano and colleagues[33] found higher odds of a Clavien-Dindo class IV complication in patients with an mFI greater than 0.2 (OR 3.7, 95% CI 2.865–4.788, P<.005). As such, when examining different populations of oncologic patients undergoing different oncologic procedures, it is the presence of the association that should be noted rather than its magnitude.

There are ongoing initiatives in surgery to improve the outcomes of all geriatric surgical patients.[34] Tailored preoperative risk assessments, prehabilitation programs, tailored anesthesia plans, team-based care pathways, delirium prevention, and early palliative care input represent efforts in the surgical community to support the frail patient through surgery.[3] Cancer-specific treatment algorithms based on frailty have been proposed but are rarely used in clinical practice.[35]

Radiation Oncology Outcomes

There are a fewer number of studies in radiation oncology than in surgery exploring the association between frailty and treatment outcomes as seen in **Table 3**. Although some analyses suggest that performing a frailty assessment may be associated with survival benefit and may be predictive of certain treatment toxicities in certain

Table 3
Frailty and radiation oncology practice pattern changes and outcomes in older patients with cancer

Cancer Type	Author, Year	Study Population	Study Outcome Measure	Frailty Assessment	Results
Breast	Denkinger et al,[43] 2015	74 women, ≥65 y, with breast cancer treated with RT	Fatigue after RT	CSGA, Fried frailty score	The CSGA and the Fried frailty score outperformed the other indices in predicting fatigue after RT
Esophageal	Bo et al,[36] 2016	239 patients, >60 y, with esophageal squamous cell cancer undergoing RT	Overall survival	GNRI	The GNRI is an independent prognostic factor for overall survival time in elderly ESCC patients undergoing RT
Glioblastoma	Giaccherinie et al,[37] 2019	34 elderly patients treated with concurrent radiation and temozolomide	Overall survival	KPS, Prognostic nutritional index, CCI, frailty index	High KPS and type of surgery, FI were associated with overall survival
Head and Neck	Neve et al,[65] 2016	35 patients, >65 y, with head and neck cancer undergoing local therapy	Treatment completion and postoperative LOS	G8	Mean length of postoperative stay was 12.2 vs 6.5 d in patients deemed vulnerable vs fit by G8 scores, respectively ($P = .46$); completion rate of radical radiotherapy was 75% vs 100% in each group, respectively ($P = .13$)

	Study	Population	Outcome	Tool	Result
Head and Neck	Pottel et al,[38] 2015	100 patients, ≥65 y with head and neck cancer eligible for RT w/without chemotherapy	Survival	G-8	G-8 indicated quality-adjusted survival
Lung	Jeppesen et al,[42] 2018	51 patients with T1-2N0M0 NSCLC treated with SBRT	QOL, survival, unplanned admissions	CGA	CGA did not affect overall QOL, unplanned admissions or survival
Multiple	Keenen et al,[41] 2017	63 patients, >70 y, upper GI, gynecologic, prostate, and head and neck	RT toxicity	EFS	Neither EFS score, age, nor ECOG performance status were predictive of radiotherapy toxicity, breaks in treatment, or hospital admissions
Multiple	Laurent et al,[66] 2014	385 patients with solid tumors, >70 y	Cancer treatment feasibility	CGA	Feasibility rates were considerably lower for chemotherapy (72.4%) than for surgery (95.7%), radiotherapy (96.4%), and hormonal therapy (97.9%) among patients with nonmetastatic cancer
Multiple	Spyropoulou et al,[39] 2014	230 patients, >75 y, undergoing radical or palliative radiotherapy	Completion of RT	VES-13	Higher VES-13 scores were associated with higher noncompletion rates of RT (VES-13 score>3 OR 2.14, 95% CI 1.01–4.53 compared with those with a score ≤3)

(continued on next page)

Table 3
(continued)

Cancer Type	Author, Year	Study Population	Study Outcome Measure	Frailty Assessment	Results
Multiple	Middelburg et al,[44] 2017	402 patients, >65 y with breast, NSCLC, prostate, head and neck, rectal, or esophageal cancer	Acute RT toxicity	TUG, G8	Type of primary tumor, chemoradiotherapy, age, and World Health Organization performance status were more strongly associated with acute toxicity than TUG and G8 tests
Multiple	Rim et al,[40] 2018	353 patients, >70 y of age undergoing RT	RT intolerance	ECOG PS, serum albumin	Eastern Cooperative Oncology Group (ECOG) performance score ($P = .004$ and $.002$), serum albumin level ($P = .016$ and $.002$), and the expected 5-y survival ($P = .033$ and $.034$) were significant factors for midphase incompletion and total interruption
Urologic	Maebayashi et al,[67] 2016	16 patients undergoing RT or IACRT for muscle-invading bladder cancer	Feasibility of IACRT	G8	The G8 screening tool is potentially applicable for determining the feasibility of performing IACRT

Abbreviations: CCI, Charlson comorbidity index; ECOG PS, Eastern Cooperative Oncology Group performance status; EFS, Edmonton Frail Scale; FI, frailty index; G8, Geriatric 8; GNRI, geriatric nutritional risk index; IACRT, intraarterial chemoradiotherapy; KPS, Karnofsky performance status; LOS, length of stay; QOL, quality of life; RT, radiotherapy; TUG, timed up and go test; VES-13, vulnerable elders survey 13.

cancers, there is no clear evidence that its incorporation into clinical use would change clinical pathways or patient counseling.

The relationship between frailty and decreased survival in patients undergoing radiation therapy (RT) has been demonstrated in patients with glioblastoma, esophageal, and head and neck cancers.[36–41] Of interest, Jeppesen and colleagues[42] found there was no association between survival and frailty in patients with lung cancer. Frailty was found to be associated with higher treatment noncompletion rates in Spyropoulou and colleagues'[39] and Rim and colleaguess'[40] analyses performed in heterogenous populations of patients with cancer. The analysis performed by Keenan and colleagues[41] in patients with multiple tumor types undergoing RT, however, did not find any association between performance on the Edmonton Frail scale and RT toxicity, breaks in treatment, or hospital admissions.

The association between frailty scores and treatment toxicities have also been mixed. Although Denkinger and colleagues[43] found that frailty scores were strongly predictive of fatigue after RT, Middelburg and colleagues[44] found that other predictors, such as primary tumor type, age, and World Health Organization performance status were more strongly associated with acute toxicity than Geriatric 8 or Timed Up and Go scores.

FRAILTY AND OUTCOMES IN SYSTEMIC THERAPY

Traditional performance measures used in medical oncology (eg, the Karnofsky performance scores and Eastern Cooperative Oncology Group Performance Status) do not accurately identify older adults who are at the highest risk of adverse outcomes from chemotherapy.[18,23] The CGA has thus been touted as a better alternative. The American Society of Clinical Oncology (ASCO) has recently released guidelines surrounding the assessment and management of older patients receiving chemotherapy and determined that at a minimum, this patient population requires an assessment of function (Instrumental Activities of Daily Living [IADLs]), comorbidity, falls (as a single question), depression (Geriatric Depression Scale), cognition (Blessed Orientation-Memory-Concentration), and nutrition (unintentional weight loss).[8] Use of either the CARG or CRASH tools can aid clinicians in assessing the risk of chemotherapy toxicity. Different measures of frailty have been explored in different cancers and the direction of association between geriatric assessment domains and mortality remain consistent despite the differences in measures (**Table 4**).[45,46] Systematic reviews of geriatric oncology studies have also confirmed this association.[47–49]

Chemotherapy toxicity is also a major concern in all oncology patients, and the aforementioned CARG and CRASH scores have been validated as useful prediction tools in adults aged 65 years and older.[22,24] Some studies have only been able to pinpoint certain factors in the CGA as being associated with chemotherapy-related toxicity, rather than using binary designations such as "frail" or "fit" as is common in surgical literature. For instance, in patients with breast cancer, Hamaker and colleagues[50] found that polypharmacy was the only factor within the CGA to be associated with treatment toxicity, whereas Falandry and colleagues[51] found that age and living situation were the only CGA factors significantly associated with nonhematologic toxicities. Systematic reviews pinpointed functional status and geriatric syndromes as the most significant predictors of toxicity risk.[47–49] However, the ASCO guidelines for Geriatric Oncology reference 2 studies that found consensus among geriatric oncology experts that all domains of the geriatric assessment are important to assess in older patients with cancer.[8]

Table 4
Frailty and medical oncology practice pattern changes and outcomes in older patients with cancer

Cancer Type	Author, Year	Study Population	Study Outcome Measure	Frailty Assessment	Results
Breast	Hamaker et al,[50] 2014	78 patients, patients with metastatic breast cancer, >65 y, ECOG PS 0–2	Chemotherapy-related toxicity (randomized to doxorubicin vs capecitabine), overall survival	CGA	No difference in chemotherapy toxicity rates or median survival between fit and frail patients. Polypharmacy was the only factor within the CGA associated with toxicity
Breast	Barthelemy et al,[68] 2011	192 patients with early stage primary breast cancer, aged ≥70 y	Adjuvant chemotherapy use	CGA	Patient CGA results not associated with trends in recommendations for adjuvant chemotherapy
Breast	Falandry et al,[51] 2013	60 patients, >70 y, with metastatic hormone-receptor negative and human-epidermal growth factor 2 (HER-2) negative breast cancer	Chemotherapy-related toxicity, survival	CGA	Age >80 y and living in residential homes was associated with nonhematologic toxicity. Age, deficiency in IADLs, cardiac dysfunction, and living in residential homes were associated with decreased PFS
Breast	Meresse et al,[69] 2017	223 patients, 65–80 y, nonmetastatic breast cancer	Chemotherapy receipt	Age	Patients aged 75–80 y received chemotherapy treatment less often than younger patients
Breast	Owusu et al,[54] 2017	123 patients, ≥65 y, with newly diagnosed stages I–III breast cancer	Functional decline	SPPB, gait speed, grip strength, and VES-13	SPPB, gait speed, grip strength and VES-13 all demonstrated excellent predictive abilities for functional decline

Breast	Owusu et al,[55] 2016	206 patients with nonmetastatic breast cancer	Functional decline and death	VES-13	VES-13 scores (OR, 1.37; 95% CI 1.18–1.57) and having a high school education or less (OR 2.47; 95% CI 1.08–5.65) were independent predictors of functional decline/death (area under the receiver operator curve, 0.79)
Colorectal	Sastre et al,[52] 2015	33 patients with colon cancer undergoing panitumumab	Biological therapy-related toxicity	CGA	No deaths or grade 4–5 adverse events in frail patients
Colorectal	Aparicio et al,[70] 2018	102 patients with metastatic colorectal cancer	Biological therapy/ chemotherapy-related outcomes	CGA	Survival without deteriorated QOL and autonomy was similar with bevacizumab and chemotherapy. On subgroup analyses, the benefit of bevacizumab seemed to be maintained in patients with baseline impaired IADL or nutritional status
Lung	Corre et al,[71] 2016	494 patients, >70 y, with stage IV non-small-cell lung cancer (NSCLC)	Treatment failure, OS, PFS, toxicity	CGA	No association between CGA and treatment failure-free survival or OS Fewer treatment failures and toxicities observed in CGA arm
Lung	Biesma et al,[72] 2011	181 patients, >70 y, chemotherapy-naïve, with stage II–IV NSCLC	QOL	CGA	No changes in QOL after treatment CGA items associated with neuropsychiatric toxicity

(continued on next page)

Table 4
(continued)

Cancer Type	Author, Year	Study Population	Study Outcome Measure	Frailty Assessment	Results
Lymphoma	Park et al,[73] 2015	70 patients, >65 y, treated with multiagent chemotherapy for aggressive non-Hodgkin lymphoma	Chemotherapy tolerance, overall survival	CGA	Poor MNA-SF, bone marrow involvement, and baseline anemia of hemoglobin <10g/dL were found to be independent factors associated with inferior overall survival
Multiple	Hurria et al,[74] 2011	500 patients, ≥65 y, with a diagnosis of cancer	Chemotherapy-related toxicity	CGA	GA variables were associated with grade 3–5 toxicity
Multiple	Caillet et al,[75] 2011	375 patients, >70 y, with diagnosis of solid cancer	Change in cancer treatment after multidisciplinary discussion	CGA	Malnutrition and functional status assessed by ADL were independently associated with changes in cancer treatment after multidisciplinary discussion
Multiple	Puts et al,[76] 2011	112 patients, ≥65 y with new cancer diagnoses	Treatment toxicity, 6-mo mortality	Frailty markers/functional status	Low grip strength predicted toxicity ECOG performance status and ADL disability predicted time to death No association between frailty markers, functional measures, and outcome measures

Multiple	Shin et al,[77] 2012	64 patients, >65 y, undergoing chemotherapy	Chemotherapy-related outcome	CGA	Baseline ECOG PS was an independent predictive factor of significant chemotherapy-related toxicity
Multiple	Extermann et al,[22] 2012	123 patients, ≥70, starting chemotherapy	Chemotherapy-related toxicity	CGA/CRASH	The CRASH score distinguished between several risk level of severe toxicity
Multiple	Aaldriks et al,[45] 2016	494 patients, >70, starting chemotherapy	Mortality, feasibility of chemotherapy	GA/GPI	Compared with patients with 0 positive items on the 3-item GPI, patients with 1, 2, or 3 items had hazard ratios (HRs) for mortality of 1.58, 2.32, and 5.58, respectively (all $P<.001$)
Multiple	Hoppe et al,[53] 2013	364 patients ≥70 y receiving first-line chemotherapy for cancer	Functional decline	Abbreviated CGA	In multivariate analyses, high baseline depression scores (GDS) (OR 2.16; 95% CI, 1.09–4.30; $P = .03$) and low IADL scores (OR, 2.87; 95% CI, 1.06–7.79; $P = .04$) were independently associated with increased risk of functional decline

Abbreviations: ECOG PS, Eastern Cooperative Oncology Group performance status; GA, geriatric assessment; GPI, geriatric prognostic index; MNA-SF, Mini Nutritional Assessment-Short Form; PFS, progression-free survival; QOL, quality of life; SPPB, short physical performance battery; VES-13, vulnerable elders survey13.

Table 5
Geriatric assessment-guided interventions per American Society of Clinical Oncology[8]

Geriatric Domain	Measures	Suggested Interventions
Function and falls	• Instrumental activities of daily living deficit • History of falls	• Physical and/or occupational therapy • Assist device evaluation • Home exercise program • Safety evaluation • Fall prevention discussion • Home safety evaluation
Comorbidities	• Comorbidities • Polypharmacy	• Assessment of therapy risk and management of comorbidities with involvement of caregivers • Consideration of a referral to geriatrician • Involvement of primary care physician and/or geriatrician in decision-making for treatment and management of comorbidities • Reduction of polypharmacy, if possible • Assessment medication adherence
Cognition	Positive screen on a validated cognitive evaluation instrument	• Consideration of psychotherapy/psychiatry referral • Consideration of cognitive behavior therapy • Involvement of social work • Consideration of pharmacologic therapy
Depression	Geriatric Depression Scale >5	• Consideration of referral for psychotherapy/psychiatry • Consideration of cognitive behavioral therapy • Social work involvement • Possible pharmacologic therapy
Nutrition	Weight loss >10%	• Referral to nutritionist/dietician • Assessment of need for meal support

Toxicity related to targeted biological therapies has been explored in a few studies; however, these studies have not compared outcomes in frail versus fit patients. Sastre and colleagues,[52] in a phase II study examining panitumumab in a cohort of 33 frail patients with colon cancer, did not report any grade 4 or 5 adverse events; however, the study did not have a "fit" cohort for comparison.

Elements of geriatric assessment have also been shown to be predictive of functional decline among older adults receiving chemotherapy.[53–55] Hoppe and colleagues[53] showed that depression and IADLs are associated with early functional decline during chemotherapy. Owusu and colleagues[55] showed worse scores on the Vulnerable Elders Survey-13, which identified older women with breast cancer at risk for functional decline within the first year after treatment. In addition, patients who identified as African American, who had a high-school education or less, or who had lower baseline ADL scores were more likely to experience functional decline. These studies suggest that vulnerable patients may be identified before treatment.

Recommendations exist for early interventions that may mitigate functional decline with treatment. Intervention recommendations by ASCO are stratified by geriatric assessment domain as seen in **Table 5**.[56,57] The ASCO recommendations are actionable steps triggered by data gathered from the geriatric assessment. Despite having ASCO recommendations, there is no evidence-based approach for integrating the ASCO recommendations into the chemotherapy decision-making process, leaving practitioners to use their best judgment.[8]

SUMMARY

Data from the geriatric assessment can be useful in tailoring cancer treatments, counseling newly diagnosed patients, and optimizing patients for their treatment course. Additional investigation is required to fully understand how to integrate these data into treatment decision-making to optimize outcomes in older oncology patients. Given that treatment strategies are multidisciplinary and interdependent, frailty assessment data must be shared among surgical, radiation, and medical oncologists. It is incumbent on all 3 specialties to understand the relationship between the baseline geriatric assessment and its potential treatment implications for oncology patients.

REFERENCES

1. Bluethmann SM, Mariotto AB, Rowland JH. Anticipating the "Silver Tsunami": prevalence trajectories and comorbidity burden among older cancer survivors in the United States. Cancer Epidemiol Biomarkers Prev 2016;25(7):1029–36.
2. Institute NC. Age and cancer risk. 2015. Available at: https://www.cancer.gov/about-cancer/causes-prevention/risk/age. Accessed December 10, 2019.
3. Robinson TN, Walston JD, Brummel NE, et al. Frailty for Surgeons: review of a National Institute on Aging conference on frailty for specialists. J Am Coll Surg 2015; 221(6):1083–92.
4. Bortz WM 2nd. A conceptual framework of frailty: a review. J Gerontol A Biol Sci Med Sci 2002;57(5):M283–8.
5. Fried LP, Tangen CM, Walston J, et al. Frailty in older adults: evidence for a phenotype. J Gerontol A Biol Sci Med Sci 2001;56(3):M146–56.
6. Lipsitz LA. Dynamics of stability: the physiologic basis of functional health and frailty. J Gerontol A Biol Sci Med Sci 2002;57(3):B115–25.
7. Rockwood K, Song X, MacKnight C, et al. A global clinical measure of fitness and frailty in elderly people. CMAJ 2005;173(5):489–95.

8. Mohile SG, Dale W, Somerfield MR, et al. Practical assessment and management of vulnerabilities in older patients receiving chemotherapy: ASCO guideline for geriatric oncology. J Clin Oncol 2018;36(22):2326–47.

9. Song X, Mitnitski A, Rockwood K. Prevalence and 10-year outcomes of frailty in older adults in relation to deficit accumulation. J Am Geriatr Soc 2010;58(4): 681–7.

10. Collard RM, Boter H, Schoevers RA, et al. Prevalence of frailty in community-dwelling older persons: a systematic review. J Am Geriatr Soc 2012;60(8): 1487–92.

11. Handforth C, Clegg A, Young C, et al. The prevalence and outcomes of frailty in older cancer patients: a systematic review. Ann Oncol 2015;26(6):1091–101.

12. Kristjansson SR, Nesbakken A, Jordhoy MS, et al. Comprehensive geriatric assessment can predict complications in elderly patients after elective surgery for colorectal cancer: a prospective observational cohort study. Crit Rev Oncol Hematol 2010;76(3):208–17.

13. Clough-Gorr KM, Thwin SS, Stuck AE, et al. Examining five- and ten-year survival in older women with breast cancer using cancer-specific geriatric assessment. Eur J Cancer 2012;48(6):805–12.

14. Kenis C, Decoster L, Van Puyvelde K, et al. Performance of two geriatric screening tools in older patients with cancer. J Clin Oncol 2014;32(1):19–26.

15. Makary MA, Segev DL, Pronovost PJ, et al. Frailty as a predictor of surgical outcomes in older patients. J Am Coll Surg 2010;210(6):901–8.

16. Tan KY, Kawamura YJ, Tokomitsu A, et al. Assessment for frailty is useful for predicting morbidity in elderly patients undergoing colorectal cancer resection whose comorbidities are already optimized. Am J Surg 2012;204(2):139–43.

17. Lu J, Cao LL, Zheng CH, et al. The preoperative frailty versus inflammation-based prognostic score: which is better as an objective predictor for gastric cancer patients 80 years and older? Ann Surg Oncol 2017;24(3):754–62.

18. Hurria A, Gupta S, Zauderer M, et al. Developing a cancer-specific geriatric assessment: a feasibility study. Cancer 2005;104(9):1998–2005.

19. Jolly TA, Deal AM, Nyrop KA, et al. Geriatric assessment-identified deficits in older cancer patients with normal performance status. Oncologist 2015;20(4): 379–85.

20. Rockwood K, Mitnitski A. Frailty in relation to the accumulation of deficits. J Gerontol A Biol Sci Med Sci 2007;62(7):722–7.

21. Guerard EJ, Deal AM, Chang Y, et al. Frailty index developed from a cancer-specific geriatric assessment and the association with mortality among older adults with cancer. J Natl Compr Canc Netw 2017;15(7):894–902.

22. Extermann M, Boler I, Reich RR, et al. Predicting the risk of chemotherapy toxicity in older patients: the chemotherapy risk assessment scale for high-age patients (CRASH) score. Cancer 2012;118(13):3377–86.

23. Hurria A, Mohile S, Gajra A, et al. Validation of a prediction tool for chemotherapy toxicity in older adults with cancer. J Clin Oncol 2016;34(20):2366–71.

24. Hurria A, Togawa K, Mohile SG, et al. Predicting chemotherapy toxicity in older adults with cancer: a prospective multicenter study. J Clin Oncol 2011;29(25): 3457–65.

25. Hurria A, Levit LA, Dale W, et al. Improving the evidence base for treating older adults with cancer: American Society of Clinical Oncology Statement. J Clin Oncol 2015;33(32):3826–33.

26. Subramaniam S, Aalberg JJ, Soriano RP, et al. New 5-factor modified frailty index using American College of Surgeons NSQIP data. J Am Coll Surg 2018;226(2): 173–81.e8.

27. Buettner S, Wagner D, Kim Y, et al. Inclusion of sarcopenia outperforms the modified frailty index in predicting 1-year mortality among 1,326 patients undergoing gastrointestinal surgery for a malignant indication. J Am Coll Surg 2016;222(4): 397–407.e2.

28. Peng P, Hyder O, Firoozmand A, et al. Impact of sarcopenia on outcomes following resection of pancreatic adenocarcinoma. J Gastrointest Surg 2012; 16(8):1478–86.

29. Peng PD, van Vledder MG, Tsai S, et al. Sarcopenia negatively impacts short-term outcomes in patients undergoing hepatic resection for colorectal liver metastasis. HPB (Oxford) 2011;13(7):439–46.

30. Courtney-Brooks M, Tellawi AR, Scalici J, et al. Frailty: an outcome predictor for elderly gynecologic oncology patients. Gynecol Oncol 2012;126(1):20–4.

31. Mogal H, Vermilion SA, Dodson R, et al. Modified frailty index predicts morbidity and mortality after pancreaticoduodenectomy. Ann Surg Oncol 2017;24(6): 1714–21.

32. Dindo D, Demartines N, Clavien PA. Classification of surgical complications: a new proposal with evaluation in a cohort of 6336 patients and results of a survey. Ann Surg 2004;240(2):205–13.

33. Lascano D, Pak JS, Kates M, et al. Validation of a frailty index in patients undergoing curative surgery for urologic malignancy and comparison with other risk stratification tools. Urol Oncol 2015;33(10):426.e1-12.

34. Mohanty S, Rosenthal RA, Russell MM, et al. Optimal perioperative management of the geriatric patient: a best practices guideline from the American College of Surgeons NSQIP and the American Geriatrics Society. J Am Coll Surg 2016; 222(5):930–47.

35. Wang SJ, Hathout L, Malhotra U, et al. Decision-making strategy for rectal cancer management using radiation therapy for elderly or comorbid patients. Int J Radiat Oncol Biol Phys 2018;100(4):926–44.

36. Bo Y, Wang K, Liu Y, et al. The geriatric nutritional risk index predicts survival in elderly esophageal squamous cell carcinoma patients with radiotherapy. PLoS One 2016;11(5):e0155903.

37. Giaccherini L, Galaverni M, Renna I, et al. Role of multidimensional assessment of frailty in predicting outcomes in older patients with glioblastoma treated with adjuvant concurrent chemo-radiation. J Geriatr Oncol 2019;10(5):770–8.

38. Pottel L, Lycke M, Boterberg T, et al. G-8 indicates overall and quality-adjusted survival in older head and neck cancer patients treated with curative radiochemotherapy. BMC Cancer 2015;15:875.

39. Spyropoulou D, Pallis AG, Leotsinidis M, et al. Completion of radiotherapy is associated with the Vulnerable Elders Survey-13 score in elderly patients with cancer. J Geriatr Oncol 2014;5(1):20–5.

40. Rim CH, Yoon WS, Lee JA, et al. Factors predicting intolerance to definitive conventional radiotherapy in geriatric patients. Strahlenther Onkol 2018;194(10): 894–903.

41. Keenan LG, O'Brien M, Ryan T, et al. Assessment of older patients with cancer: Edmonton Frail Scale (EFS) as a predictor of adverse outcomes in older patients undergoing radiotherapy. J Geriatr Oncol 2017;8(3):206–10.

42. Jeppesen SS, Matzen LE, Brink C, et al. Impact of comprehensive geriatric assessment on quality of life, overall survival, and unplanned admission in

patients with non-small cell lung cancer treated with stereotactic body radio-therapy. J Geriatr Oncol 2018;9(6):575–82.

43. Denkinger MD, Hasch M, Gerstmayer A, et al. Predicting fatigue in older breast cancer patients receiving radiotherapy. A head-to-head comparison of established assessments. Z Gerontol Geriatr 2015;48(2):128–34.

44. Middelburg JG, Mast ME, de Kroon M, et al. Timed get up and go test and geriatric 8 scores and the association with (Chemo-)Radiation therapy Noncompliance and acute toxicity in elderly cancer patients. Int J Radiat Oncol Biol Phys 2017;98(4):843–9.

45. Aaldriks AA, Maartense E, Nortier HJ, et al. Prognostic factors for the feasibility of chemotherapy and the Geriatric Prognostic Index (GPI) as risk profile for mortality before chemotherapy in the elderly. Acta Oncol 2016;55(1):15–23.

46. Palumbo A, Bringhen S, Mateos MV, et al. Geriatric assessment predicts survival and toxicities in elderly myeloma patients: an International Myeloma Working Group report. Blood 2015;125(13):2068–74.

47. Caillet P, Laurent M, Bastuji-Garin S, et al. Optimal management of elderly cancer patients: usefulness of the Comprehensive Geriatric Assessment. Clin Interv Aging 2014;9:1645–60.

48. Ramjaun A, Nassif MO, Krotneva S, et al. Improved targeting of cancer care for older patients: a systematic review of the utility of comprehensive geriatric assessment. J Geriatr Oncol 2013;4(3):271–81.

49. Puts MT, Hardt J, Monette J, et al. Use of geriatric assessment for older adults in the oncology setting: a systematic review. J Natl Cancer Inst 2012;104(15):1133–63.

50. Hamaker ME, Seynaeve C, Wymenga AN, et al. Baseline comprehensive geriatric assessment is associated with toxicity and survival in elderly metastatic breast cancer patients receiving single-agent chemotherapy: results from the OMEGA study of the Dutch breast cancer trialists' group. Breast 2014;23(1):81–7.

51. Falandry C, Brain E, Bonnefoy M, et al. Impact of geriatric risk factors on pegylated liposomal doxorubicin tolerance and efficacy in elderly metastatic breast cancer patients: final results of the DOGMES multicentre GINECO trial. Eur J Cancer 2013;49(13):2806–14.

52. Sastre J, Massuti B, Pulido G, et al. First-line single-agent panitumumab in frail elderly patients with wild-type KRAS metastatic colorectal cancer and poor prognostic factors: a phase II study of the Spanish Cooperative Group for the Treatment of Digestive Tumours. Eur J Cancer 2015;51(11):1371–80.

53. Hoppe S, Rainfray M, Fonck M, et al. Functional decline in older patients with cancer receiving first-line chemotherapy. J Clin Oncol 2013;31(31):3877–82.

54. Owusu C, Margevicius S, Schluchter M, et al. Short Physical Performance Battery, usual gait speed, grip strength and Vulnerable Elders Survey each predict functional decline among older women with breast cancer. J Geriatr Oncol 2017;8(5):356–62.

55. Owusu C, Margevicius S, Schluchter M, et al. Vulnerable elders survey and socioeconomic status predict functional decline and death among older women with newly diagnosed nonmetastatic breast cancer. Cancer 2016;122(16):2579–86.

56. Mohile SG, Velarde C, Hurria A, et al. Geriatric assessment-guided care processes for older adults: a Delphi consensus of geriatric oncology experts. J Natl Compr Canc Netw 2015;13(9):1120–30.

57. O'Donovan A, Mohile SG, Leech M. Expert consensus panel guidelines on geriatric assessment in oncology. Eur J Cancer Care (Engl) 2015;24(4):574–89.

58. Clough-Gorr KM, Stuck AE, Thwin SS, et al. Older breast cancer survivors: geriatric assessment domains are associated with poor tolerance of treatment adverse effects and predict mortality over 7 years of follow-up. J Clin Oncol 2010;28(3):380–6.

59. Extermann M, Meyer J, McGinnis M, et al. A comprehensive geriatric intervention detects multiple problems in older breast cancer patients. Crit Rev Oncol Hematol 2004;49(1):69–75.

60. Stotter A, Reed MW, Gray LJ, et al. Comprehensive Geriatric Assessment and predicted 3-year survival in treatment planning for frail patients with early breast cancer. Br J Surg 2015;102(5):525–33 [discussion: 533].

61. Okonji DO, Sinha R, Phillips I, et al. Comprehensive geriatric assessment in 326 older women with early breast cancer. Br J Cancer 2017;117(7):925–31.

62. Parks RM, Hall L, Tang SW, et al. The potential value of comprehensive geriatric assessment in evaluating older women with primary operable breast cancer undergoing surgery or non-operative treatment–a pilot study. J Geriatr Oncol 2015; 6(1):46–51.

63. Abt NB, Richmon JD, Koch WM, et al. Assessment of the predictive value of the modified frailty index for Clavien-Dindo grade IV critical care complications in major head and neck cancer operations. JAMA Otolaryngol Head Neck Surg 2016;142(7):658–64.

64. Chappidi MR, Kates M, Patel HD, et al. Frailty as a marker of adverse outcomes in patients with bladder cancer undergoing radical cystectomy. Urol Oncol 2016; 34(6):256.e1-6.

65. Neve M, Jameson MB, Govender S, et al. Impact of geriatric assessment on the management of older adults with head and neck cancer: a pilot study. J Geriatr Oncol 2016;7(6):457–62.

66. Laurent M, Paillaud E, Tournigand C, et al. Assessment of solid cancer treatment feasibility in older patients: a prospective cohort study. Oncologist 2014;19(3): 275–82.

67. Maebayashi T, Ishibashi N, Aizawa T, et al. Radiotherapy for muscle-invasive bladder cancer in very elderly patients. Anticancer Res 2016;36(9):4763–9.

68. Barthelemy P, Heitz D, Mathelin C, et al. Adjuvant chemotherapy in elderly patients with early breast cancer. Impact of age and comprehensive geriatric assessment on tumor board proposals. Crit Rev Oncol Hematol 2011;79(2): 196–204.

69. Meresse M, Bouhnik AD, Bendiane MK, et al. Chemotherapy in old women with breast cancer: is age still a predictor for under treatment? Breast J 2017;23(3): 256–66.

70. Aparicio T, Bouche O, Francois E, et al. Geriatric analysis from PRODIGE 20 randomized phase II trial evaluating bevacizumab + chemotherapy versus chemotherapy alone in older patients with untreated metastatic colorectal cancer. Eur J Cancer 2018;97:16–24.

71. Corre R, Greillier L, Le Caer H, et al. Use of a comprehensive geriatric assessment for the management of elderly patients with advanced non-small-cell lung cancer: the phase III randomized ESOGIA-GFPC-GECP 08-02 study. J Clin Oncol 2016;34(13):1476–83.

72. Biesma B, Wymenga AN, Vincent A, et al. Quality of life, geriatric assessment and survival in elderly patients with non-small-cell lung cancer treated with carboplatin-gemcitabine or carboplatin-paclitaxel: NVALT-3 a phase III study. Ann Oncol 2011;22(7):1520–7.

73. Park S, Hong J, Hwang I, et al. Comprehensive geriatric assessment in elderly patients with newly diagnosed aggressive non-Hodgkin lymphoma treated with multi-agent chemotherapy. J Geriatr Oncol 2015;6(6):470–8.

74. Hurria A, Cirrincione CT, Muss HB, et al. Implementing a geriatric assessment in cooperative group clinical cancer trials: CALGB 360401. J Clin Oncol 2011; 29(10):1290–6.

75. Caillet P, Canoui-Poitrine F, Vouriot J, et al. Comprehensive geriatric assessment in the decision-making process in elderly patients with cancer: ELCAPA study. J Clin Oncol 2011;29(27):3636–42.

76. Puts MT, Monette J, Girre V, et al. Are frailty markers useful for predicting treatment toxicity and mortality in older newly diagnosed cancer patients? Results from a prospective pilot study. Crit Rev Oncol Hematol 2011;78(2):138–49.

77. Shin DY, Lee J-O, Kim YJ, et al. Toxicities and functional consequences of systemic chemotherapy in elderly Korean patients with cancer: a prospective cohort study using Comprehensive Geriatric Assessment. J Geriatr Oncol 2012;3(4): 359–67.

Delirium Assessment in Critically Ill Older Adults

Considerations During the COVID-19 Pandemic

Maria C. Duggan, MD, MPH[a,b,*], Julie Van[c,d],
Eugene Wesley Ely, MD, MPH[b,c,d]

KEYWORDS

- Delirium • Screening • Assessment • Critical care • Intensive care unit
- Older adults • Geriatrics • Pandemic

KEY POINTS

- Delirium is common in critically ill older adults, who are more vulnerable to adverse outcomes, as was on full display in the Coronavirus disease 2019 (COVID-19) pandemic.
- Regular assessment for delirium is recommended, and many validated tools exist for detecting delirium in critically ill older adults. This assessment was a challenge amid the COVID-19 pandemic, when personnel and personal protective equipment were limited.
- Special considerations are necessary for patients with certain conditions (eg, sensory impairment, chronic neurodegenerative conditions, acute neurologic injury), which both increase risk for delirium and may be mistaken for delirium. In COVID-19, these patients proved especially vulnerable to delirium and may have greater long-term cognitive impairment as a result. Ongoing studies are pursuing this aspect of survivorship from the pandemic.

INTRODUCTION

If an experiment were designed to make delirium as big a problem as possible in an intensive care unit (ICU), Coronavirus disease 2019 (COVID-19) would be it. Delirium (an acute disturbance of consciousness with inattention accompanied by a change in cognition or perceptual disturbance that fluctuates over time) was already prevalent in the ICU before the pandemic of the novel severe acute respiratory syndrome

[a] Division of Geriatric Medicine, Vanderbilt University School of Medicine, Nashville, TN, USA;
[b] Department of Veteran Affairs, Geriatric Research Education and Clinical Center (GRECC), Tennessee Valley Healthcare System, 1310 24th Avenue South, Nashville, TN 37212, USA;
[c] Division of Allergy, Pulmonary, and Critical Care Medicine, Vanderbilt University School of Medicine, Nashville, TN, USA; [d] Center for Health Services Research (HSR), Vanderbilt University Medical Center, 2525 West End Avenue, Suite 450, Nashville, TN 37203, USA
* Corresponding author. 2525 West End Avenue, Suite 450, Nashville, TN 37203.
E-mail address: Mariu.duggan@vumc.org

Crit Care Clin 37 (2021) 175–190
https://doi.org/10.1016/j.ccc.2020.08.009
0749-0704/21/© 2020 Elsevier Inc. All rights reserved.

Coronavirus 2 (SARS-CoV-2) causing COVID-19. Before the pandemic, delirium affected up to 80% of critically ill adults, with each year more than 65 years of age increasing the odds of delirium by 2%. Older adults were already more prone to experiencing delirium because of multiple predisposing risk factors: dementia (odds ratio [OR], 2.3–4.7), hearing impairment (OR, 3.0), vision impairment (OR, 2.1–3.5), functional impairment (OR, 4.0), age greater than or equal to 75 years (OR, 4.0), and polypharmacy.[1,2] On top of all these risk factors, the COVID-19 pandemic has made that delirium risk even higher for older adults through isolation, immobilization, and removing family from the bedside.

The pandemic has raised many challenges in managing critically ill older adults, a population preferentially killed by COVID-19. Mortalities for hospitalized adults aged in their 60s, 70s, and 80s are 18.7%, 35.8%, and 60.6%, respectively.[3] Coupled with delirium, which independently increases risk for prolonged mechanical ventilation, longer ICU and hospital stay, institutionalization, functional dependence, long-term cognitive impairment, and higher mortality up to 2 years after discharge,[4–11] COVID-19 poses a huge challenge for older adults.

Even for survivors who physically recover from critical illness, delirium can have long-standing neuropsychiatric effects. It may also lead to psychiatric illnesses, including depression and posttraumatic stress disorder, and these effects are likely to be worse during the pandemic because of the restriction of family presence. Delirium itself may last for weeks to months, and for some patients it may both unmask and lead to the development of dementia with substantial declines in memory and executive functioning.[6] Delirium increases the odds for developing dementia by 12.5 times.[12] In the Bringing to Light the Risk Factors and Incidence of Neuropsychological Dysfunction in ICU Survivors (BRAIN-ICU) study, a longer duration of delirium was associated with worse long-term global cognition and executive function, independent of sedative or analgesic medication use, age, preexisting cognitive impairment, coexisting disease, and severity of illness in the ICU.[6] This finding is particularly important for older adults, who place a high value on their cognitive status and fear developing dementia.[13]

To spare this vulnerable population of older adults from these poor outcomes associated with delirium, early recognition of delirium is critical in order to best lessen the burden of delirium. This article discusses practical recommendations for delirium screening in the COVID-19 pandemic era, tips for training health care workers in delirium screening, validated tools for detecting delirium in critically ill older adults, and approaches to special populations of older adults (eg, sensory impairment, dementia, acute neurologic injury).

WHY SHOULD DELIRIUM SCREENING BE A PRIORITY DURING THE COVID-19 PANDEMIC?

The COVID-19 pandemic may increase delirium risk because of viral factors (direct central nervous system invasion, induction of central nervous system inflammatory mediators), prolonged mechanical ventilation and the deep sedation that accompanies it, immobilization, other organ failures, and environmental factors such as isolation and absence of family.

Even before the COVID-19 pandemic, up to 75% of cases of delirium were missed without formal delirium screening.[14] Delirium has been reported in up to two-thirds of patients with acute respiratory distress syndrome caused by COVID-19.[15] The number of undetected delirium cases is likely even higher now because of the challenges highlighted in **Table 1**.

Table 1 Delirium screening considerations for critically ill older adults during the COVID-19 pandemic	
Challenges	**Potential Solutions**
HCWs limit contact with patients to conserve PPE and reduce risk of COVID-19 transmission	• Equip other HCWs beyond nurses to screen for delirium through training[a] • Use brief delirium screening tools; eg, 2-min CAM-ICU[a]
Shortages of personnel caused by surge volumes	• Train other disciplines of HCWs in brief delirium screening as above[a]
Assessing a change from baseline mental status (feature 1 of CAM-ICU) is challenging with family visitation restricted	• Involve family remotely through use of smartphones or tablets during or after rounds to facilitate communication with patient • Call nursing homes for patients admitted from a nursing home to understand baseline mental status
Surgical masks on HCWs impede older adults' comprehension of delirium screening questions, especially in hearing impairment	• Reduce background noise • Speak slowly, clearly, in low pitch • Use sound amplifiers (pocket talkers) • Have hearing aid batteries available • Ask family to bring hearing aids • Use transparent surgical masks if available (https://www.theclearmask.com)
PPE may make certain patients with dementia more paranoid and not willing to participate in delirium screening	• Use large signs on gowns with pictures of providers and names/roles written in large font • Hand out baseball cards to patients for providers with picture, name, role • Allow family to visit patients with cognitive impairment[b] • Be aware that refusal to participate in CAM-ICU may be a sign of delirium
Patients with dementia or history of stroke commonly have aphasia. Families are helpful in facilitating communication, but are not present at bedside	• Speak slowly • Ask yes/no questions • Involve family remotely through use of smartphones or tablets at the bedside to facilitate communication with patient • Allow family to visit patients with cognitive impairment[b]
Delirium is unable to be assessed during deep sedation administered during neuromuscular blockade and proning to treat respiratory failure	• Assess sedation daily and limit as much as is feasible, adhering to A2F bundle

The A2F bundle stands for assess, prevent, and manage pain; both spontaneous awakening trial and spontaneous breathing trial; choice of sedation and analgesia; delirium assessment, prevention, and management; early mobility and exercise; and family engagement.

Abbreviations: CAM-ICU, Confusion Assessment Method for the ICU; HCW, health care worker; PPE, personal protective equipment.

[a] The CAM-ICU can be taught to ICU staff in less than 30 minutes and administered to patients in less than 2 minutes.

[b] Allow family visitation provided that the family member passes a health screen and wears a mask.

Delirium can be recognized early with formal screening, prompting an expedited clinical assessment that may identify problems sooner and lead to earlier treatment and resolution. In addition, early recognition of delirium can help optimize nonpharmacologic measures, which have been proven to reduce delirium days and potentially help reduce the suffering of patients and families that accompanies delirium.[16]

Many expert guidelines and professional societies and organizations have strongly recommended delirium monitoring twice daily: The ICU Pain, Agitation, and Delirium Clinical Practice Guidelines by the Society of Critical Care Medicine (grade 1B)[17] and the updated Pain, Agitation, Delirium, Immobility, and Sleep (PADIS) guidelines,[18] hospital standards for surgical care of older adults by the Coalition for Quality in Geriatric Surgery,[19] and the Age-Friendly Health Systems Initiative of the Institution for Healthcare Improvement.

Studies examining the impact of delirium screening interventions in critically ill patients have shown improvements in clinical outcomes. One of the most well-known strategies for preventing delirium in critically ill patients is the ABCDEF (A2F) bundle (assess, prevent, and manage pain; both spontaneous awakening trial and spontaneous breathing trial; choice of sedation and analgesia; delirium assessment, prevention, and management; early mobility and exercise; and family engagement). The A2F bundle was associated with lower likelihood of hospital death within 7 days, next-day mechanical ventilation, coma, delirium, physical restraint use, immobility, ICU readmission, and discharge to a facility.[20–25] Greater adherence to the bundle was associated with greater improvements in each of these outcomes. Although this bundle was implemented in patients of all ages, it is arguably most important to implement for older adults, who are predisposed to newly acquired deficits and diseases when they experience critical illness.

However, there is insufficient high-quality evidence to show that delirium screening alone is beneficial. Teasing out the effect of delirium screening is challenging because many studies, such as those involving the A2F bundle, examine the impact of delirium screening as part of a bundle of management strategies.

WHO SHOULD SCREEN FOR DELIRIUM IN THE INTENSIVE CARE UNIT?

During a pandemic where personnel may be limited, other health care workers should be trained in administering validated delirium screening tools at least once per shift and with every change in mental status. Even with adequate nursing staff, ensuring the assessment of a patient's brain health is not solely the bedside nurses' responsibility but is a shared responsibility of the interdisciplinary team. All clinicians have a role in this and should be able to screen a patient for delirium if they are caring for a patient and are the first to recognize its symptoms. Members of the interdisciplinary team should be aware of the common clinical presentation of delirium and possible contributing factors. For instance, a pharmacist performing a medication reconciliation with a patient who is unable to stay attentive should be trained to recognize this as a potential sign of delirium and to relay this information to the clinician with pertinent recommendations for possible contributing medications.

Family members and caregivers should be seen as an extension of the health care team and may be instrumental in recognizing subtle changes from a patient's baseline mental status. In addition to helping recognize delirium, family members are often most effective at reorienting patients, knowing ways to calm them down, helping with feeding and hydration, and bringing in hearing aids and glasses. This point is particularly true for individuals with dementia. Engaging caregivers as active members of the health care team improves patient care, education, and communication, but it can also facilitate the transition from hospital to home and prepare caregivers for delirium prevention and recognition after discharge. Education materials on delirium for families are available at ICUdelirium.org.[26] Although family visitation may be restricted during the COVID-19 pandemic, it is possible to involve family remotely through use of smartphones or tablets during or after rounds.

HOW TO SCREEN FOR DELIRIUM IN THE INTENSIVE CARE UNIT?

The PADIS guidelines recommend delirium screening using the Confusion Assessment Method–ICU (CAM-ICU)[27] or the Intensive Care Delirium Screening Checklist (ICDSC).[28] The CAM-ICU and the ICDSC were developed to detect delirium in nonverbal patients, primarily in the ICU. Although many tools exist to detect delirium, the CAM-ICU and the ICDSC are the most valid and reliable tools for delirium screening among adult ICU patients.[17,29,30] Both tools have been translated and validated in several other languages. They are reviewed here.

The Confusion Assessment Method–Intensive Care Unit

The CAM-ICU was adapted from the Confusion Assessment Method[31] and uses the same feature structure: (1) acute onset or fluctuations in mental status from baseline, (2) inattention, (3) disorganized thinking, and (4) an altered level of consciousness (**Fig. 1**). The CAM-ICU was validated by the Diagnostic and Statistical Manual of Mental Disorders, fourth edition (DSM-IV) criteria as gold standard, with sensitivity of 80% and specificity of 96%.[27,30]

The CAM-ICU is positive (ie, delirium present) if features 1 and 2 and either feature 3 or 4 are present. Patients who are not in a stupor or coma are assessed for these features using objective criteria and direct patient assessment. The assessment involves the following:

- Comparing the patient's current mental status with the patient's baseline (feature 1)
- Evaluating attention by asking the patient to squeeze on the letter A while reading a string of 10 letters (feature 2)
- Evaluating level of consciousness with the use of a sedation scale (eg, Richmond Agitation Sedation Scale [RASS][32,33] or Sedation-Agitation Scale [SAS][34]) (feature 3)
- A set of 4 yes/no questions followed by a 2-stage command (feature 4)

The CAM-ICU can be taught to ICU staff in less than 30 minutes and administered to patients in less than 2 minutes.[35] Ten clinical pearls related to administering the CAM-ICU are listed in **Box 1**.

Intensive Care Delirium Screening Checklist

The ICDSC is a checklist with 8 questions that allows ICU staff to observe the following delirium symptoms over a period of 8 to 12 hours: altered level of consciousness, inattention, delusion or hallucination, disorientation, inappropriate mood or speech, psychomotor agitation, sleep/wake cycle disturbance, and symptom fluctuation.[28] Patients do not have to be verbal in order to undergo the ICDSC. Scores range from 0 to 8 and are associated with a classification (0, normal; 1–3, subsyndromal delirium; 4–8, delirium). The ICDSC is a valid and reliable tool with sensitivity and specificity studies of 74% and 82%, respectively.[30]

A

RICHMOND AGITATION-SEDATION SCALE (RASS)

STEP 1   Level of Consciousness Assessment

Scale	Label	Description
+4	COMBATIVE	Combative, violent, immediate danger to staff
+3	VERY AGITATED	Pulls to remove tubes or catheters; aggressive
+2	AGITATED	Frequent nonpurposeful movement, fights ventilator
+1	RESTLESS	Anxious, apprehensive, movements not aggressive
0	ALERT & CALM	Spontaneously pays attention to caregiver
-1	DROWSY	Not fully alert, but has sustained awakening to voice (eye opening & contact >10 s)
-2	LIGHT SEDATION	Briefly awakens to voice (eyes open & contact <10 s)
-3	MODERATE SEDATION	Movement or eye opening to voice (no eye contact)

V O I C E

→ **If RASS is ≥ -3 proceed to CAM-ICU** (Is patient CAM-ICU positive or negative?)

-4	DEEP SEDATION	No response to voice, but movement or eye opening to physical stimulation
-5	UNAROUSABLE	No response to voice or physical stimulation

T O U C H

→ **If RASS is -4 or -5 → STOP** (patient unconscious), **RECHECK later**

B

Confusion Assessment Method for the ICU (CAM-ICU)

STEP 2   Content of Consciousness Assessment

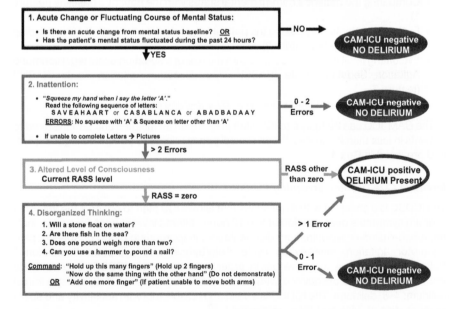

Box 1
Ten clinical pearls related to delirium assessment

1. Assessment is fast: 90% of RASS/CAM-ICU assessments take less than 1 minute. The other 10% take only a few minutes. Speed and ease of use make this feasible on a large scale multiple times daily.

2. RASS and CAM-ICU: implementing RASS without CAM-ICU (sedation scale without delirium tool) leaves only half of consciousness assessed (arousal, not content), is clinically unsatisfying, and hurts compliance.

3. Tailor examination: you do not have to do every CAM-ICU feature if you get your answers via a brief examination sooner.

4. Starting with features 1 and 3: feature 1 is comparing patients with their baseline mental status, and feature 3 is about their level of consciousness now. Because many ICUs repeat sedation scale assessment every 2 to 4 hours, these data are readily available. A quick mantra: "Is patient at the baseline or fluctuating + RASS now."

5. Inattention (feature 2): this is the cardinal feature and must be present to diagnose delirium. Feature 2 is quick and simple. Ninety percent of evaluations are done using only hand squeezes on correct letters or numbers. The picture method of screening is needed for inattention in less than 5%.

6. Hand squeezing: in the absence of other specific neurologic diagnoses, a patient who squeezes on all letters, squeezes on no letters, or misses more than 2 letters/numbers/pictures is inattentive and feature 2 positive. With a RASS other than 0, the patient is delirious.

7. Unable to assess: this term is only recorded when patients are in stupor/coma (RASS −4/−5).

8. Rare feature 4: it is only necessary to proceed to Feature 4 (disorganized thinking) when a patient is feature 2 positive (inattentive) and awake and alert (RASS 0) at the time of CAM-ICU evaluation.

9. Subsyndromal delirium: patients may have some features without the full syndrome of delirium (eg, feature 2 only or feature 1 and feature 4 only). This condition is a (subsyndromal) intermediate state between normal and delirium. Reassess with CAM-ICU frequently to determine the clinical course of the emerging brain dysfunction.

10. Key to success: physicians and nurses must work together. The team must understand the definition of delirium and its prognostic implications, modifiable causes, and treatment options. Enthusiasm is destroyed when physicians do not respond to nurses who report that a patient is CAM-ICU positive. Overcome this implementation barrier by engaging and educating all members of the ICU team and having experts.

Adapted from Top 10 Teaching Tips for Delirium Monitoring. Available at: https://uploads-ssl.webflow.com/5b0849daec50243a0a1e5e0c/5bad3d17cc14608db92dbeed_Top-10-Tips-for-Teaching-Delirium-Monitoring.pdf; with permission.

SCREENING OUTSIDE THE INTENSIVE CARE UNIT

Because delirium may initially present in nursing homes or emergency departments (EDs) and persists beyond the ICU, all health care settings that encounter acutely ill

Fig. 1. (*A*) The Richmond Agitation-Sedation Scale (RASS). (*B*) The Confusion Assessment Method for the ICU (CAM-ICU). The RASS is a valid and reliable tool to monitor level of consciousness, which is feature 3 of the CAM-ICU. The CAM-ICU is a valid and reliable tool to screen for delirium. (Copyright © 2002, E. Wesley Ely, MD, MPH, and Vanderbilt University. All rights reserved.)

adults should use appropriate delirium screening tools. Some of these tools are reviewed later. More information on optimizing delirium screening in settings outside the ICU can be found on the Age-Friendly Health Systems initiative's Web site.[36]

Delirium Triage Screen

The Delirium Triage Screen (DTS) is an ultrabrief delirium screen developed for use in a busy clinical setting, such as the ED. This approach uses a very brief (<20 seconds) delirium screen to rapidly rule out delirium if negative, and triggering a confirmatory assessment if positive. In older ED patients, the DTS is 98% sensitive and 55% specific for delirium.[37]

The DTS has only 2 components: (1) altered level of consciousness assessed by using an arousal tool; and (2) inattention, which is assessed by asking the patient to spell "lunch" backward. The DTS is considered negative if the patient has a normal level of consciousness and makes zero or 1 error when spelling "lunch" backward. If the patient has an altered level of consciousness or makes 2 or more errors during the spelling test, the examination is considered positive and a more specific test (Brief Confusion Assessment Method [bCAM] or CAM-ICU) is required to confirm a diagnosis of delirium.

The geriatric ED guidelines recommend the DTS as the first step in delirium screening.[38]

The Brief Confusion Assessment Method

The bCAM was adapted from CAM-ICU for use in verbal patients in the ED.[37] The geriatric ED guidelines recommend the bCAM as the next step in delirium screening for a positive DTS.[38] The bCAM was also validated in a geriatric ward setting.[37] The bCAM had a sensitivity of 70% to 84% and a specificity of 96% to 97%.[37]

The bCAM uses the same 4 features as the CAM-ICU. Feature 2 (inattention) is assessed by asking the patient to recite the months backward from December to July. Administration of the bCAM is otherwise identical to the CAM-ICU. Scoring varies slightly. Feature 2 is positive if 2 or more errors are made, and feature 4 is positive if any errors are made.

IDENTIFYING DELIRIUM SUPERIMPOSED ON DEMENTIA

Delirium that occurs in patients with dementia is referred to as delirium superimposed on dementia (DSD). Older adults with dementia have reduced cognitive reserve, making them more likely to develop delirium with fewer precipitating factors.[1] DSD is associated with adverse outcomes: accelerated cognitive and functional decline, institutionalization, and mortality.[12,39,40] Diagnosing DSD can be difficult for many reasons.

First, although dementia is common, affecting up to a quarter of hospitalized older adults, it often goes unrecognized.[41] Dementia may be particularly difficult to recognize in critically ill older adults who are noncommunicative because of critical illness or the treatments that accompany it. The AD8 is an 8-item proxy screening tool for dementia that has been validated in hospitalized adults with delirium[42] and in the ICU.[43] The AD8 can be administered to a family member over the phone. Recognizing dementia is important to help identify those at highest risk of delirium and ensure optimal nonpharmacologic prevention.

Second, 80% of patients with dementia experience behavioral and psychiatric symptoms at some point in the disease course. Although manifestations of dementia, these symptoms may resemble features of delirium.[44] These symptoms may include sleep disturbances, paranoia, and anxiety in earlier stages, and may progress to accusatory behavior, irritability, wandering, agitation, hallucinations, and aggression in later stages.[45] Understanding a patient's baseline behavioral and psychiatric state is key to teasing out whether a clinical presentation is likely to be caused by delirium.

In addition, certain types of dementia can have acute changes in cognition in the natural course of the disease that may be mistaken for delirium. For example, dementia with Lewy bodies, the third most common type of dementia, can have fluctuating levels of consciousness with inattention and psychosis.[46] Vascular dementia can have acute worsening of cognition caused by vascular events, and it can be difficult to ascertain whether a change is the next stepwise decline or delirium of another cause. It is safest to assume acute changes in cognition are delirium and to rule out other contributing factors before attributing changes to progression of dementia.

In addition, delirium screening tests require the participant to perform tasks that depend on multiple cognitive domains: visual and auditory processing, visual processing, language, and motor execution. Dementia does not only affect memory but can also affect other cognitive domains, making delirium screening difficult to interpret. Although mild attention deficits are common, starting in the early stages of dementia, visual attention is often preserved even in advanced stages of dementia.[47]

Assessing Baseline Mental Status

For patients with dementia, establishing the patient's baseline mental state is imperative to determining the acuity of mental status change and fluctuations that are associated with delirium. Providers should ask a proxy that is most familiar with the patient, whether a family member, personal caregivers, or nursing home provider. This requirement can be challenging with visitation restrictions if family contact information is unknown. If possible, the patient's baseline level of consciousness and ability to speak and follow commands should be elicited. In addition, any behavioral or psychiatric symptoms of dementia and triggers should be identified, as well as actions that help redirect the patient. If baseline cognition is unable to be confirmed, it should never be assumed that the patient is at baseline.

Tools Validated to Detect Delirium Superimposed on Dementia

Few studies report diagnostic validity of delirium screening tools for detecting DSD (**Table 2**). Based on available evidence, the CAM-ICU has the most support for use in the diagnosis of DSD in critically ill older adults.[48] The CAM-ICU has an option to use a visual attention form to assess feature 2, the core feature of delirium, which can be useful in identifying delirium in patients with dementia. Other screening tools validated in larger populations of patients with dementia (the 4As test,[49] 6-Item Cognitive Impairment Test,[50] 3-Item Screener[51]) require patients to be verbal, which is often a barrier to implementation in the ICU.

OTHER SPECIAL CONSIDERATIONS
Sensory Impairment

Hearing impairment can result in inappropriate answers to questions if an older adult does not correctly interpret the information communicated by the health care provider. This situation can lead to a false-positive delirium screen, which may trigger unnecessary, burdensome testing. For delirium screens to be accurate and reliable, it is

Table 2
Validation studies of screening tools for delirium superimposed on dementia

Screening Tool (Author, Year)	Setting	Total Sample (N)	Sample with Dementia, N (%)	Sensitivity (%)	Specificity (%)
Short Portable Mental Status Questionnaire (Erkinjuntti et al,[63] 1987)	Geriatric ward	282	34 (12)	7.3–98	82–100
Confusion Assessment Method (Inouye et al,[31] 1990)	Internal medicine ward	56	12 (21)	94–100	90–05
Confusion Assessment Method (Hestermann et al,[64] 2009)	Geriatric ward	39	33 (85)	77	96–100
Delirium Rating Scale (Rosen et al,[65] 1994)	Geriatric ward	791	197 (27)	94	82
Cognitive Test for Delirium (Hart et al,[66] 1996)	ICU	103	26 (25)	100	95
CAM-ICU (Ely et al,[67] 2001)	ICU	96	12 (15)	93–100	98–100
CAM-ICU (Ely et al,[35] 2001)	ICU	38	11 (29)	95–100	89–93
CAM-ICU (Mitasova et al,[54] 2011)	Stroke unit	129	41 (32)	76	98
EEG (Thomas et al,[68] 2007)	Geriatric ward	35	35 (100)	67	91
4 As Test (Bellelli et al,[49] 2014)	Geriatric ward or inpatient rehabilitation	234	74 (31)	94	65
6-Item Cognitive Impairment Test (O'Regan et al,[50] 2017)	Medicine ward	470	79 (17)	81	31
3-Item Screener (Steensma et al,[51] 2019)	General medicine or surgery ward	391	391 (100)	94	42

Abbreviation: EEG, electroencephalography.

imperative to ensure that older adults can hear. Securing hearing aids is often practically challenging because older adults rarely plan to get critically ill and thus do not bring their hearing aids to the hospital, and families may not be available to retrieve them. Hearing aids are also notorious for disappearing during hospitalizations. In the absence of hearing aids, sound amplifiers (so-called pocket talkers) can be used to amplify sound, although they do not work for all types of hearing impairment.

Surgical masks worsen comprehension for older adults with hearing impairment. Transparent surgical masks have been developed and can facilitate enhanced comprehension for those with hearing impairment.[52] Although not yet US Food and Drug Administration approved, they are in use for areas with personal protective equipment (PPE) shortages caused by COVID-19.[53] It is also important to ensure that glasses are on to facilitate communication.

Even for individuals with hearing or vision impairment that cannot be remedied, the CAM-ICU can still be used reliably. For deaf individuals, the CAM-ICU can be administered with 2 exceptions: using the visual attention form for feature 2, and written out questions and instructions for feature 4. For individuals who are blind, the CAM-ICU can be administered with 1 exception: the 2-stage command in feature 4 is not administered and any error on the 4 questions results in a positive feature 4. For individuals who are both blind and deaf, cognitive assessment is much more challenging and often relies on observing level of consciousness to inform ratings of features 1 and 3 and using family observations whenever possible.

Primary Neurologic Injury

Stroke is an emerging complication of COVID-19.[15] Delirium in neurocritically ill patients has been associated with prolonged hospital stay,[54–56] worse functional status,[56] and worse cognitive status.[55,57] Because of the neurologic nature of the primary injury, it can be difficult to determine whether a change in mental status is caused by a new condition causing delirium or a continuation of the primary neurologic insult. Changes in mental status in this population may be driven by the deterioration caused by the primary neurologic disorder (eg, brain edema, vasospasm, seizures, rebleeding, and/or ischemia in patients with acute stroke). These patients are also prone to neck-down complications that may result in delirium.

Patel and colleagues[58] performed a systematic review to identify valid and reliable tools to assess for delirium in primary neurocritically ill patients. Both the CAM-ICU and the ICDSC had fair sensitivity (62%–76%) and specificity (74%–98%) in this population.

POTENTIAL DOWNSIDES TO SCREENING

It is worth discussing the potential unintended consequences of delirium screening. As with any screening tool, false-negatives and false-positives arise. Relying too strongly on a binary result from a delirium screening tool can lead to discounting changes in mental status that do not meet criteria for delirium but still may signal an acute problem. A screen may miss a true case of delirium and more often may miss subsyndromal delirium (acute brain dysfunction that does not meet the full criteria for delirium). Missing subsyndromal delirium is particularly problematic because of its association with prolonged hospitalization,[10,59] cognitive and functional decline,[59] and institutionalization.[59,60]

In contrast, for false-positive cases, it may lead to unnecessary testing, prolonged hospitalization, and subsequently increased health care costs.

Another potential concern is that more identification of delirium may result in unnecessary pharmacologic treatment. One study in a surgical and trauma ICU found that communicating CAM-ICU screens to providers resulted in more days receiving antipsychotic medications compared with a group where the CAM-ICU was not communicated to providers, although total dose was no different.[61] However, since this study, a robust evidence base has shown that antipsychotic medications do not shorten time in delirium, reduce mortality, length of stay, or other clinical outcomes.[62] It is less likely that positive delirium screens would lead to increased prescribing of antipsychotics given the current evidence.

Despite these concerns, multiple professional societies and organizations continue to recommend delirium screening at least twice daily, especially given the large evidence base from the A2F bundle in improvements in clinical outcomes associated with the bundle's implementation. Especially in this pandemic, where the health care system is like a delirium factory, regular screening for delirium is imperative.

SUMMARY

The COVID-19 pandemic has raised many challenges in managing critically ill older adults with attention to delirium prevention and management. To spare this vulnerable population of older adults from poor outcomes associated with delirium, early recognition of delirium is critical. Despite the health care system limitations during this pandemic and the difficult clinical challenges, delirium screening and management remains an evidence-based cornerstone of critical care.

CLINICS CARE POINTS

- Older adults are particularly vulnerable during the COVID-19 pandemic, because higher age increases risk for both delirium and COVID-19–related death.
- The PADIS guidelines recommend delirium screening using the CAM-ICU[27] or the ICDSC.[28]
- Ensure communication during delirium screening is effective despite environmental barriers related to the pandemic (PPE, lack of family presence at the bedside), and restore sensory impairment as able (use hearing aids or sound amplifiers, reduce background noise, provide glasses).
- Always ask about a patient's baseline cognitive status. Never assume someone is demented because of age alone.
- Special considerations are necessary for patients with certain conditions (eg, sensory impairment, chronic neurodegenerative conditions, acute neurologic injury) that both increase risk for delirium and may be mistaken for delirium.

DISCLOSURE

E.W. Ely is currently receiving grant funding from NIA (#R01AG058639) and NIGMS (#R01GM120484) and serves as a consultant for Pfizer and Eli Lilly. The funding sources had no role in the preparation, review, or approval of the article, or in the decision to submit it for publication.

REFERENCES

1. Inouye SK, Westendorp RG, Saczynski JS. Delirium in elderly people. Lancet 2014;383(9920):911–22.
2. Hein C, Forgues A, Piau A, et al. Impact of polypharmacy on occurrence of delirium in elderly emergency patients. J Am Med Dir Assoc 2014;15(11): 850.e1-5.
3. Richardson S, Hirsch JS, Narasimhan M, et al. Presenting characteristics, comorbidities, and outcomes among 5700 patients hospitalized with COVID-19 in the New York City Area. JAMA 2020;323(20):2052–9.

4. Ely EW, Shintani A, Truman B, et al. Delirium as a predictor of mortality in mechanically ventilated patients in the intensive care unit. JAMA 2004;291(14):1753–62.
5. Salluh JI, Wang H, Schneider EB, et al. Outcome of delirium in critically ill patients: systematic review and meta-analysis. BMJ 2015;350:h2538.
6. Pandharipande PP, Girard TD, Jackson JC, et al. Long-term cognitive impairment after critical illness. N Engl J Med 2013;369(14):1306–16.
7. Girard TD, Jackson JC, Pandharipande PP, et al. Delirium as a predictor of long-term cognitive impairment in survivors of critical illness. Crit Care Med 2010; 38(7):1513–20.
8. Mehta S, Cook D, Devlin JW, et al. Prevalence, risk factors, and outcomes of delirium in mechanically ventilated adults. Crit Care Med 2015;43(3):557–66.
9. Pisani MA, Kong SY, Kasl SV, et al. Days of delirium are associated with 1-year mortality in an older intensive care unit population. Am J Respir Crit Care Med 2009;180(11):1092–7.
10. Ouimet S, Riker R, Bergeron N, et al. Subsyndromal delirium in the ICU: evidence for a disease spectrum. Intensive Care Med 2007;33(6):1007–13.
11. Ely EW, Gautam S, Margolin R, et al. The impact of delirium in the intensive care unit on hospital length of stay. Intensive Care Med 2001;27(12):1892–900.
12. Witlox J, Eurelings LS, de Jonghe JF, et al. Delirium in elderly patients and the risk of postdischarge mortality, institutionalization, and dementia: a meta-analysis. JAMA 2010;304(4):443–51.
13. Maust D, Langa K, Solway E, et al. Thinking about brain health. University of Michigan National Poll on Healthy Aging.; 2019.
14. Spronk PE, Riekerk B, Hofhuis J, et al. Occurrence of delirium is severely underestimated in the ICU during daily care. Intensive Care Med 2009;35(7):1276–80.
15. Helms J, Kremer S, Merdji H, et al. Neurologic features in severe SARS-CoV-2 infection. N Engl J Med 2020;382(23):2268–70.
16. Hshieh TT, Yue J, Oh E, et al. Effectiveness of multicomponent nonpharmacological delirium interventions: a meta-analysis. JAMA Intern Med 2015;175(4): 512–20.
17. Barr J, Fraser GL, Puntillo K, et al. Clinical practice guidelines for the management of pain, agitation, and delirium in adult patients in the intensive care unit. Crit Care Med 2013;41(1):263–306.
18. Devlin JW, Skrobik Y, Gelinas C, et al. Clinical practice guidelines for the prevention and management of pain, agitation/sedation, delirium, immobility, and sleep disruption in adult patients in the ICU. Crit Care Med 2018;46(9):e825–73.
19. Berian JR, Rosenthal RA, Baker TL, et al. Hospital standards to promote optimal surgical care of the older adult: a report from the coalition for quality in geriatric surgery. Ann Surg 2018;267(2):280–90.
20. Balas M, Olsen K, Gannon D, et al. Safety and efficacy of the abcde bundle in critically-ill patients receiving mechanical ventilation. Crit Care Med 2012; 40(12):U18.
21. Marra A, Ely EW, Pandharipande PP, et al. The ABCDEF bundle in critical care. Crit Care Clin 2017;33(2):225–43.
22. Barnes-Daly MA, Phillips G, Ely EW. Improving hospital survival and reducing brain dysfunction at seven California community hospitals: implementing PAD guidelines via the ABCDEF bundle in 6,064 patients. Crit Care Med 2017;45(2): 171–8.
23. Ely EW. The ABCDEF bundle: science and philosophy of how ICU liberation serves patients and families. Crit Care Med 2017;45(2):321–30.

24. Pun BT, Balas MC, Barnes-Daly MA, et al. Caring for critically ill patients with the ABCDEF bundle: results of the icu liberation collaborative in over 15,000 adults. Crit Care Med 2019;47(1):3–14.

25. Hsieh SJ, Otusanya O, Gershengorn HB, et al. Staged implementation of awakening and breathing, coordination, delirium monitoring and management, and early mobilization bundle improves patient outcomes and reduces hospital costs. Crit Care Med 2019;47(7):885–93.

26. Critical illness BdaSC. Delirium in the intensive care Unit: a Guide for families and patients. Available at: https://uploads-ssl.webflow.com/5b0849daec50243 a0a1e5e0c/5e7b9a2fb906fb34322404ee_CIBS-Center-Delirium-Brochure.pdf. Accessed April 16, 2020.

27. Ely EW, Truman B, May L, et al. Validation of the CAM-ICU for delirium assessment in mechanically ventilated patients. J Am Geriatr Soc 2001;49(4):S2.

28. Bergeron N, Dubois MJ, Dumont M, et al. Intensive care delirium screening checklist: evaluation of a new screening tool. Intensive Care Med 2001;27(5): 859–64.

29. Gelinas C, Berube M, Chevrier A, et al. Delirium assessment tools for use in critically ill adults: a psychometric analysis and systematic review. Crit Care Nurse 2018;38(1):38–49.

30. Gusmao-Flores D, Salluh JI, Chalhub RA, et al. The confusion assessment method for the intensive care unit (CAM-ICU) and intensive care delirium screening checklist (ICDSC) for the diagnosis of delirium: a systematic review and meta-analysis of clinical studies. Crit Care 2012;16(4):R115.

31. Inouye SK, van Dyck CH, Alessi CA, et al. Clarifying confusion: the confusion assessment method. A new method for detection of delirium. Ann Intern Med 1990;113(12):941–8.

32. Sessler CN, Gosnell MS, Grap MJ, et al. The Richmond Agitation-Sedation Scale: validity and reliability in adult intensive care unit patients. Am J Respir Crit Care Med 2002;166(10):1338–44.

33. Ely EW, Truman B, Shintani A, et al. Monitoring sedation status over time in ICU patients: reliability and validity of the Richmond Agitation-Sedation Scale (RASS). JAMA 2003;289(22):2983–91.

34. Riker RR, Picard JT, Fraser GL. Prospective evaluation of the Sedation-Agitation Scale for adult critically ill patients. Crit Care Med 1999;27(7):1325–9.

35. Ely EW, Inouye SK, Bernard GR, et al. Delirium in mechanically ventilated patients: validity and reliability of the confusion assessment method for the intensive care unit (CAM-ICU). JAMA 2001;286(21):2703–10.

36. Institute for Healthcare Improvement. Age-friendly health systems Guide to using 4Ms CAre. Available at: http://www.ihi.org/Engage/Initiatives/Age-Friendly-Health-Systems/Documents/IHIAgeFriendlyHealthSystems_GuidetoUsing4Ms Care.pdf. Accessed February 10, 2020.

37. Han JH, Wilson A, Vasilevskis EE, et al. Diagnosing delirium in older emergency department patients: validity and reliability of the delirium triage screen and the brief confusion assessment method. Ann Emerg Med 2013;62(5):457–65.

38. Physicians ACoE. Geriatric emergency departments guidelines. Available at: https://www.acep.org/globalassets/new-pdfs/policy-statements/geriatric-emergency-department-guidelines.pdf. Accessed April 16, 2020.

39. Morandi A, Davis D, Fick DM, et al. Delirium superimposed on dementia strongly predicts worse outcomes in older rehabilitation inpatients. J Am Med Dir Assoc 2014;15(5):349–54.

40. Fong TG, Jones RN, Shi P, et al. Delirium accelerates cognitive decline in Alzheimer disease. Neurology 2009;72(18):1570–5.
41. Livingston G, Sommerlad A, Orgeta V, et al. Dementia prevention, intervention, and care. Lancet 2017;390(10113):2673–734.
42. Jackson TA, MacLullich AM, Gladman JR, et al. Diagnostic test accuracy of informant-based tools to diagnose dementia in older hospital patients with delirium: a prospective cohort study. Age Ageing 2016;45(4):505–11.
43. Duggan MC, Morrell ME, Chandrasekhar R, et al. A brief informant screening instrument for dementia in the ICU: the diagnostic accuracy of the AD8 in critically ill adults suspected of having pre-existing dementia. Dement Geriatr Cogn Disord 2020;48(5–6):241–9.
44. Lyketsos CG, Lopez O, Jones B, et al. Prevalence of neuropsychiatric symptoms in dementia and mild cognitive impairment: results from the cardiovascular health study. JAMA 2002;288(12):1475–83.
45. Jost BC, Grossberg GT. The evolution of psychiatric symptoms in Alzheimer's disease: a natural history study. J Am Geriatr Soc 1996;44(9):1078–81.
46. Ballard C, Aarsland D, Francis P, et al. Neuropsychiatric symptoms in patients with dementias associated with cortical Lewy bodies: pathophysiology, clinical features, and pharmacological management. Drugs Aging 2013;30(8):603–11.
47. Brown LJ, Fordyce C, Zaghdani H, et al. Detecting deficits of sustained visual attention in delirium. J Neurol Neurosurg Psychiatry 2011;82(12):1334–40.
48. Morandi A, McCurley J, Vasilevskis EE, et al. Tools to detect delirium superimposed on dementia: a systematic review. J Am Geriatr Soc 2012;60(11):2005–13.
49. Bellelli G, Morandi A, Davis DH, et al. Validation of the 4AT, a new instrument for rapid delirium screening: a study in 234 hospitalised older people. Age Ageing 2014;43(4):496–502.
50. O'Regan NA, Maughan K, Liddy N, et al. Five short screening tests in the detection of prevalent delirium: diagnostic accuracy and performance in different neurocognitive subgroups. Int J Geriatr Psychiatry 2017;32(12):1440–9.
51. Steensma E, Zhou W, Ngo L, et al. Ultra-brief screeners for detecting delirium superimposed on dementia. J Am Med Dir Assoc 2019;20(11):1391–6.e1.
52. Atcherson SR, Mendel LL, Baltimore WJ, et al. The effect of conventional and transparent surgical masks on speech understanding in individuals with and without hearing loss. J Am Acad Audiol 2017;28(1):58–67.
53. Available at: http://www.theclearmask.com. Accessed April 22, 2020.
54. Mitasova A, Kostalova M, Bednarik J, et al. Poststroke delirium incidence and outcomes: validation of the confusion assessment method for the intensive care Unit (CAM-ICU). Crit Care Med 2012;40(2):484–90.
55. Naidech AM, Beaumont JL, Rosenberg NF, et al. Intracerebral hemorrhage and delirium symptoms. Length of stay, function, and quality of life in a 114-patient cohort. Am J Respir Crit Care Med 2013;188(11):1331–7.
56. Oldenbeuving AW, de Kort PL, Jansen BP, et al. Delirium in the acute phase after stroke: incidence, risk factors, and outcome. Neurology 2011;76(11):993–9.
57. Rosenthal LJ, Francis BA, Beaumont JL, et al. Agitation, delirium, and cognitive outcomes in intracerebral hemorrhage. Psychosomatics 2017;58(1):19–27.
58. Patel MB, Bednarik J, Lee P, et al. Delirium monitoring in neurocritically ill patients: a systematic review. Crit Care Med 2018;46(11):1832–41.
59. Cole M, McCusker J, Dendukuri N, et al. The prognostic significance of subsyndromal delirium in elderly medical inpatients. J Am Geriatr Soc 2003;51(6):754–60.

60. Brummel NE, Boehm LM, Girard TD, et al. Subsyndromal delirium and institution-alization among patients with critical illness. Am J Crit Care 2017;26(6):447–55.
61. Bigatello LM, Amirfarzan H, Haghighi AK, et al. Effects of routine monitoring of delirium in a surgical/trauma intensive care unit. J Trauma Acute Care Surg 2013;74(3):876–83.
62. Girard TD, Exline MC, Carson SS, et al. Haloperidol and Ziprasidone for treatment of delirium in critical illness. N Engl J Med 2018;379(26):2506–16.
63. Erkinjuntti T, Sulkava R, Wikstrom J, et al. Short portable mental status question-naire as a screening-test for dementia and delirium among the elderly. J Am Ger-iatr Soc 1987;35(5):412–6.
64. Hestermann U, Backenstrass M, Gekle I, et al. Validation of a German version of the Confusion Assessment Method for delirium detection in a sample of acute geriatric patients with a high prevalence of dementia. Psychopathology 2009; 42(4):270–6.
65. Rosen J, Sweet RA, Mulsant BH, et al. The Delirium Rating Scale in a psychogeri-atric inpatient setting. J Neuropsychiatry Clin Neurosci 1994;6(1):30–5.
66. Hart RP, Levenson JL, Sessler CN, et al. Validation of a cognitive test for delirium in medical ICU patients. Psychosomatics 1996;37(6):533–46.
67. Ely EW, Margolin R, Francis J, et al. Evaluation of delirium in critically ill patients: validation of the confusion assessment method for the intensive care Unit (CAM-ICU). Crit Care Med 2001;29(7):1370–9.
68. Thomas C, Hestermann U, Walther S, et al. Prolonged activation EEG differenti-ates dementia with and without delirium in frail elderly patients. J Neurol Neuro-surg Psychiatry 2008;79(2):119–25.

Dementia and the Critically Ill Older Adult

Mira Ghneim, MD, MS*, Jose J. Diaz Jr, MD, CNS

KEYWORDS

- Older adults • Dementia • Delirium • Critical illness

KEY POINTS

- Dementia is a terminal illness and a leading cause of death in the United States in adults greater than 65 years of age.
- Clinicians should develop an advanced awareness regarding disease diagnosis.
- Dementia is a risk factor for delirium and delirium is associated with an accelerated, irreversible cognitive decline in patients with dementia.
- Dementia in the setting of critical illness is associated with a decreased likelihood of discharge to preinjury residence and an increased short- and long-term mortality.
- Early establishment of goals of care is the cornerstone for care in this patient population.

INTRODUCTION

The exponential growth of the population ages 65 and older is one of the most significant demographic trends in the history of the United States. Between 2020 and 2030, the number of older adults, defined as greater than 65 years of age, is projected to increase by 18 million. Additionally, it is predicted that this same population will double to more than 98 million and will triple to 20 million for those older than 80 years of age by 2060.[1]

Dementia, an underrecognized terminal illness, is one of the greatest health care problems among adult ages 65 or older world-wide.[2] At present, 5.7 million older adults have dementia and by 2050 it is projected that dementia will result in 1.6 million deaths.[3,4] A chronic disease of aging, dementia is characterized by progressive cognitive (memory, thinking, orientation, comprehension, learning capacity, and judgment) decline that interferes with independent functioning leading to severe disability and death within 3 to 9 years after diagnosis.[5,6] The most common cause of dementia is Alzheimer disease; however, vascular, frontotemporal, and Lewy body dementias are also prevalent.[7] The most common complications associated with the progression of dementia include dysphagia, recurrent respiratory and urinary tract infections, and an increased need for hospitalization.[8]

R Adams Cowley Shock Trauma Center, The University of Maryland Medical Center, 22 South Green Street, S4D07, Baltimore, MD 21201, USA
* Corresponding author. 22 South Greene Street, P1G1, Baltimore, MD 21201.
E-mail address: mira.ghneim@som.umaryland.edu

Crit Care Clin 37 (2021) 191–203
https://doi.org/10.1016/j.ccc.2020.08.010
0749-0704/21/© 2020 Elsevier Inc. All rights reserved.
criticalcare.theclinics.com

Of persons in the United States who die with dementia, approximately 16% die in the hospital.[8] Between 2000 and 2009, 19% of nursing home patients in the United States who died with advanced dementia experienced a burdensome hospitalization near the end of life.[9,10] The hospitalization burden consisted of hospitalizations within the last 3 days of life, increased intensive care unit (ICU) use, and extended ICU lengths of stay in the last 30 to 90 days of life.[10] It has been estimated that up to 75% of such burdensome transitions are avoidable given that they are frequently medically unnecessary and may be discordant with patients' wishes.[8,11,12]

Dementia has been shown to increase the risk of death in older patients hospitalized for acute illnesses.[13] For those who survive, especially older patients with advanced dementia, mortality after discharge is even higher.[13,14] Morrison[13] reported a 53% 6-month mortality for patients with end-stage dementia and pneumonia versus 13% for cognitively intact patients. In the same cohort, there was a 55% 6-month mortality in patients with hip fractures and end-stage dementia versus 12% mortality for cognitively intact patients.[13] These findings have been attributed to a greater comorbidity burden and a higher number of adverse events during hospitalization.[15,16]

Dementia presents critical care providers with clinical and ethical dilemmas when it comes to medical management and end-of-life care. Optimally, treatments and goals of care decisions are guided by patient preferences. Although older adults with milder forms of dementia may have capacity to make decisions regarding their care, with increasing disease severity, this may no longer be feasible. Clinicians must then rely on only occasionally available advanced directives or health care proxies' judgment. Because many medical professionals fail to screen for dementia in critically ill patients, because of the unawareness of its prevalence and the patient's severity of illness, many clinicians struggle to assist health care proxies navigate end-of-life goals in the absence of advanced directives.[14]

As a result, a major concern in older adults with advanced stages of dementia is that decisions may lead to more aggressive treatment than the patient would have chosen, leading to prolongation of life without improvement of quality of life. Therefore, it is crucial for critical care practitioners to maintain a high index of suspicion for the diagnosis, develop a better understanding of dementia to guide management during critical illness, recognize the limitations in available evidence, establish goals of care with the patient or proxy early on in the course of illness, and implement palliative interventions when deemed appropriate.

DISCUSSION
Stages of Dementia

Dementia is a progressive disease with a variable clinical course and is an entity that defines an individual's life expectancy independent of other comorbidities.[16] Life expectancies are seen in **Fig. 1**. Although stages of dementia have been classically described as mild (early), moderate (middle), and severe (late), more specific grading systems exist that provide a comprehensive description of symptom progression as seen in **Tables 1** and **2**. Using these grading systems as a guide to develop a better global understanding of cognitive and functional decline allows physicians to better communicate with patients and their caregivers to determine optimal treatment options during acute and critical illness.

THE CLINICAL COURSE AND OUTCOMES OF ADVANCED DEMENTIA

Caring for the expanding population with advanced dementia is one of the most important challenges for the US health care system.[20] In patients with advanced

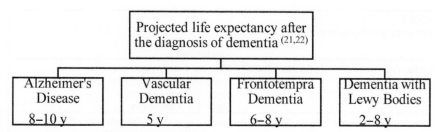

Fig. 1. Life expectancy by dementia type.

dementia, final years of life are characterized by a worsening trajectory of severe disability including: profound memory deficits, minimal verbal communication, loss of ambulatory abilities, the inability to perform activities of daily living, and urinary and fecal incontinence.[7,21]

The clinical course of advanced dementia was described in the Choices, Attitudes, and Strategies for Care of Advanced Dementia at the End-of-Life (CASCADE) study, which prospectively followed 323 nursing home residents over an 18-month period, 57% of whom were diagnosed with advanced dementia.[22] In this population, the average age was 85 ± 7 years and Alzheimer disease was the most common cause of dementia. Nursing home residents in this cohort suffered from severe cognitive and functional disabilities and the health care proxies were mainly middle-aged

Table 1
Stages of dementia

	Mild	Moderate	Severe
Duration of symptoms	2–4 y	2–10 y	1–3 y
ADLs	Problems with routine tasks	Need help with basic ADL (feeding, dressing, bathing)	Progress to total dependence on caregiver
Behavior	Changes in personality	Anxiety, suspicion, pacing, insomnia, depression, agitation, and wandering	Crying, screaming, groaning
Cognition	Confusion with memory loss Misplacing objects Forgetting names Disorientation	Difficulty recognizing family and friends Chronic loss of recent memory	Loss of speech Misidentifies or is unable to recognize familiar people
Assistance needed	Minimal and focused on daily to do lists to assist with memory loss	Hands on daily assistance with ADLs	24-h daily supervision

Abbreviation: ADL, activities of daily living.

From National Institute on Aging. National Institutes of Health; 2003. NIH publication 02-3782. Available at: http://www.alzheimers.org/unraveling/index.htm. Dementia Care Central;2020.

Table 2
Dementia grading systems

	Descriptions
Global Deterioration Scale/Reisberg Scale[17]	Most commonly used scale Seven stages based on cognitive decline Stage 1–3 = predementia Stage 4–7 = dementia
Functional Assessment Staging Test[18]	Seven stages (1–7) based on level of functioning and ability to perform ADLs Stage 4 = mild dementia Stage 5 = moderate dementia Stage 6 = moderately severe dementia Stage 7 = severe dementia (associated with the highest mortality rate)
Clinical Dementia Rating[19]	Assess cognitive and functional abilities Used mainly as a research tool

From Dementia Care Central;2020. Available at: https://www.dementiacarecentral.com/aboutdementia/facts/stages/#.

women with 67% identifying as the individual's child. Median survival was 1.3 years and the probability of death within the first 6 months was 25% for those with severe dementia. The three most common clinical complications were pneumonia, infection, and eating problems and were associated with increased risk of mortality. Within 3 months of death, many of the nursing home residents with advanced dementia underwent burdensome interventions (total parenteral nutrition, emergency room visits, hospitalizations, and placement of feeding tubes), which did not lead to improvement of outcomes or quality of life. Proxies and pre-established end-of-life goals of care were found to focus on comfort measures and relief of any physical suffering. One of the most fundamental findings in the study strengthens the concept that advanced dementia is a terminal illness: most deaths were not precipitated by any devastating events (myocardial infarctions), terminal illnesses (cancer), or acute decompensation of chronic conditions (congestive heart failure).[22]

Best practices for caring for terminally ill patients do not generally promote resuscitation with life-sustaining technologies; rather, they focus on prevention and relief of suffering and pain. Given the high mortality rate in older adults with end-stage dementia, in the setting of limited availability, high demand, and prohibitive cost of ICU services, it is essential to better establish whether critical life-sustaining procedures should be pursued in this patient population.

MANAGEMENT OF PATIENTS WITH DEMENTIA IN THE INTENSIVE CARE UNIT: WHAT DO WE KNOW SO FAR?
Updated 2019 American Geriatric Society Beer Criteria

i. Updated 2019 American Geriatric Society Beer Criteria for inappropriate medication use in adults with dementia because of drug-disease interactions that may lead to exacerbation of the disease:[23]

   a. *Anticholinergics*: Should be avoided in older adults given that their clearance is reduced with advanced age and leads to increased sedation and worsening delirium and dementia. Medications with anticholinergic properties are seen in **Table 3**.

   b. *Antipsychotics*: Avoid use in patients with behavioral problems and history of dementia and delirium unless nonpharmacologic options have failed, are not

Table 3		
Medications with anticholinergic effects that should be avoided		

Antiparkinsonian agents
  Benztropine
  Trihexyphenidyl
Antiarrhythmic
  Disopyramide
	Antihistamines (first
	  generation)
	  Brompheniramine
	  Carbinoxamine
	  Chlorpheniramine
	  Clemastine
	  Cyproheptadine
	  Dexbrompheniramine
	  Dexchlorpheniramine
	  Dimenhydrinate
	  Diphenhydramine (oral)
	  Doxylamine
	  Hydroxyzine
	  Meclizine
	  Promethazine
	  Pyrilamine
	  Triprolidine
		Antidepressants
		  Amitriptyline
		  Amoxapine
		  Clomipramine
		  Desipramine
		  Doxepin >6 mg/d
		  Imipramine
		  Nortriptyline
		  Paroxetine
		  Protriptyline
		  Trimipramine

Muscle relaxants
  Cyclobenzaprine
  Orphenadrine
Antiemetics
  Prochlorperazine
  Promethazine
	Antispasmodics
	  Atropine (excludes
	    ophthalmic)
	  Belladonna alkaloids
	  Clidinium-chlordiazepoxide
	  Dicyclomine
	  Homatropine
	  Hyoscyamine
	  Methscopolamine
	  Propantheline
	  Scopolamine
		Antimuscarinics (urinary
		  incontinence)
		  Darifenacin
		  Fesoterodine
		  Flavoxate
		  Oxybutynin
		  Solifenacin
		  Tolterodine
		  Trospium

possible, and the older adult is threatening substantial harm to self or others. Antipsychotics in older adults are associated with an increased risk of stroke and a greater rate of cognitive decline and mortality in patients with dementia (**Table 4**).

  c. *Benzodiazepines*: Older adults have an increased sensitivity to benzodiazepines and a decreased metabolism of longer acting agents. These agents increase the risk of cognitive impairment and should be avoided to treat behavioral problems in dementia and delirium. Benzodiazepines may be appropriate for seizure disorders, ethanol withdrawal, severe generalized anxiety disorders, and periprocedural anesthesia (see **Table 4**).

  d. *Nonbenzodiazepine, benzodiazepine receptor agonist hypnotics*: Lead to increased delirium and cognitive impairment. Representative agents are seen in **Table 4**.

Management of Patients with Dementia Is Variable and Lacks Practice Guidelines

Some studies comparing patients with and without dementia have found either similar rates or higher rates of aggressive treatment (mechanical ventilation [MV], central venous catheter placement, pulmonary artery catheter placement, and hemodialysis) among patients with dementia. This is attributed to lack of decision-making capacity or defined goals of care with proxies in the setting of dementia.[24–28] However, one study found that patients with dementia during the last 30 days of life, although more likely to experience an acute hospitalization, are less likely to be admitted to the ICU or undergo invasive interventions (invasive MV, cardiac catheterization,

Table 4
Antipsychotics, benzodiazepines, and the Z-drugs that should be avoided

Antipsychotics	Benzodiazepines	Nonbenzodiazepine,
Chlorpromazine	Short and	benzodiazepine
Clozapine	intermediate acting:	receptor agonist
Loxapine	Alprazolam	hypnotics ("Z-drugs")
Olanzapine	Estazolam	Eszopiclone
Perphenazine	Lorazepam	Zaleplon
Thioridazine	Oxazepam	Zolpidem
Trifluoperazine	Temazepam	
	Triazolam	
	Long acting:	
	Chlordiazepoxide	
	(alone or in	
	combination	
	with amitriptyline	
	or clidinium)	
	Clonazepam	
	Clorazepate	
	Diazepam	
	Flurazepam	
	Quazepam	

placement of pulmonary artery catheter, dialysis).[14] Moreover, Sampson and colleagues[27] retrospectively examined dying patients with and without dementia on medical wards to identify differences between their care. Patients with dementia received different end-of-life care when compared with those who are cognitively intact. Overall, there was an inadequate recognition and recording of patients' cognitive dysfunction. Patients with dementia were less likely to be intubated, undergo central venous catheter placement, or receive palliative interventions. Health care providers were less likely to perceive advanced dementia as a terminal illness and as a result, failed to recognize the barriers of cognitive dysfunction in expressing pain and therefore pain management was inadequate.

The Incidence of Dementia in the Intensive Care Unit Is Increasing

As the elderly population grows and accounts for a large proportion of patients admitted to the ICU, it has been projected that this growth will lead to an accompanying rise in dementia-associated hospitalizations.[28] Oud[29] reported that in Texas, the rate of ICU admission of elderly adults hospitalized with dementia nearly doubled over the last decade accompanied by a more than two-fold increased volume of ICU admissions. The latter change has substantially outpaced the corresponding growth rates of the elderly population. Between 2000 and 2008, although the 85 years and older population comprised less than 2% of the total US population, they represented more than 40% of all annual hospitalizations associated with dementia. According to static projections, the estimated 2050 volume of dementia hospitalizations in the 85 years and older group may be between 3 and 4 million cases, whereas the dynamic model predicted a rise to more than 7 million dementia-associated hospitalizations. This represents a 10-fold growth in the volume of these hospitalizations from the year 2000 baseline.[29]

Delirium Accelerates Cognitive Decline in the Setting of Dementia

Delirium is a syndrome that manifests as an acute change in mental status characterized by inattention and disturbances in cognition with a fluctuating course of symptoms. Delirium is most common in hospitalized older adults and one-third of general medical patients who are 70 years of age or older. It is the most common surgical complication among older adults with an incidence of 15% to 25% after major elective surgery and 50% after hip fracture repair and cardiac surgery. Additionally, there is a high incidence of delirium in mechanically ventilated patients.[30] Delirium is classified into two categories: hypoactive and hyperactive delirium. Hypoactive delirium is more prevalent in hospitalized older adults than agitated hyperactive delirium and is less frequently recognized, and as a result, is associated with a poorer prognosis.[31] Although delirium has been suggested to be transient, current evidence suggests that delirium may persist at hospital discharge in 45% of patients and in 33% of patients at 1 month thereafter.[30]

Risk factors for delirium are classified into two groups: predisposing and precipitating factors. Predisposing factors include age, dementia or preexisting cognitive dysfunction, history of delirium, functional disability, sensory impairment (hearing and vision loss), comorbidities and severity of illness, depression, transient ischemic attack or stroke, and alcohol abuse. Precipitating factors include sedative hypnotic and anticholinergic medications, surgery, trauma, anesthesia, pain, use of restraints, use of bladder catheters, infection, acute illness, and iatrogenic event.[30,31] The more predisposing factors exist, the fewer precipitating factors are needed to cause delirium. As a result, older frail adults are at much higher risk of developing delirium than younger patients. Persistent posthospitalization delirium is seen with advanced age, preexisting dementia, multiple coexisting conditions, severity of delirium, and the in-hospital use of physical restraints.[30,31] Delirium is associated with an increased length of stay, discharge to a nursing facility, increased posthospitalization mortality, and long-term cognitive dysfunction and functional decline with slow recovery.[31–33]

The interplay between dementia and delirium remains a topic of debate. Delirium might be a marker for vulnerability to dementia, might unmask unrecognized dementia, or delirium itself might lead to permanent neuronal damage that leads to dementia. Nonetheless, it has been well established that cognitive impairment and dementia are important risk factors for delirium and increase delirium risk by two to five times. Additionally, delirium is an independent risk factor for long-term cognitive decline and dementia.[31] Fong and colleagues[33] has shown that a single episode of delirium in a patient with Alzheimer disease can dramatically accelerate the trajectory of cognitive decline, increase mortality, increase rates of rehospitalization/institutionalization, and increase overall adverse outcomes. In another study, delirium in the setting of Alzheimer disease was associated with double the rate of cognitive decline in the first year following initial hospital admission. In addition, the authors found an accelerated decline that persisted over the 5-year follow-up period when comparing those with Alzheimer disease and delirium with those with Alzheimer disease and no delirium episodes. This study showed not only that delirium accelerated the cognitive decline, but that this change was irreversible.

Given that delirium is a frequent but modifiable occurrence in hospitalized older adults, and unlike other risk factors for dementia is reversible, early recognition and management is paramount to prevent further rapid and irreversible long-term decline in cognition. The first step in the diagnosis of delirium is possessing a high clinical index of suspicion based on risk factors, recognizing the possible coexistence of cognitive impairment and dementia in older adults, and using the confusion assessment method algorithm (CAM-ICU) for diagnosis. Once the diagnosis of delirium is established, reversable and modifiable risk factors must be identified and addressed. Behavioral disturbances should be managed with a nonpharmacologic approach first. Nonpharmacologic interventions include maintaining a sleep-wake cycle, frequent reorientation, encouraging family to interact with the patient, early mobilization, nursing training in de-escalation techniques, using a sitter, minimizing the use of restraints, and discontinuation of restraints in the ICU as soon as deemed appropriate. If required for patient safety, low doses of an antipsychotic agent are used but stopped as soon as safe. Proactive, multifactorial interventions, and geriatric consultations have been shown to reduce the incidence, severity, and duration of delirium.[30]

Dementia may be Associated with an Increased Risk of Organ Dysfunction

A population-based cohort study out of Taiwan showed that the presence of dementia was associated with an increased incidence of multiorgan failure (respiratory, cardiac, and neurologic), sepsis and severe sepsis, and in-hospital mortality leading to more interventions including vasopressors, MV, and ICU admission.[34] After accounting for interventions using life-sustaining treatments, dementia exhibited a minor effect on short-term mortality. This study was limited by the inability to clearly define the stages of dementia in the population evaluated leading to a possible selection bias with an underrepresentation of patients with advanced dementia.

Oud[29] showed that dementia was associated with an increasing burden of comorbidities (congestive heart failure, diabetes, and lung disease), doubling of organ failure rates from 25% to 50% (respiratory, neurologic, cardiac, and renal), decreasing use of invasive interventions (MV, new hemodialysis, and central venous catheter placement), increasing use of noninvasive ventilation, increasing mortality and discharge to hospice, and a decreasing rate in discharge to home because of increased residual morbidity among survivors.

The Relationship Between Dementia and Invasive Mechanical Ventilation Is Complex

The last few years have witnessed intense debate regarding life support in the ICU in patients with dementia, specifically regarding the topic of invasive MV.[35–40] MV is a key component in the management of critically ill patients with respiratory failure. However, MV is known to be associated with a high mortality, short- and long-term complications, and requires a high level of care with a substantial impact on hospital resources.[35] The average annual growth rate of invasive MV in patients with dementia has been estimated to be 11.4%.[36,37] Teno and colleagues[2] showed that there was a two-fold increase in MV use in patients with dementia between 2000 and 2013. Moreover, there was an association between increased ICU bed availability and MV use for patients with advanced dementia even after adjusting for multiple patient-level characteristics.[2] The underlying cause of the increase in MV in patients with dementia remains unclear but could be attributed to the growth of the elderly population over the last decade, and decision making by clinicians, patients, and families regarding the use of ICU toward the end of life in the setting of increased available beds, and the variability of palliative care resources. The aforementioned findings are in contrast to those articulated by Mitchell and colleagues[22] that found that 96% of health care proxies desire comfort to be the primary goal of care.

Although there is a trend toward increased usage of MV,[36] few studies have examined trends in MV in patients with dementia. The limited data available come from Lagu and colleagues[37] who showed that individuals with advanced dementia who underwent MV had lower costs of hospitalization, shorter length of stay, and lower mortality when compared with those without dementia. In this study, MV was less frequently used in patients with dementia, and the individuals with dementia receiving MV were less likely to have comorbidities. Most importantly, this study failed to classify patients based on severity of dementia and therefore did not provide insight on outcomes of MV in patients with end-stage dementia.

There Are Increased Rates of Cognitive and Functional Impairment, Rehospitalization, Discharge to Skilled Nursing Facilities, and Mortality in the Setting of Dementia and Hospitalization

Individuals with dementia may be especially vulnerable to accelerated cognitive and physical decline with increased mortality and shorter survival after critical illness.[41] Although the epidemiology and clinical features for hospitalization among patients with dementia have been extensively studied, the data regarding outcomes in ICU-managed older adults with dementia are conflicting.[42,43]

In 2005, a small single-center prospective observational cohort study in older patients with moderate to severe dementia evaluating in-hospital mortality and ICU length of stay showed no difference in short-term outcomes with regards to in-hospital mortality, readmission to the ICU, or discharge location when compared with patients without dementia. The ICU mortality in this cohort was 17% and overall mortality was found to be 25%. This study was limited by a small sample size (66 patients with dementia), indicating that the study lacked sufficient power to detect differences in patients with and without dementia.[44]

A longitudinal cohort study in the United Kingdom assessed mortality risk in older adults with dementia after acute hospitalization and ICU admission.[45] Admissions for pneumonia and urinary tract infections were associated with an increased incidence of cognitive impairment. Increased severity of dementia was an independent risk factor for in-hospital mortality. In addition, there was an overall increase in 6-month mortality with worsening cognitive impairment.

A review by Mukadam and Sampson[46] revealed significant associations between dementia and increased length of stay, functional decline, and discharge to institutional care. Other studies have shown that more severe cognitive impairment on admission is associated with increased institutionalization and mortality.[47,48] A prospective cohort study by Zekry and colleagues[49] showed that the best predictor of posthospitalization discharge to a skilled nursing facility was baseline moderate to severe dementia. Finally, a recent review of hospital readmission in patients with dementia showed that all-cause 30-day readmission ranged from 7% to 35%.[50]

APPROACH TO DECISION MAKING AND ESTABLISHING GOALS OF CARE IN CRITICALLY ILL OLDER ADULTS WITH ADVANCED DEMENTIA

Given that dementia is a terminal illness that is associated with an increased posthospitalization morbidity and mortality, advanced care planning is the cornerstone of care and treatment decisions for the critically ill patient. When directives have been established, treatment decisions should be based on the goals of care, and health care providers and the patients' health care proxy should share in the decision-making process.[7]

In situations where clear directives are absent, it is crucial for clinicians to guide the health care proxy through the decision-making process. This includes educating the health care proxy about the clinical course of dementia in the setting of critical illness, describing the treatment options for the specific clinical problem, describing the advantages and disadvantages of the options based on the best available evidence, and acknowledging the limitations of the available evidence in this patient population.

Discussing with the proxy what they believe the patient's goals of care would be in the setting of acute illness, which includes comfort care, aggressive management (central venous access, MV), or a middle ground (administration of antimicrobial agents only), is beneficial in the end-of-life decision-making process.[7] Early hospice and palliative involvement can assist in guiding the health care proxy in the decision process. Once the proxy has been fully informed and counseled, the health care team must respect their choice and be cognizant of ethnic and cultural preferences and beliefs. Revisiting the goals of care as the clinical status evolves is paramount to ensure proper patient management.[7]

SUMMARY

As the elderly population grows the incidence of hospitalized patients with dementia will continue to increase. It is of the utmost importance that health care providers develop a better understanding of the disease process, possess a high index of suspicion for early diagnosis, recognize the limitation in the available evidence for managing critically ill patients with dementia, establish goals of care early with the patient or health care proxy, and judiciously use health care resources and prevent any pain and suffering that can result in unwanted and futile care.

CLINICS CARE POINTS

- Dementia is a leading cause of death in the United States in adults greater than 65 years of age.
- Common clinical features as the disease progresses include profound memory deficits, minimal verbal communication, loss of ambulatory abilities, the inability to perform activities of daily living, and urinary and fecal incontinence.
- Dementia is a risk factor for delirium and delirium is associated with an accelerated, irreversible cognitive decline in patients with dementia.
- Research and evidence-based guidelines for the management of critically ill older adults with dementia are lacking and current observational studies have focused on outcomes and resource use of invasive mechanical ventilation.
- Results of the studies show that dementia in the setting of critical illness is associated with increased organ dysfunction, cognitive and functional decline, decreased likelihood of discharge to preinjury residence, and increased short- and long-term mortality.
- Early establishment of goals of care is the cornerstone for care.
- Treatment decisions should be guided by the goals of care with the patient or their health care proxies.
- More than 90% of health care proxies state that patient comfort is the primary goal.

GUIDELINES

Although no definitive population-specific guidelines exist for the management of critically ill older adults with dementia, the following societies provide resources and guidance to navigate management challenges and end-of-life care.

The American Geriatric Society (https://www.americangeriatrics.org)
The American Academy of Hospice and Palliative Medicine (http://aahpm.org)
The Alzheimer's Association (https://www.alz.org)
Dementia Care Centers (https://www.dementiacarecentral.com/about-us/)
Geriatric Care (https://geriatricscareonline.org/)

FUTURE DIRECTIONS

Designing and testing interventions that promote high-quality, goal-directed care across all health care settings is the cornerstone for future research for patients diagnosed with dementia. Future goals should focus on establishing guidelines that avoid unwanted hospitalizations of older adults with dementia whose goals of care are primarily comfort. Finally, research should focus on establishing policies that incentivize cost-effective and evidence-based care that maximizes favorable quality of life outcomes.

DISCLOSURE

The authors do not have any relevant financial conflict of interest or funding sources to disclose.

REFERENCES

1. Mather M, Jacobsen L, Pollard K. Population Bulletin. Available at: https://www.prb.org/wp-content/uploads/2016/01/aging-us-population-bulletin-1.pdf. Accessed June, 2020.
2. Teno JM, Gozalo P, Khandelwal N, et al. Association of increasing use of mechanical ventilation among nursing home residents with advanced dementia and intensive care unit beds. JAMA Intern Med 2016;176(12):1809.
3. Weuve J, Hebert LE, Scherr PA, et al. Deaths in the United States among persons with Alzheimer's disease (2010-2050). Alzheimers Demen 2014;10(2):e40–6.
4. Hurd MD, Martorell P, Delavande A, et al. Monetary costs of dementia in the United States. N Engl J Med 2013;368(14):1326–34.
5. Querfurth HW, LaFerla FM. Alzheimer's disease. N Engl J Med 2010;362(4):329–44.
6. Achterberg W, Pieper MJC, van Dalen-Kok AH, et al. Pain management in patients with dementia. Clin Interv Aging 2013;8:1471–82.
7. Mitchell SL. Advanced dementia. N Engl J Med 2015;372(26):2533–40.
8. Mitchell SL, Teno JM, Miller SC, et al. A national study of the location of death for older persons with dementia. J Am Geriatr Soc 2005;53(2):299–305.
9. Teno JM, Gozalo PL, Bynum JPW, et al. Change in end-of-life care for Medicare beneficiaries: site of death, place of care, and health care transitions in 2000, 2005, and 2009. JAMA 2013;309(5):470.
10. Gozalo P, Teno JM, Mitchell SL, et al. End-of-life transitions among nursing home residents with cognitive issues. N Engl J Med 2011;365(13):1212–21.
11. Givens JL, Selby K, Goldfeld KS, et al. Hospital transfers of nursing home residents with advanced dementia. J Am Geriatr Soc 2012;60(5):905–9.
12. Meier DE, Ahronheim JC, Morris J, et al. High short-term mortality in hospitalized patients with advanced dementia: lack of benefit of tube feeding. Arch Intern Med 2001;161(4):594.
13. Morrison RS. Survival in end-stage dementia following acute illness. JAMA 2000;284(1):47.
14. Richardson SS, Sullivan G, Hill A, et al. Use of aggressive medical treatments near the end of life: differences between patients with and without dementia. Health Serv Res 2007;42(1p1):183–200.
15. Laditka JN, Laditka SB, Cornman CB. Evaluating hospital care for individuals with Alzheimer's disease using inpatient quality indicators. Am J Alzheimers Dis Other Demen 2005;20(1):27–36.

16. Dementia Care Central. Stages of Alzheimer's & dementia: durations & scales used to measure progression (GDS, FAST & CDR) [Internet]. 2020. Available from: Stages of Alzheimer's & Dementia: Durations & Scales Used to Measure Progression (GDS, FAST & CDR). Available at: https://www.dementiacarecentral.com/aboutdementia/alzheimers/stages. Accessed June, 2020.

17. Reisberg B, Ferris SH, de Leon MJ, et al. The Global Deterioration Scale for assessment of primary degenerative dementia. Am J Psychiatry 1982;139(9): 1136–9.

18. Sclan SG, Reisberg B. Functional assessment staging (FAST) in Alzheimer's disease: reliability, validity, and ordinality. Int Psychogeriatr 1992;4(Suppl 1):55–69.

19. O'Bryant SE, Lacritz LH, Hall J, et al. Validation of the new interpretive guidelines for the clinical dementia rating scale sum of boxes score in the national Alzheimer's coordinating center database. Arch Neurol 2010;67(6):746–9.

20. Winzelberg GS, Hanson LC. Intensive care unit bed availability and use of mechanical ventilation in nursing home residents with advanced dementia: when we build it, why do they come? JAMA Intern Med 2016;176(12):1816.

21. Gill TM, Gahbauer EA, Han L, et al. Trajectories of disability in the last year of life. N Engl J Med 2010;362(13):1173–80.

22. Mitchell SL, Teno JM, Kiely DK, et al. The clinical course of advanced dementia. N Engl J Med 2009;361(16):1529–38.

23. By the 2019 American Geriatrics Society Beers Criteria® Update Expert Panel. American Geriatrics Society 2019 Updated AGS Beers Criteria® for Potentially inappropriate medication use in older adults: 2019 AGS beers criteria® update expert panel. J Am Geriatr Soc 2019;67(4):674–94.

24. Ahronheim JC, Morrison RS, Baskin SA, et al. Treatment of the dying in the acute care hospital. Advanced dementia and metastatic cancer. Arch Intern Med 1996; 156(18):2094–100.

25. Evers MM, Purohit D, Perl D, et al. Palliative and aggressive end-of-life care for patients with dementia. Psychiatr Serv 2002;53(5):609–13.

26. Mitchell SL, Kiely DK, Hamel MB. Dying with advanced dementia in the nursing home. Arch Intern Med 2004;164(3):321–6.

27. Sampson EL, Gould V, Lee D, et al. Differences in care received by patients with and without dementia who died during acute hospital admission: a retrospective case note study. Age Ageing 2006;35(2):187–9.

28. Zilberberg MD. Growth in dementia-associated hospitalizations among the oldest old in the United States: implications for ethical health services planning. Arch Intern Med 2011;171(20):1850.

29. Oud L. Evolving demand for critical care services for elderly adults with dementia in Texas: a population-based study. J Am Geriatr Soc 2016;64(2):432–4.

30. Marcantonio ER. Delirium in hospitalized older adults. N Engl J Med 2017; 377(15):1456–66.

31. Fong TG, Davis D, Growdon ME, et al. The interface between delirium and dementia in elderly adults. Lancet Neurol 2015;14(8):823–32.

32. Fong TG, Jones RN, Marcantonio ER, et al. Adverse outcomes after hospitalization and delirium in persons with Alzheimer disease. Ann Intern Med 2012; 156(12):848–56. W296.

33. Fong TG, Jones RN, Shi P, et al. Delirium accelerates cognitive decline in Alzheimer disease. Neurology 2009;72(18):1570–5.

34. Shen H-N, Lu C-L, Li C-Y. Dementia increases the risks of acute organ dysfunction, severe sepsis and mortality in hospitalized older patients: a national population-based study. Oreja-Guevara C, editor. PLoS One 2012;7(8):e42751.
35. Bouza C, Martínez-Alés G, López-Cuadrado T. Effect of dementia on the incidence, short-term outcomes, and resource utilization of invasive mechanical ventilation in the elderly: a nationwide population-based study. Crit Care 2019; 23(1):291.
36. Lagu T, Zilberberg MD, Tjia J, et al. Use of mechanical ventilation by patients with and without dementia, 2001 through 2011. JAMA Intern Med 2014;174(6): 999–1001.
37. Lagu T, Zilberberg MD, Tjia J, et al. Dementia and outcomes of mechanical ventilation. J Am Geriatr Soc 2016;64(10):e63–6.
38. Quill CM, Ratcliffe SJ, Harhay MO, et al. Variation in decisions to forgo life-sustaining therapies in US ICUs. Chest 2014;146(3):573–82.
39. Ward NS, Chong DH. Critical care beds and resource utilization: current trends and controversies. Semin Respir Crit Care Med 2015;36(6):914–20.
40. Barnato AE, Tate JA, Rodriguez KL, et al. Norms of decision making in the ICU: a case study of two academic medical centers at the extremes of end-of-life treatment intensity. Intensive Care Med 2012;38(11):1886–96.
41. Iwashyna TJ, Ely EW, Smith DM, et al. Long-term cognitive impairment and functional disability among survivors of severe sepsis. JAMA 2010;304(16):1787.
42. Bynum JPW, Rabins PV, Weller W, et al. The relationship between a dementia diagnosis, chronic illness, Medicare expenditures, and hospital use: Medicare use for dementia and chronic illness. J Am Geriatr Soc 2004;52(2):187–94.
43. Phelan EA, Borson S, Grothaus L, et al. Association of incident dementia with hospitalizations. JAMA 2012;307(2):165.
44. Pisani MA, Redlich CA, McNicoll L, et al. Short-term outcomes in older intensive care unit patients with dementia. Crit Care Med 2005;33(6):1371–6.
45. Sampson EL, Blanchard MR, Jones L, et al. Dementia in the acute hospital: prospective cohort study of prevalence and mortality. Br J Psychiatry 2009; 195(1):61–6.
46. Mukadam N, Sampson EL. A systematic review of the prevalence, associations and outcomes of dementia in older general hospital inpatients. Int Psychogeriatr 2011;23(3):344–55.
47. Joray S, Wietlisbach V, Büla CJ. Cognitive impairment in elderly medical inpatients: detection and associated six-month outcomes. Am J Geriatr Psychiatry 2004;12(6):639–47.
48. Jónsson PV, Noro A, Finne-Soveri H, et al. Admission profile is predictive of outcome in acute hospital care. Aging Clin Exp Res 2008;20(6):533–9.
49. Zekry D, Herrmann FR, Grandjean R, et al. Does dementia predict adverse hospitalization outcomes? A prospective study in aged inpatients. Int J Geriatr Psychiatry 2009;24(3):283–91.
50. Ma C, Bao S, Dull P, et al. Hospital readmission in persons with dementia: a systematic review. Int J Geriatr Psychiatry 2019;34(8):1170–84.

Nutritional Assessment

A Primary Component of the Multidimensional Geriatric Assessment in the Intensive Care Unit

Randeep S. Jawa, MD, FCCM[a],*, Rajeev B. Patel, MD[b],
David H. Young, MD, FCCM[c]

KEYWORDS

- Intensive Care Unit • Nutrition • Geriatric • Critically ill • Malnutrition • Sarcopenia
- Frailty • Elderly

KEY POINTS

- Nutritional screening of geriatric intensive care unit patients on admission or shortly thereafter, to facilitate intervention, is recommended.
- Various nutritional screening tools exist. The optimal tool may vary by patient condition and institutional logistics.
- Assessment of muscle mass and strength can identify malnutrition and sarcopenia.
- Malnutrition, sarcopenia, and frailty are inter-related.

INTRODUCTION

Nutritional awareness was revolutionized by Dudrick and colleagues'[1] paper describing the long-term beneficial effects of parenteral nutrition in 1968. After this publication, options for improving and maintaining nutrition took on new dimensions. The importance of assessing and adjusting the nutritional state of patients has become a core principle of patient care both in and out of the intensive care unit (ICU).

Nutritional evaluation of the geriatric ICU patient encompasses 3 closely related and overlapping domains: malnutrition, sarcopenia, and frailty. According to the World Health Organization, malnutrition encompasses undernutrition (ie, stunting, wasting, underweight status, and micronutrient deficiencies), as well as overweight conditions

[a] Division of Trauma, Surgical Critical Care, and Emergency Surgery, Department of Surgery, Stony Brook University Renaissance School of Medicine, HSC Level 18, Room 040, Stony Brook, NY 11794-8191, USA; [b] Division of Pulmonary, Critical Care, and Sleep Medicine, Department of Medicine, Stony Brook University Renaissance School of Medicine, HSC Level 17, Room 040, Stony Brook, NY 11794-8172, USA; [c] Division of Trauma/Critical Care, Department of Surgery, University of Nebraska Medical Center, Omaha, NE 68198, USA
* Corresponding author.
E-mail address: Randeep.jawa@stonybrookmedicine.edu

Crit Care Clin 37 (2021) 205–219
https://doi.org/10.1016/j.ccc.2020.08.011
0749-0704/21/© 2020 Elsevier Inc. All rights reserved.
criticalcare.theclinics.com

and noncommunicable diet-related diseases.[2] Malnutrition affects over 1 billion people globally.[3] However, as there is no single approach to malnutrition diagnosis, reported rates of malnutrition in adults vary from 15% to 60%.[4] Up to two-thirds of hospitalized or inpatient rehabilitation older adults are malnourished.[5] According to a multinational retrospective pooled analysis of studies since 2000 utilizing the Mini Nutritional Assessment (MNA) tool, the prevalence of malnutrition in the geriatric population was 5.8% in the community, 13.8% in nursing homes, 38.7% in hospitalized patients, and 50.5% in rehabilitation facilities.[6] In addition to the 38.7% malnutrition rate in hospitalized geriatric patients, an additional 46.3% of geriatric hospitalized patients are at risk for malnutrition, suggesting that only 14% of hospitalized geriatric patients are well-nourished.[6]

Several major societies provide guidance for adult nutritional status assessment. The American Society for Parenteral and Enteral Nutrition (ASPEN)/Academy of Nutrition and Dietetics consensus statement recommends the presence of at least 2 of the following 6 variables for the diagnosis of adult malnutrition:

Insufficient energy intake
Weight loss
Muscle mass loss
Subcutaneous fat loss
Decreased functional status as assessed by hand grip strength
Local or generalized fluid accumulation that may be masking weight loss[4]

In contrast, according to the European Society for Parenteral and Enteral Nutrition (ESPEN) consensus definition, malnutrition is diagnosed if any of the following are present:

Body mass index (BMI) is under 18.5 kg/m^2
Weight loss with reduced BMI is present
Weight loss with reduced fat free mass index is identified[7]

This article examines tools for the nutritional assessment of geriatric ICU patients, including a review of imaging and other standardized techniques for evaluation of muscle mass that are indicators of malnutrition and sarcopenia. In addition, the authors discuss the interplay of malnutrition, reduced muscle mass/sarcopenia, and frailty. The goal of these assessments is to identify those with or at risk for malnutrition and subsequently initiate interventions to improve outcomes.

NUTRITIONAL ASSESSMENT TOOLS

Several dozen tools have been validated for nutritional assessment in older adults. Many are geared toward the hospitalized patient, although not all of them are specifically designed for the elderly.[8] Some tools identify those at an increased risk of undernutrition/malnutrition, while others identify malnourished patients. ESPEN 2018 guidelines recommend that all elderly patients should be assessed for malnutrition with a validated tool. Elderly patients with a positive screen should undergo a systematic assessment, planned intervention, and reassessment after interventions.[5] According to ESPEN 2019 guidelines, all critically ill patients with ICU hospital length of stay (LOS) over 48 hours should be considered as at risk for malnutrition.[9]

Although there are no well-established tools for the assessment for malnutrition in the elderly ICU patient, 4 scoring systems (**Table 1**) and 1 consensus recommendation are available. The Subjective Global Assessment (SGA) includes components of the history (weight change, dietary intake change, gastrointestinal symptoms, functional

Table 1
Summary of 4 (SGA, MNA, NUTRIC, NRS2002) nutritional assessment tools that may be utilized in the evaluation of the intensive care unit patient

	SGA	MNA	NUTRIC[a]	NRS 2002
History	Yes	Yes	No[b]	Yes
Weight loss/dietary intake	Yes	Yes[e]	No	Yes
Physical examination	Yes (fat loss, muscle loss, edema)	Yes	No	No
Laboratory tests	No	No	Yes[c]	No
Anthropometric	Yes	Yes	No	Yes
Imaging/BIA	No	No	No	No
Subjective component	Yes	Yes	No	No
Age	No	No	Yes	Yes
Disease severity	Yes	No	Yes (APACHE II, SOFA)	Yes (eg chronic illness, injury, APACHE II)
Mobility	Yes (history)	Yes (history)	No	No
Other considerations	-	-	Hospital LOS before ICU admission	-
Score	B-moderate malnutrition C-severe malnutrition	17–23.5: at risk for malnutrition <17: malnutrition	≥5 or ≥6: high-risk adverse outcome[d]	>3: at risk for malnutrition ≥5: high-risk for malnutrition

Two of these tools (SGA, MNA) require elements of a patient history that may not be obtainable in all geriatric ICU patients.
[a] Designed to performed entirely from EMR.
[b] But includes comorbidities.
[c] IL-6 level is optional.
[d] ≥ 5 without interleukin IL-6, ≥6 with IL-6 is high risk for adverse outcome.
[e] Detailed history of diet composition.
Data from Refs.[6,10,18,22]

capacity, and disease) and physical examination (eg, evaluation for loss of subcutaneous fat, muscle wasting, ankle edema, sacral edema, and ascites) to derive an overall subjective rating of well nourished, moderately malnourished or suspicion thereof, or severely malnourished.[10] Given the SGA's heavy reliance on the patient's subjective historical data, this assessment is perhaps less easily applied in the ICU setting. A systematic review indicated that SGA performed similar or better than anthropometric measurements and laboratory data; meanwhile, it was comparable or inferior to other screening tools that varied by the population being studied.[11]

Per ESPEN, the most commonly used and validated screening tool for older adults is the MNA.[5] The MNA was designed for evaluation of the elderly in hospitals, nursing homes, and outpatient settings, and has been employed in hundreds of studies.[6,12] The MNA is comprised of anthropometric measurements (ie, BMI, midarm and calf circumference, and weight loss), a general assessment of lifestyle/medications/neuropsychologic issues and mobility, a dietary questionnaire, and a subjective patient self-assessment of nutritional status. An MNA score of at least 24 indicates good nutritional status; 17 to 23.5 indicates those at risk for malnutrition, and a score less than 17 indicates protein-calorie malnutrition. The MNA is reported to have sensitivity, specificity, and positive predictive values in the 96% to 98% range. Of note, there are 3 versions of the MNA.[8]

The Nutritional Risk Screening 2002 (NRS 2002), espoused by ESPEN, was compiled by analyzing data from 128 randomized clinical trials.[13,14] It includes 4 screening variables: BMI less than 20.5 kg/m2, weight loss over 3 months, reduced dietary intake in the previous week, and critical illness. If the answers to any of these questions are positive, then a final screen is performed that examines nutritional impairment (as assessed by BMI/food intake/weight loss), disease severity (eg, chronic illness, ICU Acute Physiologic and Chronic Health Evaluation II (APACHE II) score greater than 10, major abdominal surgery), and age less than 70 versus greater than or equal to 70. A score of no more than 3 indicates low risk, and a score greater than 3 indicates hospitalized patients at risk of malnutrition.[13] A high-risk cutoff of at least 5 was added by expert opinion.[15] NRS 2002 has a sensitivity of 52% to 100% for malnutrition detection.[8] An international trial at 26 hospitals encompassing medical, surgical, geriatric, and ICUs, identified that 32.6% of patients were at nutritional risk, with a range of 13% to 100% that varied by department/institution.[16] Patients at nutritional risk had increased hospital length of stay, complications, and mortality compared with those who were not at nutritional risk. A study of 185 adult ICU patients demonstrated a higher ICU mortality rate in high-risk patients ($\geq$5), but no difference in ICU LOS, hospital LOS, or duration of mechanical ventilation.[15] The multicenter EFFORT trial with 2088 hospitalized medical inpatients in Switzerland screened with NRS 2002 found that all patients screened were at nutritional risk (31% had a score = 3; 38% had a score = 4, and 31% had a score $\geq$ 5).[17] Individualized nutritional support was associated with decreased mortality, better functional status, and improved quality of life at 30 days.

The NUTRIC score, developed for ICU patients, is comprised of age (<50, 50 to <75, $\geq$75 years), APACHE II score (<15, 15 to <20, 20 to 28, $\geq$28), Sequential Organ Failure Assessment score (SOFA <6, 6 to <10, $\geq$10), number of comorbidities (0 to 1, 2 or more), days from hospital admit to ICU admission (0 to <1, 1 or more), and interleukin (IL)-6 levels (0 to <400, 400 or more).[18] The NUTRIC score ranges from 0 to 10. C-reactive protein, procalcitonin, BMI, oral intake, and weight loss were excluded from the final model because of a lack of statistical significance or failure to improve model-fit. Of note, the NUTRIC does not include patient history or physical examination. The authors further commented in the initial validation article that although IL-6 was included in the final model, given its minimal improvement of the C-statistic, it may be excluded where not readily available. This has been termed as the modified NUTRIC score. In the original study, an increasing NUTRIC score was significantly associated with an increased duration of mechanical ventilation and 28-day mortality.[18] Furthermore, adequate nutritional intake significantly reduced mortality in patients with high NUTRIC scores (ie, 6–10).

NUTRIC is advantageous as the relevant information is routinely available in medical records.[19] As such, it overcomes a common limitation of other scoring systems relying on patient history, as the elderly critically ill may have impaired cognition and/or otherwise impaired abilities to communicate.[19] However, the utility of the NUTRIC score in affecting outcomes was questioned in a post hoc analysis of 894 patients enrolled in the PermiT trial (Permissive Underfeeding vs Target Enteral Feeding in Adult Critically Ill Patients), using the modified NUTRIC score, no association was noted between standard and permissive underfeeding and categorization as either high or low risk with 90-day mortality.[20] Neither BMI nor select laboratory measures of malnutrition (transferrin, 24 hour urine urea nitrogen, phosphate), other than perhaps prealbumin (also known as transthyretin), showed an association with outcomes.

Comparisons of studies using various screening tools reveal differing incidences of nutritional risk and associations with outcomes. In a study of 294 ICU patients, 47% of patients were deemed at nutritional risk by at least 1 of 3 scoring systems (SGA, modified NUTRIC, and standard hospital metrics).[21] However, there was poor agreement among the tools, as only 9% of nutritional risk patients met at-risk or malnutrition criteria by all 3 scoring systems: 63% by institutional screening tool, 80% by SGA, and 26% by NUTRIC. Those identified as at risk had the longest ICU and hospital LOS. A retrospective study comparing the NUTRIC and NRS2002 in ICU patients indicated that an increasing NUTRIC score, but not NRS2002 score, was associated with increased protein and calorie deficits.[22] A study comparing SGA, MNA, MNA-SF, and NRSstat (an adaptation of NRS2002 that excludes age) in 260 mixed medical and surgical ICU patients aged at least 65 years noted malnutrition rates of 23% to 34% with a dichotomized definition that included at-risk patients.[23] Malnutrition was associated with adverse outcomes on univariate analyses but was not a significant factor in multivariate analyses. Another study identified a 52% to 64.9% malnutrition rate in elderly ICU patients in India with associated increased in-hospital and 1-year mortality rates.[24]

Of note, with MNA, NRS 2002, and NUTRIC, age influences the overall score. NRS 2002 and NUTRIC specifically consider critical illness and may be well suited for the geriatric ICU population. Calculators for the listed scores are available online. ASPEN/Society of Critical Care Medicine guidelines favor the NRS2002 and NUTRIC tools, citing their use in randomized controlled trials to identify nutrition risk and nonrandomized studies to demonstrate that early enteral nutrition reduces complications and mortality in high nutritional risk patients.[25] In contrast, ESPEN guidelines indicate that no specific scoring system has been validated in the critical care setting.[9] Regardless of the assessment used, it is imperative to perform early nutritional assessment of the geriatric ICU patient to facilitate nutritional intervention to potentially improve outcomes.

A CONSENSUS DEFINITION FOR MALNUTRITION

Noting the differences among screening tools, the Global Leadership Initiative on Malnutrition (GLIM) convened to establish a global consensus for the diagnosis of malnutrition.[3] GLIM proposed a multistep process for the diagnosis of malnutrition.

The first step in the diagnosis of malnutrition is an initial screen using one of several available tools (including NRS 2002, MNA-SF, and SGA, among others) to identify those at risk for malnutrition. For patients with a positive screen, a diagnostic assessment is performed using phenotypic criteria including

Nonvolitional weight loss
Low BMI adjusted for age (<70 or ≥70 years)
Race (Asian vs non-Asian)
Reduced muscle mass adjusted for race (Asian vs non-Asian)

Etiologic criteria include decreased food intake/assimilation and disease burden. Reduced food intake may be secondary to psychological causes, physiologic aberrations, and medications, among others. Disease burden/inflammation may be recognized by severity and acuity of underlying illness/injury; inflammatory markers such as CRP, albumin, or prealbumin may be utilized as a proxy measure. Malnutrition is diagnosed when at least 1 phenotypic criterion and 1etiologic criterion are met. Following diagnosis, the severity of malnutrition (moderate vs severe) is determined by the phenotypic criteria (ie, percentage of weight lost and timeframe thereof, low BMI, and reduced muscle mass). GLIM recommends imaging, bioimpedance (BIA), or other standardized/validated methods to assess muscle mass. If not available or regionally acceptable, anthropometric measurements, physical examination, or handgrip strength are acceptable alternatives. Cutoffs for reduced muscle mass are reported by the European Working Group on Sarcopenia in Older People (EWGSOP).

ASSESSMENT OF MUSCLE MASS, STRENGTH, AND SARCOPENIA

GLIM uses reduced muscle mass as a diagnostic phenotypic criterion for malnutrition and its severity.[3] After age 50, muscle mass and strength decrease progressively.[26] Fatty degeneration and/or fatty infiltration of muscle, a part of the aging process, is associated with disability and decreased strength.[27] Muscle is biologically active. It secretes mediators that play roles in metabolism, neurologic function, endocrine function, and cardiovascular system function, among other things.[27] Reduction in muscle mass impairs metabolism and nutrient uptake, and increases susceptibility to malnutrition and frailty, further reducing muscle mass in a vicious cycle.[28]

A closely related concept is sarcopenia. While often described as age-associated loss of skeletal muscle mass and function, it has since been recognized to be multifactorial, beginning much earlier in life, and possibly even related to birthweight.[26,29,30] Factors contributing to its development and progression include loss of mobility and independence, comorbidities, depression, and financial hardships. Estimates of sarcopenia prevalence vary widely by population studied.[31] Sarcopenia has been reported in 10% of hospitalized adults and has been associated with mortality, complications, prolonged hospitalization, falls, fractures, and physical disability.[31,32] GLIM considers reduced muscle strength as a supportive metric in the diagnosis of malnutrition; however, for the diagnosis of sarcopenia, muscle strength is the dominant criteria.

In the 2019 revision of EWGSOP guidelines, decreased muscle strength is the primary identifying characteristic of sarcopenia.[26] (**Table 2**) EWGSOP suggests a 4-step diagnostic approach:

1. SARC-F (strength, assistance in walking, rise from chair, climb stairs, falls) questionnaire or clinical suspicion to find cases
2. Muscle strength assessment by grip strength or chair stand test

Table 2
Stepwise assessment of sarcopenia according to EWGSOP guidelines

Tool		Components			
SARC-F (subjective) questionnaire	Strength	Assistance in walking	Rise from chair	Climb stairs	Falls
Muscle strength assessment	Grip strength	Chair stand/rise test	—	—	
Confirmation of decreased muscle quantity or quality	DXA	Bioimpedance analysis	CT scan	MRI	Others
Severity	Gait speed	Timed up and go	Short performance physical battery	400 m walk	—

Clinical suspicion or SARC-F questionnaire can be used to identify cases. If muscle strength is noted to be low, then sarcopenia is considered probable in the absence of mitigating factors such as stroke. Confirmation requires assessment of muscle quantity or quality via a variety of modalities. Severity is determined by physical performance; low performance indicates severe sarcopenia.

Data from Cruz-Jentoft AJ, Bahat G, Bauer J, et al. Sarcopenia: revised European consensus on definition and diagnosis [published correction appears in Age Ageing. 2019 Jul 1;48(4):601]. Age Ageing. 2019;48(1):16-31.

3. Confirmation of sarcopenia via decreased muscle quantity or quality on dual-energy X-ray (DXA) (preferable for clinical use), BIA, CT, or MRI
4. Severity assessment by physical performance (ie, locomotion-related whole-body function-as measured by gait speed, timed up and go, short physical performance battery, or 400 m walk).[26] These cutoffs for these measures of sarcopenia are −2 to −2.5 standard deviations from reference values in young healthy European adults.[26]

Criticisms of these criteria include: (1) grip strength assesses only a single muscle group and (2) gait speed may be limited by osteoarthritis.[33] Heart, lung, or peripheral vascular disease may also influence gait speed.

A discussion follows of recommended standardized tools to assess muscle mass. Although correlations exist between various methods (eg, DXA, bioimpedance spectroscopy, creatine [methyl-d3] dilution), the absolute quantity of muscle mass derived varies between them.[33] Not all modalities are feasible for critically ill patients, and even fewer are specifically validated in geriatric critically ill patients.

Dual Energy X-ray Absorptiometry

DXA scanning, given its precision, has been endorsed as a reference standard by several societies.[32,34,35] Although commonly used for the evaluation of bone density, it can be utilized to evaluate soft tissue mass. DXA employs low-dose x-rays at 2 different energy levels and measures the amount of energy absorbed in soft tissues and bone.[27,32] Limitations of DXA include overestimation of lean soft tissue compartments with increased hydration, underestimation of fat mass with increased body thickness, inability to distinguish various types of lean soft tissue (ie, muscles and organs) and fat (ie, visceral, subcutaneous, and intramuscular) mass, and susceptibility to artifact from orthopedic hardware.[27] Furthermore, inconsistencies between machine hardware and software make comparison of results unreliable between machines and institutions.[32] Because intra-abdominal organs decrease truncal fat and muscle measurement accuracy, estimations of total body muscle and fat mass are derived from measurements in the extremities.[27] Instead of using an absolute value of appendicular skeletal muscle mass, various indices adjusting for body size are available, such as the appendicular skeletal muscle (ASM)/height squared (skeletal muscle index).[27] Other indices include ASM/weight and ASM/BMI.[26] DXA scanning of ICU patients is seldom performed.

Computed Tomography Scan

The abdominal computed tomography (CT) scan is also considered a gold standard for body composition analysis, especially truncal composition analysis.[27,32] CT examines muscle quantity and also quality as assessed by the degree of fatty infiltration.[27,35] Body composition can be assessed with specialized open-source segmentation software.[36,37] Unlike DXA scanning, the CT scan may have been or often will be performed as part of the routine care of an ICU patient. Given the high dose of radiation required, its use is largely pragmatic.[32] To reduce radiation exposure, there has been investigation into low-dose and single-slice scanning.[27] Use of the L3 vertebra as the landmark for body composition assessment has been well established, as this area is found to best correlate with whole-body skeletal muscle mass.[32] Others argue for muscle assessment at the L4 level.[35] Another alternative is a peripheral quantitative CT scan, which uses lower doses of radiation.[27]

In a retrospective study of 687 ICU patients, age greater than 70 versus less than or equal to 70, sarcopenia (as measured by CT scan at lumbar vertebrae L3), and simplified nutritional appetite questionnaire scores (SNAQ) were associated with in-hospital mortality in univariate but not multivariate analyses.[36] However, at 6 months, the mortality rate was significantly higher (42%) in the sarcopenic group than the non-sarcopenic group (24%).[36] A study of 149 elderly, severely injured trauma patients examined sarcopenia, as measured by muscle mass using specialized CT software, at L3 on admission CT scan.[37] To adjust for patient height, a muscle index was derived. Sarcopenia was present in 71% of patients and predictive of increased mortality, decreased ICU-free days, and decreased number of ventilator-free days. Of sarcopenic patients, 47% were obese/overweight, 44% normal weight, and 9% underweight, demonstrating that sarcopenia and hence malnutrition may be present regardless of body weight.

MRI

With MRI, as with CT, 3 areas of measurement are commonly used: L3 for total abdominal muscle area, the psoas muscle at lumbar spine level, and musculature at midthigh level.[27] MRI is superior to CT in terms of distinguishing between fat and muscle tissue. With diffusion tensor imaging and MRI spectroscopy, microstructure, fatty infiltration, and the quantity of intracellular fat can be appreciated.[27,35] Conventional (qualitative) and quantitative MRI are commercially available. The primary advantage of MRI over CT is the absence of ionizing radiation; however, there is substantial added cost and transportation and monitoring concerns in the critically ill. As with CT, consideration can be given for its utilization in muscle mass assessment when it is planned for other reasons, and cutoffs for normal values are debated.[26]

Ultrasound

Given limited availability, feasibility, and practicality of DXA, MRI, and CT as tools for the critically ill patient, portable ultrasound offers a viable alternative for assessing muscle quantity and quality. A major limitation is its operator dependence.[32] Ultrasound may also be used to measure intramuscular glycogen and fat content.[38] As muscle quality has been correlated with muscle strength, the evaluation for both quality and quantity is important.[38] Assessment of lower limb muscles, which comprise 75% of total muscle mass, is especially important because of their primacy in determining functional independence in older individuals.[39,40] In older adults, functional capacity and nutritional status have been correlated with ultrasonographic muscle thickness and muscle echo intensity.[39]

A pilot study of 19 elderly institutionalized adults demonstrated that ultrasonographic gastrocnemius and tibialis anterior muscle thickness was significantly correlated with nutritional status as measured by the MNA.[39] A 2019 Brazilian study evaluating maximal compressible quadriceps femoris thickness in 55 adult patients with ICU stay greater than 48 hours demonstrated significant association with the modified NUTRIC score.[41] A 2016 study of 102 surgical ICU patients noted a 43.1% incidence of sarcopenia, as measured by rectus femoris cross-sectional area on ultrasound, a 38.2% incidence of frailty, as measured by the Frailty Index Questionnaire, and noted that both were predictive of discharge to a nursing home and in-hospital mortality.[42]

Bioimpedance/Bioimpedance Spectroscopy

Bioimpedance measures body water and estimates muscle and fat mass based on impedance to electrical current flow. Intracellular water (ICW) decreases with age, but extracellular water (ECW) does not; hence, the ECW to total body water (TBW) ratio increases with age, masking muscular atrophy, making traditional bioimpedance analysis, which uses a single electrical current frequency, less useful.[33,43] However, bioimpedance spectroscopy, which uses a spectrum of electrical frequencies, overcomes these limitations.[33] Segmental bioelectrical impedance spectroscopy measures ICW (reflective of muscle mass), ECW, and the ECW/ICW ratio, which suggests the ratio of nonmuscle tissue to muscle tissue.[38] Of note, bioimpedance values are calibrated to lean-body mass as assessed by DXA scanning; the Sergi conversion equation is European population based.[26] When evaluating different populations, ethnicity, age, and hydration status should be considered.[26] As with DXA scanning, values can be adjusted for weight, height, and BMI.[26]

Other Techniques for Assessment of Nutritional Status and Muscle Mass

Anthropometric measurements

Anthropometric measurements such as BMI, calf circumference, and triceps skin fold thickness have long been utilized for nutritional and sarcopenia assessments. However, their reliability in the elderly is unclear because of altered body composition and height loss associated with aging.[5,40] Further, anthropometric measurements depend on several assumptions:

Extremity modeling of concentric cylinders is accurate
Manual caliper measurements accurately reflect subcutaneous fat thickness
Bone atrophy remains in constant proportion to muscle[40]

When compared with MRI measurements in elderly patients, anthropometric measurements significantly overestimated muscle mass with proportion of error in line with increasing adiposity.[40] Utility of anthropometric measurements in other populations is also questionable. A study of ARDS survivors demonstrated that anthropomorphic measurements (eg, upper arm percent muscle area) had poor precision compared with DXA scanning.[44] Because weight loss can result in further muscle loss and lacks mortality benefit, ESPEN recommends, in absence of obesity-related comorbidities or adverse health effects, the avoidance of weight loss/weight reduction diets in obese older adults.[5]

Laboratory markers

Various laboratory indices have been and continue to be used to assess nutritional status including, albumin, prealbumin, transferrin, C-reactive protein (CRP), total cholesterol, and total lymphocyte count.[45] However, metabolic changes in critical illness raise concerns about their reliability, as their levels can decrease with injury and/or illness.[19,46] In a systematic review of albumin levels in calorie-restricted individuals without disease, serum albumin and prealbumin did not identify malnourishment until extreme starvation.[46] In a consensus statement, ASPEN and the Academy of Nutrition and Dietetics did not endorse any particular marker of inflammation for diagnostic purposes.[4] According to the consensus statement, albumin and prealbumin are markers of inflammation with limited response to feeding and have little relevance to the diagnosis of malnutrition.[4] Finally, several laboratory parameters have been suggested as markers for sarcopenia, including sclerostin, IGF-1, myostatin, skeletal muscle troponin T, creatine (methyl-d3) dilution method, and serum creatinine to cystatin C ratio.[33,47] However, the most recent laboratory markers have not gained widespread acceptance.

Following the identification of sarcopenia, intervention is indicated. Exercise programs in the general population have demonstrated improvements in muscle strength and performance.[31] A recommendation is therefore made for early mobility programs in the ICU. Although they may not affect ICU mortality, mobility programs do improve mobility, strength, and postdischarge hospital free-days.[48]

FRAILTY

Aging, disease, decreased reserve, malnutrition, sarcopenia with attendant decreased strength and physical activity are interrelated in the generation of frailty.[49] Frailty is "a multidimensional syndrome of loss of reserves (energy, physical ability, cognition, health) that gives rise to vulnerability".[50] A diagnostic measure that stands out, given its simplicity, is the Clinical Frailty Scale for the elderly, which ranges from 1 to 7, where a score of 7 indicates a severely frail individual. A patient who is severely frail is one who is fully dependent on others for activities of daily living or is terminally ill.[50] Higher frailty scores are associated with medium-term (70-month) mortality and institutionalization. A detailed frailty index based on 70 dichotomous variables is also employed.[50,51] Alternatively, frailty as a phenotype has also been characterized by the presence of any 3 of the following 5 criteria: unintentional weight loss by direct measurement, self-reported exhaustion, grip strength, slow 15-foot walking speed, and low physical activity level as measured by kcal expended per week.[52] The presence of 1 or 2 of these criteria identifies those who are pre-frail.

Of note, frailty, sarcopenia, and malnutrition are closely related (**Fig. 1**). The presence of 1 finding affects the others. Aging and malnutrition contribute to sarcopenia, which results in decreased physical performance and dependence. The effects of frailty can then exacerbate undernutrition and sarcopenia.[52] A systematic review revealed substantial associations and overlap between the 3 domains when including prefrailty and at-risk of malnutrition in older hospitalized adults.[53] Perhaps unsurprisingly, parameters assessed for each overlap, ie, the Frailty Index, Subjective Global Assessment for malnutrition, and the EWGSOP sarcopenia criteria. Muscle mass and locomotion play an important role in all three. Indeed, per ESPEN, malnutrition encompasses starvation-related underweight, cachexia/disease-related malnutrition, sarcopenia, and frailty.[7]

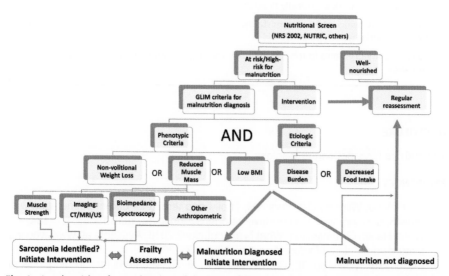

Fig. 1. An algorithm for evaluation of the inter-related concepts of nutritional status, sarcopenia, and frailty.

SUMMARY

The geriatric patient faces several nutritional challenges in the ICU and on the ward. Decreasing muscle mass, impaired mobility, malnutrition, comorbidities with attendant medications, and frailty make this patient population worthy of specialized knowledge and attention. The admission of a geriatric patient to the ICU should prompt early nutritional screening (see **Fig. 1**). Tools that may be particularly feasible to use at bedside include NRS2002 and NUTRIC. In patients identified as at risk for malnutrition, nutritional support is initiated, and assessment for malnutrition severity is indicated. Along with etiologic criteria, referencing the GLIM criteria of reduced muscle mass will also identify sarcopenia. Hence, consideration should be given to evaluating the muscle mass of patients who have undergone or would otherwise undergo a torso CT scan. For other patients, consider bedside ultrasound or bioimpedance evaluations. If these modalities are unavailable, handgrip strength can be assessed by way of an inexpensive dynamometer. Recognition of sarcopenia should prompt initiation of early mobility and muscle-strengthening programs. Confirmation of malnutrition should prompt nutritional support via an appropriate route (eg, oral, enteral, or parenteral) followed by reassessment. These determinations individually or in conjunction with the frailty evaluation can help in the assessment, outcome prognostication, and multidisciplinary management of the geriatric ICU patient. Attention to and prevention of worsening sarcopenia, malnutrition, and immobilization may be rewarded with lower morbidity and mortality.

Clinics care points

- An adult ICU length of stay >48 hours should be considered a risk factor for malnutrition.
- Early nutritional assessment and intervention of the geriatric ICU patient can improve outcomes.
- A variety of nutritional assessment tools are available, with varying degrees of dependence on patient's ability to participate in the assessment.
- ASPEN/Society of Critical Care Medicine guidelines favor the NRS2002 and NUTRIC tools to identify nutrition risk in critically ill adults.
- Sarcopenia is associated with mortality, complications, prolonged hospitalization, falls, fractures, and physical disability.
- Early mobility programs in the ICU improve mobility, strength, and post-discharge hospital free-days.

DISCLOSURE

The authors have nothing to disclose.

REFERENCES

1. Dudrick SJ, Wilmore DW, Vars HM, et al. Long-term total parenteral nutrition with growth, development, and positive nitrogen balance. Surgery 1968;64(1):134–42.
2. World Health Organization. What is malnutrition? 2016. Available at: www.who.int/features/qa/malnutrition/en. Accessed June 06, 2019.
3. Cederholm T, Jensen GL, Correia MITD, et al. GLIM criteria for the diagnosis of malnutrition - a consensus report from the global clinical nutrition community. Clin Nutr 2019;38(1):1-9.

4. White JV, Guenter P, Jensen G, et al. Consensus statement of the Academy of Nutrition and Dietetics/American Society for Parenteral and Enteral Nutrition: characteristics recommended for the identification and documentation of adult malnutrition (undernutrition). J Acad Nutr Diet 2012;112(5):730–8 [Erratum appears in J Acad Nutr Diet. 2012 Nov;112(11):1899].

5. Volkert D, Beck AM, Cederholm T, et al. ESPEN guideline on clinical nutrition and hydration in geriatrics. Clin Nutr 2019;38(1):10–47.

6. Kaiser MJ, Bauer JM, Rämsch C, et al. Frequency of malnutrition in older adults: a multinational perspective using the mini nutritional assessment. J Am Geriatr Soc 2010;58(9):1734–8.

7. Cederholm T, Bosaeus I, Barazzoni R, et al. Diagnostic criteria for malnutrition - an ESPEN consensus statement. Clin Nutr 2015;34(3):335–40.

8. Power L, Mullally D, Gibney ER, et al. A review of the validity of malnutrition screening tools used in older adults in community and healthcare settings - a MaNuEL study. Clin Nutr ESPEN 2018;24:1–13.

9. Singer P, Blaser AR, Berger MM, et al. ESPEN guideline on clinical nutrition in the intensive care unit. Clin Nutr 2019;38(1):48–79.

10. Detsky AS, McLaughlin JR, Baker JP, et al. What is subjective global assessment of nutritional status? JPEN J Parenter Enteral Nutr 1987;11(1):8–13.

11. da Silva Fink J, Daniel de Mello P, Daniel de Mello E. Subjective global assessment of nutritional status – a systematic review of the literature. Clin Nutr 2015; 34(5):785–92.

12. Vellas B, Guigoz Y, Garry PJ, et al. The Mini Nutritional Assessment (MNA) and its use in grading the nutritional state of elderly patients. Nutrition 1999;15(2): 116-122.

13. Kondrup J, Rasmussen HH, Hamberg O, et al, Ad Hoc ESPEN Working Group. Nutritional risk screening (NRS 2002): a new method based on an analysis of controlled clinical trials. Clin Nutr 2003;22(3):321–36.

14. Kondrup J, Allison SP, Elia M, et al. Educational and clinical Practice Committee, European society of parenteral and enteral nutrition (ESPEN). ESPEN guidelines for nutrition screening 2002. Clin Nutr 2003;22(4):415–21.

15. Maciel LRMA, Franzosi OS, Nunes DSL, et al. Nutritional risk screening 2002 cut-off to identify high-risk is a good predictor of ICU mortality in critically ill patients. Nutr Clin Pract 2019;34(1):137–41.

16. Sorensen J, Kondrup J, Prokopowicz J, et al. EuroOOPS: an international, multi-centre study to implement nutritional risk screening and evaluate clinical outcome. Clin Nutr 2008;27(3):340–9.

17. Schuetz P, Fehr R, Baechli V, et al. Individualised nutritional support in medical inpatients at nutritional risk: a randomised clinical trial. Lancet 2019; 393(10188):2312–21.

18. Heyland DK, Dhaliwal R, Jiang X, et al. Identifying critically ill patients who benefit the most from nutrition therapy: the development and initial validation of a novel risk assessment tool. Crit Care 2011;15(6):R268.

19. Teixeira V, Morimoto I. Parameters for nutritional status monitoring in critically ill older adults: an integrative review. Geriatr Gerontol Aging 2018;12(2):113–20.

20. Arabi YM, Aldawood AS, Al-Dorzi HM, et al. Permissive underfeeding or standard enteral feeding in high- and low-nutritional-risk critically ill adults. post hoc analysis of the PermiT Trial. Am J Respir Crit Care Med 2017;195(5):652–62.

21. Coltman A, Peterson S, Roehl K, et al. Use of 3 tools to assess nutrition risk in the intensive care unit. JPEN J Parenter Enteral Nutr 2015;39(1):28–33.

22. Canales C, Elsayes A, Yeh DD, et al. Nutrition risk in critically ill versus the nutritional risk screening 2002: are they comparable for assessing risk of malnutrition in critically ill patients? JPEN J Parenter Enteral Nutr 2019;43(1):81–7.
23. Sheean PM, Peterson SJ, Chen Y, et al. Utilizing multiple methods to classify malnutrition among elderly patients admitted to the medical and surgical intensive care units (ICU). Clin Nutr 2013;32:752e7.
24. Tripathy S, Mishra JC. Assessing nutrition in the critically ill elderly patient: a comparison of two screening tools. Indian J Crit Care Med 2015;19(9):518–22.
25. McClave SA, Taylor BE, Martindale RG, et al. Guidelines for the Provision and assessment of nutrition support therapy in the adult critically ill patient: society of critical care medicine (SCCM) and American society for parenteral and enteral nutrition (A.S.P.E.N.). JPEN J Parenter Enteral Nutr 2016;40(2):159–211 [Erratum appears in JPEN J Parenter Enteral Nutr. 2016 Nov;40(8):1200].
26. Cruz-Jentoft AJ, Bahat G, Bauer J, et al. Sarcopenia: revised European consensus on definition and diagnosis. Age Ageing 2019;48(1):16–31 [Erratum appears in Age Ageing. 2019 Jul 1;48(4):601].
27. Lee K, Shin Y, Huh J, et al. Recent issues on body composition imaging for sarcopenia evaluation. Korean J Radiol 2019;20(2):205–17.
28. Cruz-Jentoft AJ, Kiesswetter E, Drey M, et al. Nutrition, frailty, and sarcopenia. Aging Clin Exp Res 2017;29(1):43–8.
29. Fielding RA, Vellas B, Evans WJ, et al. Sarcopenia: an undiagnosed condition in older adults. Current consensus definition: prevalence, etiology, and consequences. International working group on sarcopenia. J Am Med Dir Assoc 2011;12(4):249–56.
30. Sayer AA, Syddall HE, Gilbody HJ, et al. Does sarcopenia originate in early life? Findings from the Hertfordshire cohort study. J Gerontol A Biol Sci Med Sci 2004; 59(9):M930–4.
31. Cruz-Jentoft AJ, Landi F, Schneider SM, et al. Prevalence of and interventions for sarcopenia in ageing adults: a systematic review. Report of the International Sarcopenia Initiative (EWGSOP and IWGS). Age Ageing 2014;43(6):748–59.
32. Prado CM, Heymsfield SB. Lean tissue imaging: a new era for nutritional assessment and intervention. JPEN J Parenter Enteral Nutr 2014;38(8):940–53 [published correction appears in JPEN J Parenter Enteral Nutr. 2016 Jul;40(5):742].
33. Buehring B, Siglinsky E, Krueger D, et al. Comparison of muscle/lean mass measurement methods: correlation with functional and biochemical testing. Osteoporos Int 2018;29(3):675–83.
34. Buckinx F, Landi F, Cesari M, et al. Pitfalls in the measurement of muscle mass: a need for a reference standard. J Cachexia Sarcopenia Muscle 2018;9(2):269–78.
35. Messina C, Maffi G, Vitale JA, et al. Diagnostic imaging of osteoporosis and sarcopenia: a narrative review. Quantitative Imaging Med Surg 2018;8(1):86–99.
36. de Hoogt PA, Reisinger KW, Tegels JJW, et al. Functional compromise cohort study (FCCS): sarcopenia is a strong predictor of mortality in the intensive care unit. World J Surg 2018;42(6):1733–41.
37. Moisey LL, Mourtzakis M, Cotton BA, et al. Skeletal muscle predicts ventilator-free days, ICU-free days, and mortality in elderly ICU patients. Crit Care 2013;17(5): R206.
38. Wischmeyer P, Molinger J. Objective malnutrition diagnosis and personalised nutrition delivery in the ICU. ICU Management and Practice 2019;19(3):167–73.
39. Mateos-Angulo A, Galán-Mercant A, Cuesta-Vargas AI. Ultrasound muscle assessment and nutritional status in institutionalized older adults: a pilot study. Nutrients 2019;11(6):1247.

40. Baumgartner RN, Rhyne RL, Troup C, et al. Appendicular skeletal muscle areas assessed by magnetic resonance imaging in older persons. J Gerontol 1992; 47(3):M67–72.
41. Özdemir U, Özdemir M, Aygencel G, et al. The role of maximum compressed thickness of the quadriceps femoris muscle measured by ultrasonography in assessing nutritional risk in critically-ill patients with different volume statuses. Rev Assoc Med Bras (1992) 2019;65(7):952–8.
42. Mueller N, Murthy S, Tainter CR, et al. Can sarcopenia quantified by ultrasound of the rectus femoris muscle predict adverse outcome of surgical intensive care unit patients as well as frailty? a prospective, observational cohort study. Ann Surg 2016;264(6):1116–24.
43. Yamada Y, Schoeller DA, Nakamura E, et al. Extracellular water may mask actual muscle atrophy during aging. J Gerontol A Biol Sci Med Sci 2010;65(5):510–6.
44. Chan KS, Mourtzakis M, Aronson Friedman L, et al. Upper arm anthropometrics versus DXA scan in survivors of acute respiratory distress syndrome. Eur J Clin Nutr 2018;72(4):613–7.
45. Bharadwaj S, Ginoya S, Tandon P, et al. Malnutrition: laboratory markers vs nutritional assessment. Gastroenterol Rep (Oxf) 2016;4(4):272–80.
46. Lee JL, Oh ES, Lee RW, et al. Serum albumin and prealbumin in calorically restricted, nondiseased individuals: a systematic review. Am J Med 2015; 128(9):1023.e1-22.
47. Kashani KB, Frazee EN, Kukrálová L, et al. Evaluating muscle mass by using markers of kidney function: development of the sarcopenia index. Crit Care Med 2017;45(1):e23–9.
48. Tipping CJ, Harrold M, Holland A, et al. The effects of active mobilisation and rehabilitation in ICU on mortality and function: a systematic review. Intensive Care Med 2017;43(2):171–83.
49. McDermid RC, Stelfox HT, Bagshaw SM. Frailty in the critically ill: a novel concept. Crit Care 2011;15(1):301.
50. Rockwood K, Song X, MacKnight C, et al. A global clinical measure of fitness and frailty in elderly people. CMAJ 2005;173(5):489–95.
51. Rockwood K, Howlett SE. Fifteen years of progress in understanding frailty and health in aging. BMC Med 2018;16(1):220.
52. Fried LP, Tangen CM, Walston J, et al. Frailty in older adults: evidence for a phenotype. J Gerontol A Biol Sci Med Sci 2001;56(3):M146–56.
53. Ligthart-Melis GC, Luiking YC, Kakourou A, et al. Frailty, sarcopenia, and malnutrition frequently (co-)occur in hospitalized older adults: a systematic review and meta-analysis. J Am Med Dir Assoc 2020;21(9):1216–28.

Rehabilitation Concerns in the Geriatric Critically Ill and Injured - Part 2

Brittany Nowak, MD, Cherisse Berry, MD*

KEYWORDS

- Rehabilitation • Disability • Frailty • Trauma • Intensive care unit • Disposition
- Geriatric • Elderly

KEY POINTS

- Geriatric patients are prone to sustain more severe injuries after seemingly minor events, due to their baseline characteristics and co-morbidities.
- These baseline conditions must be recognized early during hospitalization using screening tools, in order to intervene and optimize disposition from the hospital.
- The responsibility cannot fall on a single provider. A multidisciplinary team is critical to address every aspect of care and get patients on a path to meaningful recovery.

INTRODUCTION

As life expectancy increases and birth rates decline, the geriatric population continues to grow faster than any other age group.[1] In fact, by 2030, the number of Americans aged 65 years or older will double to 70 million and nearly 18 million will be 85 years or older.[2,3] Aging is characterized by a progressive physiologic decline that promotes the onset of functional limitation and disability.[4] With the increasing geriatric population, more elderly patients are presenting to emergency departments after trauma, and intensive care units (ICUs) are being met with increasing demand. In fact, elderly patients aged 80 years or older represent 20% to 30% of all ICU admissions[5,6] with long-term mortality rates ranging from 55% to 90% at 3 years.[7–9] For those patients who survive to discharge, the degree of disability acquired after critical illness and resultant health-related quality of life varies based on prehospital functional status, burden of comorbidities, physiologic reserve, cognitive impairments, malnutrition, frailty, sarcopenia, the duration of critical illness, and hospital-associated disability (HAD).[10,11] Thus, rehabilitation is critical in improving quality of life by maximizing physical, cognitive, and psychological recovery from injury or disease.

Department of Surgery, Division of Acute Care Surgery, New York University Grossman School of Medicine, 550 First Avenue, NBV 12 East 36, New York, NY 10016, USA
* Corresponding author.
E-mail address: cherisse.berry@nyulangone.org

Crit Care Clin 37 (2021) 221–231
https://doi.org/10.1016/j.ccc.2020.08.008
0749-0704/21/© 2020 Elsevier Inc. All rights reserved.

Injury

Elderly trauma patients have higher rates of functional impairment because of injury, requiring rehabilitation or placement in skilled care facilities.[12] Falls are by far the most common mechanism of injury in severely injured geriatric patients and account for almost three-quarters of severe geriatric traumas, followed by motor vehicle collision.[13] Even a low mechanism injury such as a fall from standing can result in severe injury and mortality in the elderly when compared with the younger patient population.[14] These patients were on average older, more frequently women, had a higher inpatient mortality, and were less likely to return home after discharge when compared with other blunt trauma patients. Postdischarge, elderly patients sustaining a low-level fall also had a decreased rate of independence and a higher mortality rate.[15] Many elderly patients are frequent fallers and should undergo rehabilitation to help mitigate the risk of additional falls. In a review of national Medicare patients, high-risk fall patients were more likely to use rehabilitation services when compared with lower risk patients. Among the high-risk patients, those who used rehabilitation services had lower self-reported physical capacity when compared with those who did not but had similar physical performance, and this indicates that many patients may be unaware of their risk and could also benefit from rehabilitation services for which they may consider themselves too high functioning to utilize.[16] In patients who had already sustained a fall, a dedicated home exercise program with a physical therapist including strength and balance training helped to prevent additional falls when compared with standard care from a geriatrician.[17] Patients who have been injured after falls had lower readmission rates after undergoing rehabilitation compared with those who had not.[18]

Traumatic brain injury

Elderly patients have the highest rate of traumatic brain injury (TBI) when compared with other age groups[19] and tend to have less severe head injuries that result in worse mortality and functional outcomes.[20,21] Close monitoring must be undertaken to prevent secondary injury in these patients. Elderly patients with TBI were more likely to require inpatient rehabilitation rather than being discharged home and were slower to regain function than the younger cohort. However, elderly patients with isolated mild TBI continue to recover over time.[22] Providers must be diligent in managing elderly patients with TBI by implementing rehabilitation early in order to help them return to their baseline function. After TBI, elderly patients were found to have a shorter length of stay in acute rehabilitation, and received fewer hours of therapy, especially from psychology and therapeutic recreation, and subsequently had less regain of function.[23] Geriatric neurorehabilitation should address excess disability or functional loss not from the brain injury itself, but from other underlying disease processes including sleep disorders, mood disorders or depression, acute and chronic pain, medication side effects, poor social support, and vision or hearing loss. Goals to focus on neurorehabilitation include life satisfaction, longevity, freedom from distractibility, mastery, growth, active engagement in life, independent functioning, and positive adaptation.[24] After rehabilitation from TBI, focus should turn to reintegration of elderly adults into their community.[25]

Hip fracture

Hip fracture is one of the most studied traumatic injuries in elderly patients and can be truly devastating. It has the potential to cause severe and long-lasting decline in a patient's health with a mortality rate of 14% to 58%.[26] Early implementation of a hip fracture pathway including involvement of a multidisciplinary team before surgery helps get patients to the operating room quickly but safely, with the goal of minimizing deconditioning while patients are relatively immobile before repair. The standard is to operate within a day of admission, but if there are medical comorbidities that can be optimized within a day or two, such as dehydration, electrolyte abnormalities, poorly controlled diabetes, or pulmonary decompensation, those should be quickly addressed before proceeding with surgery.[27] Reduced time to surgery and avoidance of delirium have been shown to decrease hospital length of stay.[28] A dedicated team that addresses the geriatric needs of elderly patients with hip fracture can help improve outcomes such as decreased length of stay and can also increase rates of patients going to rehabilitation.[29] Postoperatively, weight-bearing restrictions should be liberalized as much as possible, as greater restrictions were associated with high rates of adverse events including delirium, infection, need for transfusion, length of stay, and 30-day mortality in frail patients.[30] Geriatric comanagement teams can also help to address and reduce rates of adverse clinical events and delirium in the acute rehabilitation setting.[31]

Rib fracture

Rib fractures can be particularly devastating in geriatric patients. Of those who were admitted to the hospital with one or more rib fractures, less than two-thirds were able to return home immediately posthospitalization. Higher risk of discharge to a facility was seen with increased age, 4 or more rib fractures, white race, female gender, and chronic medical conditions such as renal failure, diabetes mellitus, obesity, and heart failure.[32] In elderly patients with rib fractures, it has also been shown that delirium leads to prolonged hospitalization and discharge to nursing home or rehabilitation instead of home.[33] These needs should be anticipated early during hospitalization so appropriate planning can be instituted.

Hospital-Associated Disability

HAD is described as a new or additional disability in activities of daily living (ADL) at hospital discharge compared with preadmission baseline.[11] It is estimated that 35% of geriatric patients and 50% of patients 85 years and older decline in ADL function between baseline and discharge.[34,35] Boyd and colleagues[36] found that by 1 year, 41% of geriatric patients with HAD died, 29% remained disabled, and 30% returned to their baseline level of function. Palleschi and colleagues[34] describe age, cognitive impairment, depression, limited social support, lower preadmission functional level (before acute illness), severity of acute illness, and comorbidities as risk factors for the development of HAD. In addition, in-hospital patient immobility, polypharmacy, complications such as infections, decline in nutritional status, and hospital length of stay can accelerate functional decline.

Early Mobility

ICU-acquired weakness affects 25% to 60% of critically ill patients and is characterized as a polyneuropathy and/or myopathy primarily affecting the lower extremities, shoulders, hip girdle, and respiratory muscles, which prolongs mechanical ventilation.[37] Thus, strategies to increase mobility in critically ill patients have been implemented nationally among ICUs in order to minimize ICU-acquired weakness and long-term disability. Although historically the culture of ICU care was bedrest and immobility, it is now overwhelmingly apparent that minimizing sedation and early mobilization of patients in the ICU is beneficial, feasible, and safe.[38,39] Schaller and colleagues[40] performed a multicenter international randomized control trial to determine if the early mobilization of surgical critically ill patients resulted in improved outcomes. They found that early mobilization resulted in decreased ICU length of stay and increased functional independence at hospital discharge. Liu and colleagues[41] found that early mobilization of critically ill patients not only resulted in decreased mortality but also decreased total hospital costs. Thus, guidelines such as the ICU Liberation Bundle (*ABCDEF*—Assess/Prevent/and Manage Pain; *B*oth Spontaneous Awakening Trials and Spontaneous Breathing Trials; *C*hoice of Analgesia and Sedation; *D*elirium: Assess, Prevent, and Manage; *E*arly Mobility and Exercise; and *F*amily Engagement and Empowerment) as described by the Society of Critical Care Medicine can help decrease delirium, improve functional outcomes, and prevent adverse outcomes.[42] Before the implementation of Early Mobility and Exercise, adult patients who are mechanically ventilated in an ICU must be assessed by objective clinical criteria to ensure safety. A consensus group of 23 multidisciplinary experts developed a standard traffic light system of recommendations to assist health care providers in evaluating safety criteria[43]: red would indicate the need for caution when the risk of an adverse event is high; yellow would indicate that mobilization is possible, but only after further consideration among the ICU multidisciplinary team; and green would indicate that the patient is safe to be mobilized. The safety criteria as described by Hodgson and colleagues[43] were divided into 4 categories: (1) respiratory considerations, including intubation status, ventilatory parameters, and the need for adjunctive therapies; (2) cardiovascular considerations, including the presence of devices, cardiac arrhythmias, and blood pressure; (3) neurologic considerations, including level of consciousness, delirium, and intracranial pressure; and (4) other considerations, including lines and surgical or medical conditions.

Cognitive Impairments

Impaired sensorium
Elderly patients are at much greater risk of having hearing impairments, decreased visual acuity, dark adaptation, contrast sensitivity, and visual processing speed impairments, increasing the risk for falls. Elderly patients with TBI may also have a decreased ability to process visual and auditory cues. Thus, in the rehabilitation setting, it is important to mitigate these impairments by using a variety of assistive devices such as hearing aids, improved lighting, and magnifiers for reading.[44]

Cognitive decline, depression, dementia, delirium
Aging can lead to cognitive decline and dementia and in the acute inpatient setting, elderly patents are at risk for developing delirium. In the hip fracture patient population, cognitive and mood disorders have been shown to increase the risk of poor outcomes, including decline in the ability to perform tasks of daily living, worsening ambulation, need for nursing home, and mortality.[45]

Malnutrition

Malnutrition is associated with decreasing functional status and increasing dependency and disability.[46–48] Although malnutrition is reported to be as high as 50% among all geriatric patients,[49–53] the prevalence among geriatric patients in rehabilitation/subacute facilities is 29%.[49] Malnutrition results from loss of body protein, impaired immune status, and loss of muscle mass, leading to frailty and impeding recovery from disease, trauma, and surgery.[46,52]

Frailty

Frailty is characterized by age-associated declines in physiologic reserve and function across multiorgan systems, leading to increased vulnerability for adverse health outcomes.[49] Assessment of frailty in geriatric patients is essential. Frailty phenotype defines frailty as a distinct clinical syndrome: (1) more than 4.5-kg weight loss over the past year, (2) self-reported exhaustion, (3) grip strength weakness, (4) slow walking speed, and (5) low physical activity. If patients have 3 or more of these characteristics, they are deemed frail, which was predictive of falls, worsening mobility and ADL, high rates of hospitalization, and higher risk of death.[54] The FRAIL questionnaire is a 5-question self-report survey that has also been shown to predict functional status and mortality. This questionnaire includes Fatigue; Resistance, which is measured as walking upstairs; Ambulation over a distance; Illness; and Loss of weight.[55] Frail patients have decreased ability to return to their baseline after an event and have greater vulnerability to stressors such as injury or critical illness.[56] Frailty has been validated in the geriatric trauma patient population specifically, similar to the general, nonsurgical patient population, and was associated with less favorable discharge disposition from the hospital.[57] The clinical frailty scale, a simple 9-point scale from "very fit" to "terminally ill" scale was able to predict mortality in elderly ICU patients.[58] Although not included within the definition of frailty, it is associated with delirium, another complication that happens frequently in elderly patients while hospitalized.[59] With regard to longer term outcomes, frail patients are less likely to recover to their baseline functional status postrehabilitation. Frail patients must be identified early during their hospitalization in order to begin intervention as early as possible to improve their functional status. Based on severity of injuries, baseline frailty can also be used in advanced care planning discussions. In the rehabilitation setting, frail patients have lower functional independence both at admission and discharge, as well as slower progress with each day, which must be considered when determining the duration of rehabilitation for these patients. Male patients and those who spent more days in rehabilitation had greater improvement in their functional independence.[60] Clinicians must recognize and assess frailty on admission to the hospital so that these high-risk patients can receive appropriate care.

Sarcopenia

Along with the functional marker of frailty, elderly patients have normal muscle loss as they age. Thirty to fifty percent of lean muscle mass is lost from 50 to 80 years of age, and a 3% decrease is seen per year after age 60 years.[61] Sarcopenia is associated with greater risk for falls and fractures, which are frequently seen in the geriatric trauma population, and also increases mortality risk. The best method to mitigate sarcopenia is with resistance training and nutritional supplementation, which should be implemented as early as possible during hospitalization. Resistance training should also be encouraged in a preventative setting for elderly sarcopenic patients identified in the primary care setting.[61] Sarcopenic patients have been found to have similar functional improvement during hospitalization but then did not improve with home rehabilitation when compared with nonsarcopenic patients.[62]

Multidisciplinary Team

It is imperative to have a robust multidisciplinary team in order to care for the complexity of geriatric patients. These teams are often composed of the trauma surgeon, geriatrician, physical therapist, occupational therapist, social worker, physiatrist, and frequently a psychiatrist, speech and language pathologist, and dietician. The physical therapists help to mobilize patients in the setting of new limitations from injury. The occupational therapists help patients regain the ability to perform activities of daily living. Social workers and care managers help arrange and coordinate various dispositions from the hospital. The physiatrist helps to determine a long-term plan for recovery. Psychiatrists can help manage psychiatric comorbidities seen frequently in geriatric patients. Speech and language pathologists help with swallowing and speaking after TBI or prolonged hospitalization requiring intubation or tracheostomy. Dieticians help to optimize nutrition in a patient population that is frail at baseline and requires supplemental nutrition to recover from an injury. Each member of the team plays a critical role in addressing acute issues while hospitalized, returning patients back to their baseline function as quickly as possible, whether that is directly home with or without outpatient services or to an acute rehabilitation setting. The earlier these team members are involved, the more efficiently decisions regarding the next steps of rehabilitation for patients can take place. A geriatric-specific multidisciplinary team can decrease medical complications and inpatient mortality.[63,64]

Geriatrician

Having a geriatrician involved in the care of elderly patients helps to address and optimize their baseline characteristics in the setting of acute injury. Geriatricians can help with managing existing medical conditions and identifying new ones, assist with advanced care planning, disposition, and medications, including pain management. Involving a geriatrician can help improve outcomes of elderly trauma patients by decreasing functional decline, falls, delirium, and death.[65] A geriatric trauma consult service was shown to decrease delirium and discharge to long-term care facilities and give more comprehensive care, thereby decreasing the need for consultation with internal medicine and psychiatry.[66] Geriatricians are a critical member of the team and improve outcomes for elderly trauma patients.

Rehabilitation Assessment and Disposition

The functional independence measure is a scoring tool to help measure functional status of patients before and on discharge from a rehabilitation facility and is used by the center for Medicare and Medicaid services (CMS) in the rehabilitation setting. This tool includes the motor tasks such as eating, grooming, bathing, upper body dressing, lower body dressing, toileting, bladder management, bowel management, bed to chair transfer, toilet transfer, shower transfer, locomotion, and stairs and cognitive tasks such as comprehension, expression, and social. Pretrauma Functional Independence Measure score has been shown to correlate with survival in elderly trauma patients.[67]

Hershkovitz and colleagues[68] found that hand grip strength was associated with outcomes and that grip strength screening on admission could help to identify those patients at higher risk for requiring intense rehabilitation. Individualized rehabilitation should be undertaken in order to address the patient's living situation and optimize their ability to return home.[26] Home rehabilitation physical therapy services have been shown to improve patient's mobility, activity, and balance but did not improve walking outdoors, walking speed, or risk of return to the emergency department.[69] The recovery process can be slow and arduous, and subjective recovery takes an average 9 months, which may lag behind objective recovery at approximately 6 months postinjury.[70]

In the United States, a patient's posthospitalization final disposition is determined by their predicted functional outcome and available insurance resources. CMS determines what criteria must be met in order to go to an acute rehabilitation facility versus subacute rehabilitation or long-term assisted care facility. Acute rehabilitation is the most rigorous environment, but in order to qualify, patients must require ongoing multidisciplinary therapy, 3 hours per day 5 days per week of physical or occupational therapy, actively participate in and be deemed to benefit from intense rehabilitation therapy, require a physiatrist to continue to follow 3 days per week, and require an interdisciplinary team to deliver rehabilitation care.[55] In order to meet these require-ments, patients must have the opportunity to work with a rehabilitation team soon after injury to minimize deconditioning.

SUMMARY

Elderly trauma patients have an increasing presence in ICUs and pose a challenge to clinicians to minimize disability on their ultimate discharge from the hospital. These pa-tients frequently require disposition to a rehabilitation facility, which is critical to a re-turn to their baseline level of function. Common injuries sustained include TBI, hip fractures, and rib fractures, all of which can occur with relatively low-energy mecha-nisms and cause significant morbidity in this population. Elderly patients often present with baseline conditions and comorbidities including cognitive impairment, malnutri-tion, frailty, and sarcopenia, which contribute to both the initial injury mechanism and the subsequent recovery. These comorbidities must be identified on presentation and addressed during the rehabilitation process. Early mobilization is critical in improving functional outcomes at discharge, and a multidisciplinary team is crucial in optimizing the care of these complex patients and ultimately progressing them to-ward an appropriate discharge from the hospital.

Clinics care points

- Seemingly minor ground level falls lead to decreased independence and high mortality in elderly patients.
- Conditions associated with aging such as sleep disorders, mood disorders, and pain must be acknowledged and addressed during geriatric TBI rehab.
- Hospital-Associated Disability is highly prevalent and is significantly associated with poor outcomes.
- A simple traffic-light grading system can help identify critically ill patients who are able to mobilize while in the ICU.
- Frail patients can be identified by various screening tools. Doing this early in hospitalization allows providers to improve on modifiable factors to expedite recovery.
- A geriatrician can be a valuable resource in managing co-morbidities in elderly patients.

REFERENCES

1. Cerreta F, Eichler HG, Rasi G. Drug policy for an aging population–the European Medicines Agency's geriatric medicines strategy. N Engl J Med 2012;367(21): 1972–4.
2. Brummel NE, Ferrante LE. Integrating geriatric principles into critical care medi-cine: the time is now. Ann Am Thorac Soc 2018;15(5):518–22.
3. Ortman J, Velkoff V, Hogan H. An aging nation: the older population in the United States. Washington, DC: U.S. Census Bureau; 2014.
4. Intiso D, Di Rienzo F, Russo M, et al. Rehabilitation strategy in the elderly. J Nephrol 2012;25(Supp 19):S90–5.
5. Bagshaw SM, Webb SAR, Delaney A, et al. Very old patients admitted to intensive care in Australia and New Zealand: a multi-centre cohort analysis. Crit Care 2009; 13(2):R45.
6. Docherty AB, Anderson NH, Walsh TS, et al. Equity of access to critical care among elderly patients in Scotland: a national cohort study. Crit Care Med 2016;44(1):3–13.

7. Heyland DK, Garland A, Bagshaw SM, et al. Recovery after critical illness in patients aged 80 years or older: a multi-center prospective observational cohort study. Intensive Care Med 2015;41:1911–20.

8. Kaarlola A, Tallgren M, Pettilä V. Long-term survival, quality of life, and quality-adjusted life-years among critically ill elderly patients. Crit Care Med 2006;34:2120–6.

9. Boumendil A, Maury E, Reinhard I, et al. Prognosis of patients aged 80 years and over admitted in medical intensive care unit. Intensive Care Med 2004;30:647–54.

10. Detsky ME, Herridge MS. Physical function, disability and rehabilitation in the elderly critically ill. In: Personnes âgées et réanimation. Références en réanimation. Collection de la SRLF. Paris: Springer; 2012. p. 123–36. https://doi.org/10.1007/978-2-8178-0287-9_12.

11. Covinsky KE, Pierluissi E, Johnston CB. Hospitalization-associated disability: "she was probably able to ambulate, but I'm not sure'. JAMA 2011;306:1782–93.

12. Lui F, Davis K. Trauma and musculoskeletal system dysfunction in the critically Ill elderly. In: Akhtar S, Rosenbaum S, editors. Principles of Geriatric Critical Care. Cambridge: Cambridge University Press; 2018. p. 126–37.

13. Labib N, Nouh T, Winocour S, et al. Severely injured geriatric population: morbidity, mortality, and risk factors. J Trauma 2011;71(6):1908–14.

14. Sterling DA, O'Connor JA, Bonadies J. Geriatric falls: injury severity is high and disproportionate to mechanism. J Trauma 2001;50(1):116–9.

15. Gerrish AW, Hamill ME, Love KM, et al. Postdischarge mortality after geriatric low-level falls: a five-year analysis. Am Surg 2018;84(8):1272–6.

16. Gell NM, Patel KV. Rehabilitation services use of older adults according to fall-risk screening guidelines. J Am Geriatr Soc 2019;67(1):100–7.

17. Liu-Ambrose T, Davis JC, Best JR, et al. Effect of a home-based exercise program on subsequent falls among community-dwelling high-risk older adults after a fall: a randomized clinical trial. JAMA 2019;321(21):2092–100.

18. Wong TH, Wong YJ, Lau ZY, et al. Not all falls are equal: risk factors for unplanned readmission in older patients after moderate and severe injury-a national cohort study. J Am Med Dir Assoc 2019;20(2):201–7.

19. Taylor CA, Bell JM, Breiding MJ, et al. Traumatic brain injury–related emergency department visits, hospitalizations, and deaths — United States, 2007 and 2013. MMWR Surveill Summ 2017;66(9):1–16.

20. Susman M, DiRusso SM, Sullivan T, et al. Traumatic brain injury in the elderly: increased mortality and worse functional outcome at discharge despite lower injury severity. J Trauma 2002;53(2):219–23.

21. Mosenthal AC, Lavery RF, Addis M, et al. Isolated traumatic brain injury: age is an independent predictor of mortality and early outcome. J Trauma 2002;52(5):907–11.

22. Mosenthal AC, Livingston DH, Lavery RF, et al. The effect of age on functional outcome in mild traumatic brain injury: 6-month report of a prospective multi-center trial. J Trauma 2004;56(5):1042–8.

23. Dijkers M, Brandstater M, Horn S, et al. Inpatient rehabilitation for traumatic brain injury: the influence of age on treatments and outcomes. NeuroRehabilitation 2013;32(2):233–52.

24. Uomoto JM. Older adults and neuropsychological rehabilitation following acquired brain injury. NeuroRehabilitation 2008;23(5):415–24.

25. Ritchie L, Wright-St Clair VA, Keogh J, et al. Community integration after traumatic brain injury: a systematic review of the clinical implications of measurement and service provision for older adults. Arch Phys Med Rehabil 2014;95(1):163–74.

26. Hack J, Buecking B, Aigner R, et al. What are the influencing factors in self-rated health status after hip fracture? A prospective study on 402 patients. Arch Osteoporos 2019;14(1):92.

27. Kulshrestha V, Sood M, Kumar S, et al. Outcomes of fast-track multidisciplinary care of hip fractures in veterans: a geriatric hip fracture program report. Clin Orthop Surg 2019;11(4):388–95.

28. Hecht G, Slee CA, Goodell PB, et al. Predictive modeling for geriatric hip fracture patients: early surgery and delirium have the largest influence on length of stay. J Am Acad Orthop Surg 2019;27(6):e293–300.

29. Murphy RP, Reddin C, Murphy EP, et al. Key service improvements after the introduction of an integrated orthogeriatric service. Geriatr Orthop Surg Rehabil 2019; 10. 2151459319893898.

30. Ottesen TD, McLynn RP, Galivanche AR, et al. Increased complications in geriatric patients with a fracture of the hip whose postoperative weight-bearing is restricted: an analysis of 4918 patients. Bone Joint J 2018;100-B(10):1377–84.

31. Morandi A, Mazzone A, Bernardini B, et al. Association between delirium, adverse clinical events and functional outcomes in older patients admitted to rehabilitation settings after a hip fracture: a multicenter retrospective cohort study. Geriatr Gerontol Int 2019;19(5):404–8.

32. Halevi AE, Mauer E, Saldinger P, et al. Predictors of dependency in geriatric trauma patients with rib fractures: a population study. Am Surg 2018;84(12): 1856–60.

33. Janssen TL, Hosseinzoi E, Vos DI, et al. The importance of increased awareness for delirium in elderly patients with rib fractures after blunt chest wall trauma: a retrospective cohort study on risk factors and outcomes. BMC Emerg Med 2019;19(1):34.

34. Palleschi L, Galdi F, Pedone C. Acute medical illness and disability in the elderly. Geriatric Care 2018;4(3):62-4.

35. Covinsky KE, Palmer RM, Fortinsky RH. Loss of independence in activities of daily living in older adults hospitalized with medical illnesses: increased vulnerability with age. J Am Geriatr Soc 2003;51:451–8.

36. Boyd CM, Landefeld CS, Counsell SR. Recovery of activities of daily living in older adults after hospitalization for acute medical illness. J Am Geriatr Soc 2008;56:2171–9.

37. Kress JP, Hall JB. ICU acquired weakness and recovery from critical illness. N Engl J Med 2014;370(17):1626–35.

38. Schweickert WD, Pohlman MC, Pohlman AS, et al. Early physical and occupational therapy in mechanically ventilated, critically ill patients: a randomised controlled trial. Lancet 2009;373(9678):1874–82.

39. Bailey P, Thomsen GE, Spuhler VJ. Early activity is feasible and safe in respiratory failure patients. Crit Care Med 2007;35(1):139–45.

40. Schaller SJ, Anstey M, Blobner M, et al. Early, goal-directed mobilization in the surgical intensive care unit: a randomized controlled trial. Lancet 2016;388: 1377–88.

41. Liu K, Ogura T, Nakamura M, et al. A progressive early mobilization program is significantly associated with clinical and economic improvement: a single center quality comparison study. Crit Care Med 2019;47(9):744–52.

42. Marra A, Ely EW, Pandharipande PP, et al. The ABCDEF bundle in critical care. Crit Care Clin 2017;33(2):225–43.

43. Hodgson CL, Stiller K, Needham DM, et al. Expert consensus and recommendations on safety criteria for active mobilization of mechanically ventilated critically ill adults. Crit Care 2014;18(6):658.

44. Whitson HE, Cronin-Golomb A, Cruickshanks KJ, et al. American Geriatrics Society and national institute on aging bench-to-bedside conference: sensory impairment and cognitive decline in older adults. J Am Geriatr Soc 2018;66(11):2052–8.

45. Givens JL, Sanft TB, Marcantonio ER. Functional recovery after hip fracture: the combined effects of depressive symptoms, cognitive impairment, and delirium. J Am Geriatr Soc 2008;56(6):1075–9.

46. Volkart D, Beck AM, Cederholm T, et al. Management of malnutrition in older patients – Current approaches, evidence, and open questions. J Clin Med 2019; 8:974.

47. Kaiser MJ, Bauer JM, Rämsch C, et al. Frequency of malnutrition in older adults: a multinational perspective using the mini nutritional assessment. J Am Geriatr Soc 2010;58:1734–8.

48. Clarke DM, Strauss BG, Wahlqvist ML. Undereating and undernutrition in old age: Integrating bio-psychosocial aspects. Age Ageing 1998;27:527–34.

49. Cereda E, Pedrolli C, Klersy C, et al. Nutritional status in older persons according to healthcare setting: a systematic review and meta-analysis of prevalence data using MNA. Clin Nutr 2016;35:1282–90.

50. Lacau S, Guily JLS, Bouvard É, et al. NutriCancer: a French observational multi-centre cross-sectional study of malnutrition in elderly patients with cancer. J Geriatr Oncol 2018;9:74–80.

51. Cereda E, Veronese N, Caccialanza R. The final word on nutritional screening and assessment in older persons. Curr Opin Clin Nutr Metab Care 2018;21:24–9.

52. Norman K, Pichard C, Lochs H, et al. Prognostic impact of disease-related malnutrition. Clin Nutr 2008;27:5–15.

53. Chen X, Mao G, Leng Sx. Frailty syndrome: an overview. Clin Interv Aging 2014;9: 433–41.

54. Fried LP, Tangen CM, Walston J, et al. Frailty in older adults: evidence for a phenotype. J Gerentol 2001;56:M146–57.

55. Maxwell CA, Dietrich MS, Miller RS. The FRAIL questionnaire: a useful tool for bedside screening of geriatric trauma patients. J Trauma Nurs 2018;25(4):242–7.

56. Waltson J, Hadley EC, Ferrucci L. Research agenda for frailty in older adults: toward a better understanding of physiology and etiology: summary from the american geriatrics society/national institute on aging research conference on frailty in older adults. J Am Geriatr Soc 2006;54(6):991–1001.

57. Joseph B, Pandit V, Rhee P, et al. Predicting hospital discharge disposition in geriatric trauma patients: is frailty the answer? J Trauma Acute Care Surg 2014;76(1):196–200.

58. Guidet B, de Lange DW, Boumendil A, et al. The contribution of frailty, cognition, activity of daily life and comorbidities on outcome in acutely admitted patients over 80 years in European ICUs: the VIP2 study. Intensive Care Med 2020; 46(1):57–69.

59. Persico I, Cesari M, Morandi A, et al. Frailty and delirium in older adults: a systematic review and meta-analysis of the literature. J Am Geriatr Soc 2018;66(10): 2022–30.

60. Hamidi M, Zeeshan M, O'Keeffe T, et al. Prospective evaluation of frailty and functional independence in older adult trauma patients. Am J Surg 2018;216(6): 1070–5.

61. Marty E, Liu Y, Samuel A, et al. A review of sarcopenia: Enhancing awareness of an increasingly prevalent disease. Bone 2017;105:276–86.
62. Sanchez-Rodriguez D, Marco E, Miralles R, et al. Sarcopenia, physical rehabilitation and functional outcomes of patients in a subacute geriatric care unit. Arch Gerontol Geriatr 2014;59(1):39–43.
63. Vidan M, Serra JA, Moreno C, et al. Efficacy of a comprehensive geriatric intervention in older patients hospitalized for hip fracture: a randomized, controlled trial. J Am Geriatr Soc 2005;53(9):1476–82.
64. Losh J, Duncan TK, Diaz G, et al. Multidisciplinary patient management improves mortality in geriatric trauma patients. Am Surg 2019;85(2):230–3.
65. Fallon WF, Rader E, Zyzanski S, et al. Geriatric outcomes are improved by a geriatric trauma consultation service. J Trauma 2006;61(5):1040–6.
66. Lenartowicz M, Parkovnick M, McFarlan A, et al. An evaluation of a proactive geriatric trauma consultation service. Ann Surg 2012;356(6):1098–101.
67. Fletcher B, Bradburn E, Baker C, et al. Pretrauma functional independence measure score predicts survival in geriatric trauma. Am Surg 2017;83(6):559–63.
68. Hershkovitz A, Yichayaou B, Ronen A, et al. The association between hand grip strength and rehabilitation outcome in post-acute hip fractured patients. Aging Clin Exp Res 2019;31(10):1509–16.
69. Wu D, Zhu X, Zhang S. Effect of home-based rehabilitation for hip fracture: a meta-analysis of randomized controlled trials. J Rehabil Med 2018;50(6):481–6.
70. Fischer K, Trombik M, Freystaetter G, et al. Timeline of functional recovery after hip fracture in seniors aged 65 and older: a prospective observational analysis. Osteoporos Int 2019;30(7):1371–81.

Evidence-Based Communication with Critically Ill Older Adults

JiYeon Choi, PhD, RN[a], Judith A. Tate, PhD, RN[b],*

KEYWORDS

- Communication • Mechanical ventilation
- Augmentative and alternative communication • Communication disorders
- Patient-centered care • Patient participation • Older adults

KEY POINTS

- Mechanical ventilation prohibits speech in critically ill patients.
- Being unable to communicate is frightening, frustrating and stressful for critically ill patients.
- Evidence-based methods to assess communication ability and select strategies to improve patient-clinician communication are important components of patient-centered care.

NATURE OF THE PROBLEM

Effective communication is the foundation of patient-centered care. Effective communication occurs when both the sender and receiver of messages achieve shared meaning and understanding.[1] Patient-centered communication builds on effective communication and includes patient perspectives, preferences, and choices. Furthermore, the patient's social and psychological context is valued as shared decision-making unfolds.[2]

The value of effective communication between health care providers and patients is acknowledged in health care accreditation standards as both a quality metric and as a fundamental patient right.[3] Communication failure is a critical factor in medical errors and in patient safety incidents.[4,5] Patients with communication impairments are at threefold risk for adverse events.[4] Despite the importance of communication to

[a] Yonsei University College of Nursing, Mo-Im Kim Nursing Research Institute, 50-1 Yonsei-Ro, Seodaemun-Gu, Seoul 03722, Korea; [b] Center of Healthy Aging, Self-Management and Complex Care, Undergraduate Nursing Honors Program, The Ohio State University College of Nursing, 386 Newton Hall, 1585 Neil Avenue, Columbus, OH 43210, USA
* Corresponding author.
E-mail address: tate.230@osu.edu

Crit Care Clin 37 (2021) 233–249
https://doi.org/10.1016/j.ccc.2020.09.002
0749-0704/21/© 2020 Elsevier Inc. All rights reserved.

improve patient care and outcomes, health care providers receive little or no training in evidence-based approaches in communication assessment and accommodation.[6]

In addition to preexisting communication disorders, patients may acquire communication impairments because of therapeutic interventions, such as mechanical ventilation, sedation, and neuromuscular blockade during critical illness. Endotracheal intubation or tracheostomy prevents patients' ability to vocalize, which is frightening, frustrating, and stressful.[7,8] Communication difficulty is one of the most common and most bothersome symptoms reported by patients undergoing mechanical ventilation (MV).[7,9–13] The inability to speak limits accurate identification of symptoms and can restrict participation in treatment decision-making.[7,8,11,12,14–16] The inability to communicate contributes to physical and emotional distress and predicts psychological distress in the post–intensive care unit (ICU) period.[17,18] Despite known communication difficulties in critically ill patients, interventions to support nonvocal patients with critical illness are poorly and inconsistently applied.[13,19,20]

Older adults, defined as older than 65 years, comprise approximately 50% of ICU admissions annually and as the aging population increases, this percentage is expected to grow.[21] Critically ill older adults present communication challenges based on their unique vulnerabilities such as burden of underlying chronic conditions, sensory impairment, frailty, and cognitive dysfunction[22–26] Most ICU health care providers learn how to communicate with impaired patients by trial and error or by observing others.[6]

This article presents an overview of evidence-based strategies to improve communication during the critical illness with older adults who have preexisting and acquired communication disorders due to hearing loss, vision impairment, limited English proficiency, health literacy, cognition, and limited upper extremity mobility.

Epidemiology of Preexisting Communication Disorders

- One in 6 people in the United States have a communication disorder.[27]
- Of these, 28 million have communication disorders associated with hearing loss.[28]
- 14 million people have disorders of speech, voice, and/or language not associated with hearing loss.[29]
- 90% of adults older than 50 require corrective lenses[30]
- 1 in 3 adults older than 65 has a hearing loss[24]

Communication disorders often occur concomitantly with other chronic disorders, such as diabetes, heart failure, stroke, renal disease, and dementia, contributing to a decreased ability to engage in self-management and resulting in high rates of disability.[30–35]

Hearing loss

Hearing loss is a common but underrecognized and undertreated problem in older adults.[36,37] Few studies provide direction for improving communication with patients who have hearing impairment.[33,38] Even with mild hearing loss, low levels of ambient noise competes with one-on-one communication.[38] Higher than normal noise levels in the ICU compound the effects of hearing loss.[39] During hospitalization, hearing aids are often removed and sent home because of their cost, which worsens communication and limits patient engagement.[25,40] Preexisting hearing impairment is associated with delirium and poor recovery following an ICU stay.[41,42] The use of hearing aids in the ICU both reduces the incidence of delirium and facilitates mobility.[43]

Health care professionals are often unaware of patients' hearing impairment and routine screening for hearing loss at the bedside lacks sensitivity.[26] Clinicians report difficulty communicating with patients with hearing loss, yet few receive formal training to develop skills necessary to resolve communication barriers.[38,44] Hearing loss is not always documented in the medical record and furthermore, few health care professionals are aware of how to access services for patients with hearing loss.[44]

A hearing assessment is necessary for all older patients admitted to the ICU. Evidence of hearing loss may be subtle and overlap with signs of other problems such as delirium. For instance, patients with hearing loss may not respond to verbal stimulus, which may be confused with inattention. Patients with hearing loss may be more responsive when they can see the communication partner's face. Clinicians may compound communication problems by rapid speech and/or use of medical jargon.[38]

An audiologist should evaluate patients with suspected or diagnosed preexisting hearing loss and can recommend simple strategies to accommodate patients with uncorrected hearing loss. Audiologists can troubleshoot problems with hearing aids and can provide brief bedside instructions to staff for appropriate use and care of hearing aids. In addition, audiologists can provide temporary hearing amplification devices if patients' own hearing aids are not available or if the hearing loss is uncorrected by hearing aids. Hearing aids should be available and inserted during the day to facilitate comprehension.[38,43,44]

Vision impairment

Given the high rates of visual impairment in all age groups and the increased prevalence of vision problems with aging, many patients require corrective lenses for reading or for distance vision correction. In older adults, visual impairment is associated with ICU delirium and poor recovery outcomes.[41] During hospitalization, patients are often expected to review educational materials, consent forms, and personal messages. Despite this, corrective lenses are not frequently made available for patients in the ICU.[45] Corrective lenses provide patients a way to make sense of their environment, identify caregivers, and compensate for hearing loss using lip-reading.

Limited English proficiency

Older adults in whom English is not their primary language may experience language barriers, making communication as well as comprehending medical terminology more difficult. Currently 1 in 15 adults are identified as Limited English Proficient (LEP) and with projected increases in immigration, this number is expected to increase.[46–48] Fifteen million older adults are LEP resulting in poor health and disparate health care access.[48,49] For any patients who are LEP, language access such as interpreter services and written materials in patients' native language are mandated now by the Affordable Care Act.

Cognitive impairment

Many patients with critical illness experience changes in their level of consciousness. Changes in cognitive function or delirium can result in changes in communication initiation and symptom communication.[16] Use of a standardized assessment tool such as the Confusion Assessment Method - ICU or Intensive Care Delirium Screening Checklist provide important data about the presence of delirium, acute confusion experienced by many ICU patients and common in older adults.[50,51] provide. Features common to delirium that may influence patient communication are impaired sustained attention, distorted thinking, inability to follow verbal commands, and changes in level of consciousness.[50,51]

Communicating with older adults may be further complicated by preexisting cognitive impairment. Impaired attention and focus are hallmark features of both delirium and dementia. Patients with delirium superimposed on dementia may have unpredictable communication patterns.[52] For instance, patients with dementia may have verbal fluency difficulties that the patient with delirium may not exhibit. Patients with dementia have slower cognitive processing speed making it difficult to understand and react to verbal input. Patients receiving sedating medications may also exhibit slower cognitive processing speed.

Because many patients experience delirium during their ICU stay, communication strategies directed at key features of delirium are imperative. To compensate for inattention, the clinician should initiate attention by facing the patient, establishing eye contact, and maintaining the face-to-face position.[53,54] Locking eyes can provide useful information for both the speaker and the patient.[53] The speaker can monitor patient engagement while the patient can see the speaker's mouth movement. Delays in comprehension may be due to cognitive impairment, sedation, fatigue, neurologic deficits, or hearing impairment.[55] Slowing the clinician's pace of speech and limiting ideas to one at a time can help to overcome delays in processing.[56] Increasing the duration of pauses between the sent message and the patient's response will allow the patient time to formulate a response. This technique can be useful in cases in which patients have motor slowing, as seen in Parkinson disease. Asking patients to confirm the sender's message or repeat the message may increase message accuracy and retention.[56]

Limited upper motor ability

ICU-acquired weakness (ICUAW) is profound neuromuscular dysfunction associated with critical illness and its treatment.[57,58] Preexisting functional impairment or frailty, common in older adults, is a risk factor for development of ICUAW.[57] Prolonged mechanical ventilation, sedation, and immobility are common and increase risk for ICUAW.[58] Patients with ICUAW exhibit decreased strength, muscle atrophy and decreased muscle mass, fatigue, weakness, and poor grip strength.[59] Effective communication strategies are limited by ICUAW. For instance, to write a message, patients should be able to sit upright, holding their head up, grip the pen, and produce a legible written message, ICUAW may prohibit use of writing as a strategy.

Pointing or gesturing is a common method of augmenting communication efforts and is an essential component for use of many communication strategies. If the patient can point, supportive communication strategies such as alphabet boards, picture boards or touch screens may be appropriate. Unfortunately, patients with critical illness may experience upper extremity edema, which can impair the ability to point or gesture. Use of sedating medications or paralytics will prevent use of pointing and writing. In addition, vascular access may make it difficult to move their extremities.[60,61]

Augmentative and Alternative Communication Strategies

Augmentative and alternative communication (AAC) strategies are a set of tools, technologies, and approaches used to overcome communication challenges that can be used to improve communication for voiceless patients in the ICU.[62] AAC strategies were originally developed to assist patients with acquired neurologic problems to communicate deficits but have been adapted by communication scientists to meet the needs of critically ill patients.[63] AAC strategies include unaided strategies (gestures, facial expressions, mouthing words), low-tech strategies (writing, letter boards) and high-tech strategies (computer-assisted devices, apps, speech-generating devices), as seen in **Table 1**.[19,63]

Adoption of AAC strategies in the ICU can lead to improved patient satisfaction with communication.[6,64,65] There are a variety of evidence-based methods to facilitate the

Table 1
Augmentative and alternative communication strategy classifications

Unaided *Nonspoken, natural*	Aided *Require external support*
Gestures Facial expression Body language Sign language	Communication boards Handheld devices Electronic devices

Low-tech strategies
 Strategy that does not
  require battery operated
  or electronic device
	High-tech strategies
	 Require energy source, electronic

Writing Picture boards Letter boards	Speech-generating devices Communication Apps VidaTalk LiveVoice Speak for Myself ICUTalk

use of AAC, including access to communication materials, and improving clinician knowledge and skills.[6,19,66–68] Barriers to use of AAC in the ICU include competing priorities for clinicians, as using AAC takes time away from other clinical activities.[6,67–69] Many clinicians limit communication exchanges with patients, as they have experienced frustration with communication breakdowns with nonspeaking patients.[70]

Low-tech strategies
Low-tech AAC include methods that enhance communication efforts using strategies and tools that do not require battery-operated devices. Communication boards include symbols, letters, pictures, icons, or a combination to facilitate messages by pointing by the patient or the clinician, as seen in **Fig. 1**. Communication boards can increase communication effectiveness and speed, decrease frustration, and improve patient satisfaction in communication with clinicians.[71,72] Communication boards, although the most restrictive option, are inexpensive, downloadable, and can be constructed on paper or purchased.

High-tech strategies
High-tech strategies include devices that use an electronic interface, as seen in **Fig. 2**.[64,73,74] Although more costly than low-tech strategies, some high-tech devices are able to generate speech in response to patients touching letters or symbols on the screen.[64,73–75] Some high-tech AACs use an application downloaded onto an electronic tablet.[76] Using the lettering feature enables patients to spell messages. To optimize effectiveness, patients should be alert and cognitively intact, unrestrained, and have the muscle strength and ability to point to icons.

Voice-enabling strategies
Several methods have been tested to enable speech generation by patients on MV. In their review of communication strategies for critically ill patients, Ten Hoorn and colleagues constructed an algorithm of voice-enabling strategies to guide clinical decision making when considering individualized communication interventions.[77]

The talking trach was designed to enable patients to generate vocal tones in a whisper, as seen in **Fig. 3**.[78] The cuff on the talking trach remains inflated, enabling

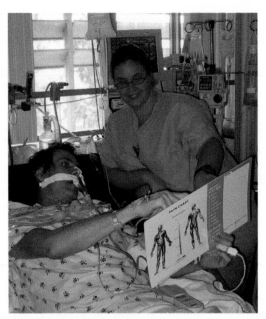

Fig. 1. Using low-tech communication board.

ventilation and vocalization as separate and safe functions. A talking trach tube necessitates a change in tube conferring a degree of risk of an airway exchange. Issues with secretion management with this device also make it a less desirable method.[78,79]

An inline speaking valve is a one-way airflow valve to enable vocalization. Use of an inline speaking valve requires deflation of the tracheostomy tube or the presence of a cuffless tracheostomy. The Passy-Muir valve improves vocal communication and cough, as illustrated in **Fig. 4**.[79] Use of the Passy-Muir valve is precluded in patients

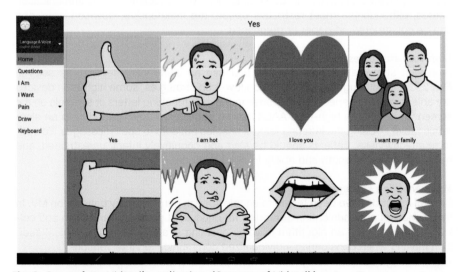

Fig. 2. Screen from Vidatalk application. (Courtesy of Vidatalk)

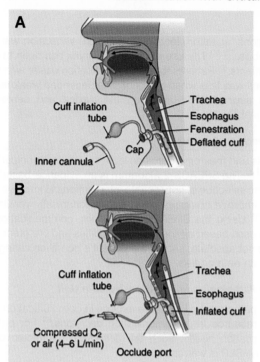

Fig. 3. (*A*, *B*) Talking Trach. (*A*) Fenestrated tracheostomy tube with cuff deflated, inner cannula removed, and tracheostomy tube capped to allow air to pass over the vocal cords. (*B*) Speaking tracheostomy tube. One tube is used for cuff inflation. (*From* Mathers, DM. Nursing Management. In: Heitkemper MM, Bucher Lin, Lewis SL, et al. (eds) Medical-Surgical Nursing: Assessment and Management of Clinical Problems, Ninth Edition, Philadelphia: Elsevier, 2014; with permission.)

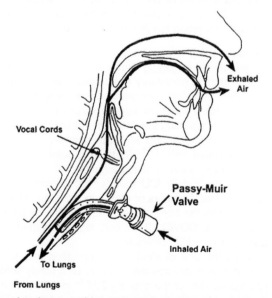

Fig. 4. Passy-Muir valve. (*From* Hodder RV. A 55-year-old patient with advanced COPD, tracheostomy tube, and sudden respiratory distress. Chest. 2002;121(1):279-280. https://doi.org/10.1378/chest.121.1.279; with permission.)

with heavy secretions, agitation, inability to maintain ventilation with a deflated cuff, and medical instability.[79,80] The use of an electrolarynx has been tested in mechanically ventilated patients.[81] Patients rated communication easier with the electrolarynx but its effectiveness was less when the patient experienced weakness.[81] In addition, patients required support for positioning the device and sentence intelligibility remained suboptimal.[81]

Communication Decision Support

Critically ill patients and their providers can learn to use communication aids in a systematic manner.[65,66] The SPEACS-2 algorithm is an evidence-based tool that guides patient assessment, selection of appropriate interventions to improve comprehension, and strategies to improve communication with mechanically ventilated patients, as seen in **Fig. 5**.[67,68] Using the SPEACS-2 algorithm, communication strategies can be attempted and used based on the patient's abilities and preferences. Communication strategies are not absolute, and as the patient's condition changes, communication approaches can be modified.

Speech Language Pathologists in the Intensive Care Unit

Speech language pathologists (SLPs) are experts in communication science and can be an invaluable resource for communication decisions.[82] For patients with more complex communication needs, such as those with neurologic disorders, expert consultation with an SLP is warranted.

Family Communication

Families often provide support and advocacy when patients are unable to speak for themselves.[83] Families experience distress when they are unable to communicate with the patient.[10,84,85] Patients on MV often appreciate the efforts of close relatives to understand them while they were unable to speak and families are likewise often interested in learning how to improve communication.[84,86] Studies have neither rigorously described patient-family communication in the ICU nor systematically tested communication strategies targeting families of the critically ill.

Engaging family members using telehealth

In the ICU setting, effectively engaging family members is essential. Information shared from family members is necessary to integrate data on a patient's medical, psychosocial, and behavioral history relevant to current illness. Support from family members can be represented a variety of ways, from providing silent companionship to actively responding and supporting patients' emotional and social needs.[86] Family members can be both surrogates and advocates, especially when the patient's communication ability is limited.[10,83,87,88] Efforts have been made to increase family presence in the ICU settings, such as using extended or open vitiation hours and inviting family to participate in daily ICU rounds.[89,90] However, family presence in the ICU is not always feasible. Decades of efforts to increase family presence in the ICU face a major barrier with the coronavirus 2019 (COVID-19) pandemic. Deprived access to family visits due to COVID-19 not only worsens suffering of patients and families but also adds stress to ICU clinicians.[91,92]

Telehealth, defined as the use of electronic information and telecommunication technologies to support health services delivery may be a timely solution to continue and improve family engagement for the critically ill.[93,94] In critical care, telehealth was initially introduced as a tool to reduce disparities in access to critical care workforces in rural areas.[95,96] Recently, family engagement has proven to be another area that

Low Tech Communication Strategies

STEP 1 – ASSESS

1. COGNITION
Is the patient alert?
Can they follow commands?
Can you raise your arm/make a fist?
Blink your eyes twice.

2. ORAL MOTOR MOVEMENT
Are the patient's mouth movements clear when
mouthing speech?
Count from 1 to 10.
Tell me about your first job in a sentence.

3. COMPREHENSION
Does the patient need help with comprehension?
Do they wear glasses/hearing aids?
Are they available?
Any language barriers?

4. EXPRESSIVE COMMUNICATION
Does the patient have a reliable yes/no signal?
How does the patient signal yes?
How does the patient signal no?

Can the patient point?
Can the patient write?

Assess language and literacy
Engage SLP or translation services if non-English
speaking or unable to read.

STEP II - PROVIDE COMPREHENSION STRATEGIES

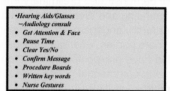

- *Hearing Aids/Glasses*
  - *Audiology consult*
- *Get Attention & Face*
- *Pause Time*
- *Clear Yes/No*
- *Confirm Message*
- *Procedure Boards*
- *Written key words*
- *Nurse Gestures*

STEP III – CHOOSE STRATEGY BASED ON ORAL MOTOR SKILL

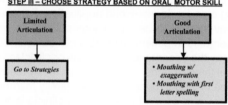

STEP IV – CHOOSE STRATEGIES FOR EXPRESSIVE COMMUNICATION

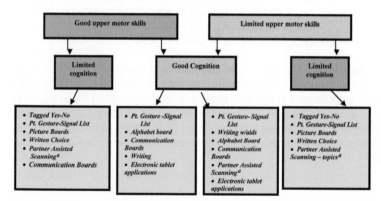

Fig. 5. SPEACS-2 algorithm.[a] Consult speech language pathologist (SLP) for complex strategies or if selected strategies are unsuccessful. (©Garret, Happ, Tate 2006 (Revised 2009: SPEACS-2; 2016) R01 HD043988.)

may benefit from telehealth. Telehealth is a solution to help family members maintain connections with patients and participate in both communication and decision making with the health care team.

A simple approach, for example, playing the audio-recorded voice of family members, can benefit both patients and families. Munro and colleagues[97] developed and pilot-tested a cognitive reorientation intervention to prevent delirium in critically ill patients. In their intervention, family members were instructed to read and record a scripted 2-minute message and the recorded message was played in the patient's room. Reorientation messages include orientation of the patient's current location and reasons for physical limitations (eg, endotracheal tube). Results of this randomized controlled trial demonstrated preliminary efficacy in reducing delirium.

Video-conferencing and Web-based portals may be the most popular technologies considered for family engagement. Video-conferencing sets up real-time interactions between 2 or more parties, whereas Web-based portals may have conferencing capabilities but also have pre-posted information or patient centered apps, for example, VidaTalk. Various commercial online platforms are now Health Insurance Portability and Accountability Act (HIPAA)-compliant. Despite their potential to promote family engagement, establishing evidence specific to gero-critical care settings is a remaining step for its real-world application. For example, video-conferencing technologies may appear to be an obvious solution to promote real-time engagement of family members in patient visits, ICU clinical team rounds, and family meetings.[98–102] However, the acceptance by families or clinicians of the use of video conferencing for virtual family rounds, varies.[103] Most family members and clinicians are supportive of the idea of virtual rounds; however, family members have varying levels of technology literacy and comfort levels. Some clinicians expressed concerns of adding burden to their clinical workload.[103]

Another example of using telehealth to engage family members includes interactive online decision-support programs to guide complex surrogate decision making, such as goals of treatment.[104,105] Guided by theories addressing both cognitive and emotional aspects of decision making, online decision-support programs have made rapid developments.[104] Although the initial program was mainly based on the cognitive aspects of surrogate decision making, a recent development added a tool to support the emotional and psychological challenges that families experience during decision making.[104,105] These programs were suggested as an adjunct to help families prepare for complex conversations during in-person meetings with the ICU clinical team.[105]

The aforementioned technologies, from the use of a voice recording device to communication and/or decision-aid software, highlight the different media available to improve family engagement in the ICU. In the process of adopting these technologies, attention should also be paid to disparities in access to the technology, digital literacy, and Internet access among the family members. Efforts to resolve these disparities are important to ensure people with fewer resources and access are included.

Box 1
Communication resources

Communication resources
  Patient-Provider Communication Organization
  https://www.patientprovidercommunication.org/

Communication training
  https://nucleus.con.ohio-state.edu/media/speacs2/project_desc.htm

Organizations
  US Society for Augmentative and Alternative Communication
  https://ussaac.org/
  International Society for Augmentative and Alternative Communication
  https://www.isaac-online.org/english/home/
  American Speech Language Hearing Association
  https://www.asha.org/

SUMMARY

Losing the ability to speak while on MV can be a frightening and frustrating experience for patients. Effective communication with mechanically ventilated patients is a critical component of patient-centered care. Given the number of older adults in the ICU with preexisting communication disorders and cognitive impairment, older adults are at greater risk for communication breakdown in the ICU. Communication assessment and selection of appropriate strategies should be approached systematically. Additional resources can be found in **Box 1**.

CLINICS CARE POINTS

Recommendations for ICU Practice Change Related to Communication
- *ICU rounds*: During ICU rounds, the clinicians should be able to answer: (1) Is the patient communicating effectively? If yes, using what mechanism? (2) Is a sign posted in the patient's room denoting communication difficulty? (3) Has a speech language pathologist been consulted? If so, what are their recommendations? and (4) Has there been a change in the patient's condition that might affect their communication ability?
- *Documentation*: Nurses should systematically and routinely chart the patient's communication function: (1) How are they communicating overall, and specifically their ability to communicate "yes" and "no"? and (2) Are there changes in patient's condition that might affect their communication ability?
- *Communication plans:* A communication plan should be posted by the patient's bed that lists how the patient is able to both (1) convey thoughts, needs, and symptoms accurately to their providers, and (2) understands what care providers are communicating, including sensory aids (eg, glasses, hearing aids).

DISCLOSURE

JiYeon Choi was supported by National Research Foundation (NRF) of Korea (2019R1F1A1057941). The other author have no conflicts to disclose.

REFERENCES

1. Fleischer S, Berg A, Zimmermann M, et al. Nurse-patient interaction and communication: a systematic literature review. J Public Health 2009;17(5):339–53.
2. Slatore CG, Hansen L, Ganzini L, et al. Communication by nurses in the intensive care unit: qualitative analysis of domains of patient-centered care. Am J Crit Care 2012;21(6):410–8.
3. JCAHO. Patient-centered communication standards for hospitals. 2011.
4. Bartlett G, Blais R, Tamblyn R, et al. Impact of patient communication problems on the risk of preventable adverse events in acute care settings. CMAJ 2008;178(12):1555–62.
5. Hemsley B, Georgiou A, Hill S, et al. An integrative review of patient safety in studies on the care and safety of patients with communication disabilities in hospital. Patient Educ Couns 2016;99(4):501–11.
6. Magnus VS, Turkington L. Communication interaction in icu—patient and staff experiences and perceptions. Intensive Crit Care Nurs 2006;22(3):167–80.
7. Rotondi AJ, Chelluri L, Sirio C, et al. Patients' recollections of stressful experiences while receiving prolonged mechanical ventilation in an intensive care unit. Crit Care Med 2002;30(4):746–52.

8. Guttormson JL, Bremer KL, Jones RM. "Not being able to talk was horrid": a descriptive, correlational study of communication during mechanical ventilation. Intensive Crit Care Nurs 2015;31(3):179–86.

9. Nelson JE, Meier DE, Litke A, et al. The symptom burden of chronic critical illness. Crit Care Med 2004;32(7):1527–34.

10. Happ MB. Interpretation of nonvocal behavior and the meaning of voicelessness in critical care. Social Sci Med 2000;50(9):1247–55.

11. Danielis M, Povoli A, Mattiussi E, et al. Understanding patients' experiences of being mechanically ventilated in the intensive care unit: Findings from a meta-synthesis and meta-summary. J Clin Nurs 2020;29(13–14):2107–24.

12. Fink RM, Makic MBF, Poteet AW, et al. The ventilated patient's experience. Dimensions Crit Care Nurs 2015;34(5):301–8.

13. Freeman-Sanderson A, Morris K, Elkins M. Characteristics of patient communication and prevalence of communication difficulty in the intensive care unit: an observational study. Aust Crit Care 2019;32(5):373–7.

14. Karlsen MMW, Ølnes MA, Heyn LG. Communication with patients in intensive care units: a scoping review. Nurs Crit Care 2019;24(3):115–31.

15. Tate JA, Seaman JB, Happ MB. Overcoming barriers to pain assessment: communicating pain information with intubated older adults. Geriatr Nurs (New York, NY). 2012;33(4):310–3.

16. Tate JA, Sereika S, Divirgilio D, et al. Symptom communication during critical illness: the impact of age, delirium, and delirium presentation. J Gerontol Nurs 2013;39(8):28–38.

17. Wade DM, Howell DC, Weinman JA, et al. Investigating risk factors for psychological morbidity three months after intensive care: a prospective cohort study. Crit Care 2012;16(5):R192.

18. Parker AM, Sricharoenchai T, Raparla S, et al. Posttraumatic stress disorder in critical illness survivors: a metaanalysis. Crit Care Med 2015;43(5):1121–9.

19. Istanboulian L, Rose L, Gorospe F, et al. Barriers to and facilitators for the use of augmentative and alternative communication and voice restorative strategies for adults with an advanced airway in the intensive care unit: a scoping review. J Crit Care 2020;57:168–76.

20. Hurtig RR, Downey D. Augmentative and alternative communication in acute and critical care settings. San Diego (CA): Plural Publishing; 2008.

21. Zilberberg MD, de Wit M, Shorr AF. Accuracy of previous estimates for adult prolonged acute mechanical ventilation volume in 2020: Update using 2000–2008 data. Crit Care Med 2012;40(1):18–20.

22. Ferrante LE, Pisani MA, Murphy TE, et al. The association of frailty with post-icu disability, nursing home admission, and mortality: a longitudinal study. Chest. 2018;153(6):1378–86.

23. He Z, Bian J, Carretta HJ, et al. Prevalence of multiple chronic conditions among older adults in Florida and the United States: Comparative analysis of the one-florida data trust and national inpatient sample. J Med Internet Res 2018;20(4):e137.

24. National Institute on Deafness and Other Communication Disorders. Hearing loss and older adults. 2016. Available at: https://www.nidcd.nih.gov/health/hearing-loss-older-adults.

25. Funk A, Garcia C, Mullen T. Ce: Original research understanding the hospital experience of older adults with hearing impairment. AJN The Am J Nurs 2018;118(6):28–34.

26. Mormer E, Bubb KJ, Alrawashdeh M, et al. Hearing loss and communication among hospitalized older adults: prevalence and recognition. J Gerontol Nurs 2020;46(6):34–42.

27. Healthy People.gov. Hearing and other sensory or communication disorders. 2014. Available at: https://www.healthypeople.gov/2020/topics-objectives/topic/hearing-and-other-sensory-or-communication-disorders. Accessed July 31, 2020.

28. Hoffman HJ, Dobie RA, Losonczy KG, et al. Declining prevalence of hearing loss in us adults aged 20 to 69 years. JAMA Otolaryngol Head Neck Surg 2017;143(3):274–85.

29. Blackwell DL, Lucas JW, Clarke TC. Summary health statistics for us adults: national health interview survey, 2012. Vital Health Stat Ser 10 2014;(260):1–161.

30. The National Eye Institute. Eye health data and statistics. 2019. Available at: https://www.nei.nih.gov/learn-about-eye-health/resources-for-health-educators/eye-health-data-and-statistics. Accessed July 31, 2020.

31. Flowers HL, Skoretz SA, Silver FL, et al. Poststroke aphasia frequency, recovery, and outcomes: a systematic review and meta-analysis. Arch Phys Med Rehabil 2016;97(12):2188–201.e8.

32. Froehlich-Grobe K, Jones D, Businelle MS, et al. Impact of disability and chronic conditions on health. Disabil Health J 2016;9(4):600–8.

33. Moore S. Scientific reasons for including persons with disabilities in clinical and translational diabetes research. J Diabetes Sci Tech 2012;6(2):236–41.

34. Nantsupawat A, Wichaikhum OA, Abhichartibutra K, et al. Nurses' knowledge of health literacy, communication techniques, and barriers to the implementation of health literacy programs: a cross-sectional study. Nurs Health Sci 2020;22(3):577–85.

35. Mirza M, Harrison EA, Roman M, et al. Walking the talk: understanding how language barriers affect the delivery of rehabilitation services. Disabil Rehabil 2020;1–14.

36. Goman AM, Reed NS, Lin FR. Addressing estimated hearing loss in adults in 2060. JAMA Otolaryngol Head Neck Surg 2017;143(7):733–4.

37. Lin FR, Niparko JK, Ferrucci L. Hearing loss prevalence in the United States. Arch Intern Med 2011;171(20):1851–3.

38. Cohen JM, Blustein J, Weinstein BE, et al. Studies of physician-patient communication with older patients: how often is hearing loss considered? A systematic literature review. J Am Geriatr Soc 2017;65(8):1642–9.

39. Konkani A, Oakley B. Noise in hospital intensive care units—a critical review of a critical topic. J Crit Care 2012;27(5):522.e1-9.

40. Hardin SR. Hearing loss in older critical care patients: participation in decision making. Crit Care Nurse 2012;32(6):43–50.

41. Ferrante LE, Pisani MA, Murphy TE, et al. Factors associated with functional recovery among older intensive care unit survivors. Am J Respir Crit Care Med 2016;194(3):299–307.

42. Inouye SK, Viscoli CM, Horwitz RI, et al. A predictive model for delirium in hospitalized elderly medical patients based on admission characteristics. Ann Intern Med 1993;119(6):474–81.

43. Vidán MT, Sánchez E, Alonso M, et al. An intervention integrated into daily clinical practice reduces the incidence of delirium during hospitalization in elderly patients. J Am Geriatr Soc 2009;57(11):2029–36.

44. Shukla A, Nieman CL, Price C, et al. Impact of hearing loss on patient–provider communication among hospitalized patients: a systematic review. Am J Med Qual 2019;34(3):284–92.

45. Zhou Q, Walker NF. Promoting vision and hearing aids use in an intensive care unit. BMJ Open Qual 2015;4(1). u206276.w2702.

46. Passel J, Rohal M. Modern immigration wave brings 59 million to US, driving population growth and change through 2065: Views of immigration's impact on US society mixed. Washington, DC: Pew Research Center; 2015. Available at: https://www.pewresearch.org/hispanic/wp-content/uploads/sites/5/2015/09/2015-09-28_modern-immigration-wave_REPORT.pdf.

47. US Census Bureau. Language use. 2019. Available at: https://www.census.gov/topics/population/language-use.html. Accessed September 18, 2020.

48. LEP.gov. Limited English proficiency (LEP) frequently asked questions. Available at: https://www.lep.gov/faqs/faqs.html#OneQ1. Accessed September 20, 2020.

49. Derose KP, Escarce JJ, Lurie N. Immigrants and health care: sources of vulnerability. Health Aff 2007;26(5):1258–68.

50. Devlin JW, Fong JJ, Schumaker G, et al. Use of a validated delirium assessment tool improves the ability of physicians to identify delirium in medical intensive care unit patients. Crit Care Med 2007;35(12):2721–4.

51. Ely EW, Margolin R, Francis J, et al. Evaluation of delirium in critically ill patients: validation of the confusion assessment method for the intensive care unit (CAM-ICU). Crit Care Med 2001;29(7):1370–9.

52. Fick DM, Agostini JV, Inouye SK. Delirium superimposed on dementia: a systematic review. J Am Geriatr Soc 2002;50(10):1723–32.

53. Frischen A, Bayliss AP, Tipper SP. Gaze cueing of attention: visual attention, social cognition, and individual differences. Psychol Bull 2007;133(4):694.

54. Poliakoff E, Ashworth S, Lowe C, et al. Vision and touch in ageing: Crossmodal selective attention and visuotactile spatial interactions. Neuropsychologia. 2006; 44(4):507–17.

55. Savundranayagam MY, Orange JB. Matched and mismatched appraisals of the effectiveness of communication strategies by family caregivers of persons with alzheimer's disease. Int J Lang Commun Disord 2014;49(1):49–59.

56. Eccles DR. Communicating with the cognitively impaired patient. Florida Board of Nursing. Tallahassee (FL): Advance Nursing Institute INC; 2013.

57. Vanhorebeek I, Latronico N, Van den Berghe G. ICU-acquired weakness. Intensive Care Med 2020;150(5):1129–40.

58. Fan E, Cheek F, Chlan L, et al. An official American Thoracic Society clinical practice guideline: the diagnosis of intensive care unit–acquired weakness in adults. Am J Respir Crit Care Med 2014;190(12):1437–46.

59. Chlan LL, Tracy MF, Guttormson J, et al. Peripheral muscle strength and correlates of muscle weakness in patients receiving mechanical ventilation. Am J Crit Care 2015;24(6):e91–8.

60. Beukelman DR, Garrett KL, Yorkston KM. Augmentative communication strategies for adults with acute or chronic medical conditions. Baltimore (MD): Paul H. Brookes Publishing Company; 2007.

61. Happ MB, Seaman JB, Nilsen ML, et al. The number of mechanically ventilated ICU patients meeting communication criteria. Heart & Lung 2015;44(1):45-9.

62. International society for augmentative and alternative communication.What is AAC? 2014. Available at: https://www.isaac-online.org/english/what-is-aac/. Accessed July 31, 2020.

63. Carruthers H, Astin F, Munro W. Which alternative communication methods are effective for voiceless patients in intensive care units? A systematic review. Intensive Crit Care Nurs 2017;42:88–96.
64. Rodriguez CS, Rowe M, Koeppel B, et al. Development of a communication intervention to assist hospitalized suddenly speechless patients. Technology Health Care 2012;20(6):519–30.
65. Happ MB, Garrett KL, Tate JA, et al. Effect of a multi-level intervention on nurse-patient communication in the intensive care unit: results of the speacs trial. Heart Lung. 2014;43(2):89–98.
66. Happ MB, Sereika SM, Houze MP, et al. Quality of care and resource use among mechanically ventilated patients before and after an intervention to assist nurse-nonvocal patient communication. Heart & Lung. 2015;44(5):408–15.e2.
67. Trotta RL, Hermann RM, Polomano RC, et al. Improving nonvocal critical care patients' ease of communication using a modified speacs-2 program. J Healthc Qual (Jhq) 2020;42(1):e1–9.
68. Radtke JV, Tate JA, Happ MB. Nurses' perceptions of communication training in the icu. Intensive Crit Care Nurs 2012;28(1):16–25.
69. Dithole K, Thupayagale-Tshweneagae G, Akpor OA, et al. Communication skills intervention: promoting effective communication between nurses and mechanically ventilated patients. BMC Nurs 2017;16(1):74.
70. Holm A, Dreyer P. Use of communication tools for mechanically ventilated patients in the intensive care unit. CIN: Comput Inform Nurs 2018;36(8):398–405.
71. Otuzoğlu M, Karahan A. Determining the effectiveness of illustrated communication material for communication with intubated patients at an intensive care unit. Int J Nurs Pract 2014;20(5):490–8.
72. Patak L, Gawlinski A, Fung NI, et al. Communication boards in critical care: patients' views. Appl Nurs Res 2006;19(4):182–90.
73. Happ MB, Roesch TK, Garrett K. Electronic voice-output communication aids for temporarily nonspeaking patients in a medical intensive care unit: a feasibility study. Heart & Lung. 2004;33(2):92–101.
74. Koszalinski RS, Tappen RM, Viggiano D. Evaluation of speak for myself with patients who are voiceless. Rehabil Nurs J 2015;40(4):235–42.
75. Miglietta MA, Bochicchio G, Scalea TM. Computer-assisted communication for critically ill patients: a pilot study. J Trauma 2004;57(3):488–93.
76. Happ MB, Von Visger T, Weber ML, et al. Iterative development, usability, and acceptability testing of a communication app for mechanically ventilated patients. Am J Resp Crit Care Med 2016;193:A1096.
77. Ten Hoorn S, Elbers P, Girbes A, et al. Communicating with conscious and mechanically ventilated critically ill patients: a systematic review. Crit Care 2016;20(1):333.
78. Hess DR. Facilitating speech in the patient with a tracheostomy. Respir Care 2005;50(4):519–25.
79. Zaga CJ, Berney S, Vogel AP. The feasibility, utility, and safety of communication interventions with mechanically ventilated intensive care unit patients: a systematic review. Am J speech-language Pathol 2019;28(3):1335–55.
80. O'Connor LR, Morris NR, Paratz J. Physiological and clinical outcomes associated with use of one-way speaking valves on tracheostomised patients: a systematic review. Heart & Lung. 2019;48(4):356–64.
81. Rose L, Istanboulian L, Smith OM, et al. Feasibility of the electrolarynx for enabling communication in the chronically critically ill: the eeccho study. J Crit Care 2018;47:109–13.

82. Blackstone SW, Pressman H. Patient communication in health care settings: new opportunities for augmentative and alternative communication. Augment Altern Commun 2016;32(1):69–79.

83. Happ MB, Swigart VA, Tate JA, et al. Family presence and surveillance during weaning from prolonged mechanical ventilation. Heart & Lung. 2007;36(1): 47–57.

84. Broyles LM, Tate JA, Happ MB. Use of augmentative and alternative communication strategies by family members in the intensive care unit. Am J Crit Care 2012;21(2):e21–32.

85. Alasad J, Ahmad M. Communication with critically ill patients. J Adv Nurs 2005; 50(4):356–62.

86. Engstrom A, Soderberg S. The experiences of partners of critically ill persons in an intensive care unit. Intensive Crit Care Nurs 2004;20(5):299–308 [quiz: 309–210].

87. Scheunemann LP, Ernecoff NC, Buddadhumaruk P, et al. Clinician-family communication about patients' values and preferences in intensive care units. JAMA Intern Med 2019;179(5):676–84.

88. Shin JW, Tate JA, Happ MB. The facilitated sensemaking model as a framework for family-patient communication during mechanical ventilation in the intensive care unit. Crit Care Nurs Clin North Am 2020;32(2):335–48.

89. Liu V, Read JL, Scruth E, et al. Visitation policies and practices in us icus. Crit Care 2013;17(2):1–7.

90. Au SS, des Ordons ALR, Leigh JP, et al. A multicenter observational study of family participation in ICU rounds. Crit Care Med 2018;46(8):1255–62.

91. Kotfis K, Williams Roberson S, Wilson JE, et al. Covid-19: ICU delirium management during sars-cov-2 pandemic. Crit Care 2020;24:1–9.

92. Greenberg N, Docherty M, Gnanapragasam S, et al. Managing mental health challenges faced by healthcare workers during covid-19 pandemic. BMJ 2020;368.

93. HealthIT. gov. What is telehealth? How is telehealth different from telemedicine?. Available at: https://www.healthit.gov/faq/what-telehealth-how-telehealth-different-telemedicine. Accessed July 31, 2020.

94. Calton B, Abedini N, Fratkin M. Telemedicine in the time of coronavirus. J Pain Symptom Management. 2020;60(1):e12–4.

95. Lilly CM, Zubrow MT, Kempner KM, et al. Critical care telemedicine: evolution and state of the art. Crit Care Med 2014;42(11):2429–36.

96. Kahn JM, Cicero BD, Wallace DJ, et al. Adoption of intensive care unit telemedicine in the United States. Crit Care Med 2014;42(2):362.

97. Munro CL, Cairns P, Ji M, et al. Delirium prevention in critically ill adults through an automated reorientation intervention–a pilot randomized controlled trial. Heart & Lung. 2017;46(4):234–8.

98. Olanipekun T, Ezeagu R, Oni O, et al. Improving the quality of family participation in ICU rounds through effective communication and telemedicine. Read Online Crit Care Med Soy Cril Care Me 2019;47(2):e159.

99. Menon PR, Stapleton RD, McVeigh U, et al. Telemedicine as a tool to provide family conferences and palliative care consultations in critically ill patients at rural health care institutions: a pilot study. Am J Hosp Palliat Medicine®. 2015; 32(4):448–53.

100. Østervang C, Vestergaard LV, Dieperink KB, et al. Patient rounds with video-consulted relatives: qualitative study on possibilities and barriers from the perspective of healthcare providers. J Med Internet Res 2019;21(3):e12584.

101. Yager PH, Clark M, Cummings BM, et al. Parent participation in pediatric intensive care unit rounds via telemedicine: feasibility and impact. J Pediatr 2017; 185:181–6.e3.
102. de Havenon A, Petersen C, Tanana M, et al. A pilot study of audiovisual family meetings in the intensive care unit. J Crit Care 2015;30(5):881–3.
103. Stelson EA, Carr BG, Golden KE, et al. Perceptions of family participation in intensive care unit rounds and telemedicine: a qualitative assessment. Am J Crit Care 2016;25(5):440–7.
104. Cox CE, White DB, Hough CL, et al. Effects of a personalized web-based decision aid for surrogate decision makers of patients with prolonged mechanical ventilation: a randomized clinical trial. Ann Intern Med 2019;170(5):285–97.
105. Suen AO, Butler RA, Arnold R, et al. Developing the family support tool: an interactive, web-based tool to help families navigate the complexities of surrogate decision making in icus. J Crit Care 2020;56:132–9.

Printed and bound by CPI Group (UK) Ltd, Croydon, CR0 4YY

03/10/2024

01040477-0004